Chlamydia Infections

Vsevolod Zinserling • Aleksey Poznyak
Sergei Sidorchuk • Katharina Wassilew

Chlamydia Infections

Clinical, Laboratory and Pathological Aspects

Springer

Vsevolod Zinserling
Institute of Experimental Medicine
Federal Almazov North-West Medical Research
Saint Petersburg, Russia

Aleksey Poznyak
Department of Indectology
II Mechnikov North-West Medical University
Saint-Petersburg, Russia

Sergei Sidorchuk
Department of Infectology
Kirov Military Medical Academy
Saint Petersburg, Russia

Katharina Wassilew
Institute for Pathology
Kantonsspital Baselland
Liestal, Switzerland

ISBN 978-3-031-99641-2 ISBN 978-3-031-99642-9 (eBook)
https://doi.org/10.1007/978-3-031-99642-9

This Springer imprint is published by the registered company Springer Nature Switzerland AG
The registered company address is: Gewerbestrasse 11, 6330 Cham, Switzerland

Contents

Taxonomy of *Chlamydia* 1

Chlamydiae are parasites of a large number of hosts: from amoebae to mammals. Currently, more than 400 species of susceptible animals are known. These include birds, reptiles, amphibians, fish, placental animals (mainly ungulates) and marsupials. The prevalence of microorganisms and their aetiological significance in the development of a wide range of nosologies have long been underestimated. Studies of molecular diversity have revealed an unexpectedly high diversity, wide distribution, and abundance of chlamydiae in various microbiomes and environments. Some chlamydiae species are specific to their hosts, whilst others are able to cross interspecies barriers (Fig. 1.1).

Unlike other free-living representatives of *the Planctomycetes–Verrucomicrobia–Chlamydiae* (PVC) superphylum, evolutionarily separated from related groups ~1–2 billion years ago, the modern phylum Chlamydiae is represented by obligate endosymbionts of animals and protozoa. They can act as pathogens or benefit the host (mutualism) [2, 3].

Chlamydiae of *the Parachlamydiaceae family* protect protozoa from viruses and other bacteria (e.g. Legionella pneumophila), and therefore have more genes and a more adaptive energy metabolism system compared to animal pathogens, *Chlamydiaceae* [4–6]. Representatives of the *Chlamydia family*, on the contrary, are socially significant pathogens. *Chlamydia trachomatis* causes eye diseases (trachoma) and sexually transmitted diseases, and *Chlamydia pneumoniae* is the causative agent of acute respiratory infections in humans and animals [7].

Due to the difficulty of cultivation, the presence of chlamydial infection in clinical material is detected by polymerase chain reaction (PCR). To enhance the signal, increase the specificity and objectivity of the interpretation of results, PCR with hybridization-fluorescence detection in real time is also used. When choosing a test system for molecular diagnostics, the key criterion is the sensitivity of the reagents.

The question of how and when free-living microorganisms became endosymbionts was answered by the authors of an article in the journal *Nature Microbiology* [6]. Based on data on differences in so-called marker genes (single-copy marker genes), scientists modelled the evolution of 180 representatives of the PVC supertype, including 91 from the *Chlamydiae group*.

Marker genes are orthologous genes (homologous genes of phylogenetically related organisms) that participate in the regulation of vital processes in the cell. A striking example is the 16S ribosomal RNA gene in prokaryotes and 18S in eukaryotes [8–10].

Reconstruction of the genetic sequence of almost 12,000 gene families made it possible to find the last common ancestor of *Chlamydiae with other PVC types*—a motile facultative anaerobic bacterium. Most of the acquired genes (401 of 1118) were associated with metabolism, such as glycogen synthesis and degradation.

V. Zinserling et al., *Chlamydia Infections*, https://doi.org/10.1007/978-3-031-99642-9_1

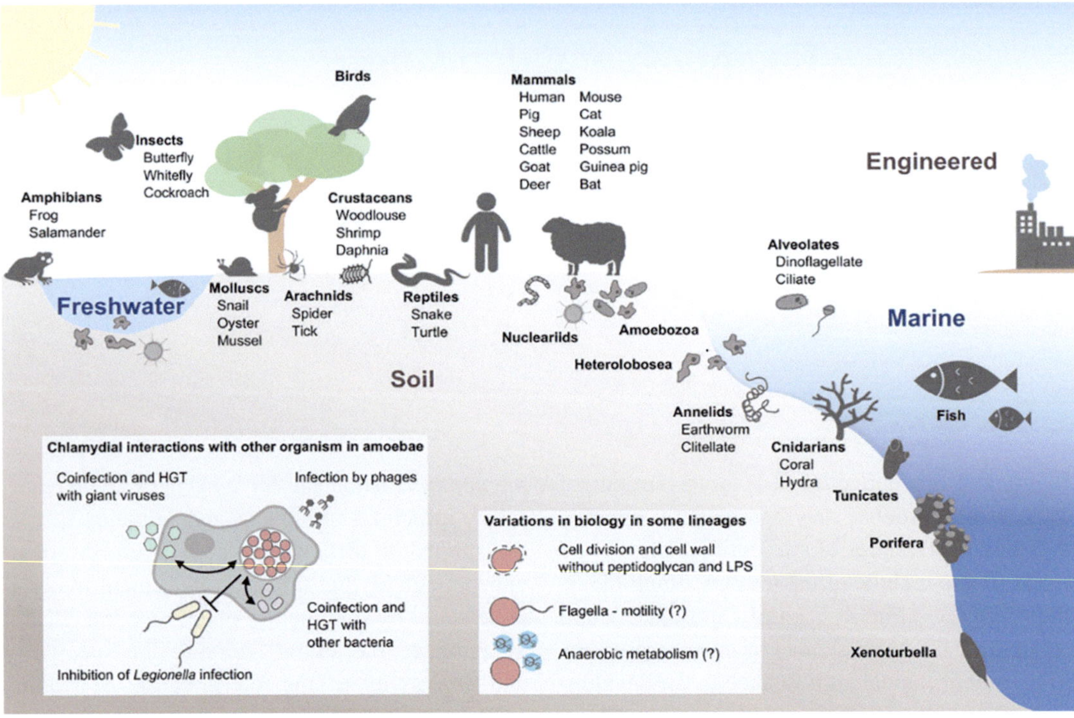

Fig. 1.1 Kingdom chlamydia. (From Ref. [1])

Genes necessary for interaction with the host and life cycle phase changes were inherited from earlier ancestral forms (Fig. 1.2).

Later, chlamydiae were divided into two groups, G1 and G2, which differed in their oxygen tolerance. G1 lived mainly in an oxygen-free environment, whilst the latter in an oxygen-containing environment. Group G2 included typical animal pathogens of the order Chlamydiales and bacteria of the order Amoebachlamydiales, which infect protozoa. Genetic differences in energy metabolism and aerobiosis (metabolic reactions in the presence of oxygen) between modern representatives of Chlamydiae arose much later [11, 12].

The detailed electron microscopic studies in experiment proved tropism of Chlamydia to different cells in brain. The peptidoglycan-based cell wall is located between the inner and outer membranes. PDH—pyruvate dehydrogenase; PFO—pyruvate: ferredoxin oxidoreductase; PFL—pyruvate formate-lyase; T4P—type IV pili; MOMP—major outer membrane protein; T3SS—type III secretory system (injectosome); Hyd—[FeFe]-hydrogenase; Rnf—membrane-bound enzyme of the simple respiratory chain, exhibits ATPase activity, participates in NAD oxidation and reduction, acts as a molecular pump and Na transporter; CI–V—electron transport chain complexes I–V; AK—amino acids; NTT—nucleotide transporters; NTP—nucleoside triphosphates; TCA—tricarboxylic acid cycle; EUO—transcription repressor protein, selectively regulates gene promoters and participates in the control of expression of late genes (genes of structural viral proteins); DsbB—disulfide bond formation protein B, an element of the respiratory chain (participates in the transfer of electrons from the reduced protein substrate to molecular oxygen) [6].

In protozoan endosymbionts, along with an increase in genome size as a whole, the number of

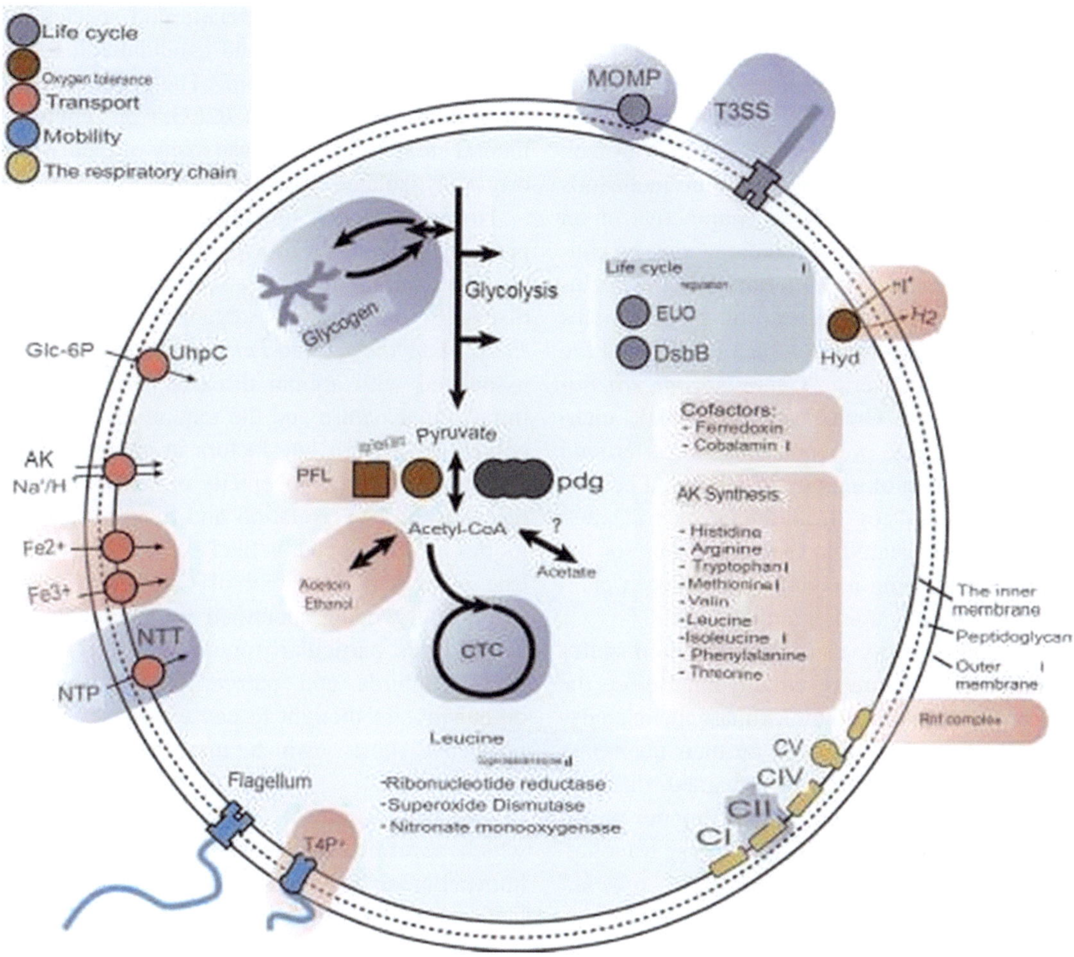

Fig. 1.2 Scheme of reconstructed gene content. (From Ref. [6])

genes providing for a more "flexible" metabolism increased: for example genes of the respiratory chain complex of electron transport. The lifestyle of the common ancestor probably included transitions between oxygen and anoxic environments.

The evolution of chlamydia is a clear example of the transition of free-living microorganisms to endosymbiosis. Phylogenomic analysis has allowed us to reconstruct key features of the genome of the ancestor *of Chlamydiae*, a mobile facultative anaerobe capable of infecting eukaryotic cells. Contrary to the expected "simplification" of the genome and the exclusion of unnecessary genes, the transition from free-living to symbiotic forms was accompanied by an increase in the number of genes, metabolic potential and complexity of bacterial organization.

1.1 Taxonomy of Chlamydiales

The development of a generally accepted nomenclature of chlamydia began more than 100 years ago and continues till now, having undergone serious disagreements amongst microbiologists concerning not only the correct determination of the position of microorganisms in the corresponding families, but also the names of these bacteria. The introduction of molecular methods has revolutionized the study of chlamydia, expanding the range of hosts of known chlamydia species, as well as discovering new species and even new families of bacteria of the order *Chlamydiales*.

In 1907, L. Halberstädter and S. von Prowazek were the first to discover cytoplasmic inclusions in the epithelial cells of the conjunctiva of an orangutan infected with a scraping from the conjunctiva of a person with trachoma. The inclusions contained a scattering of tiny particles wrapped in a kind of veil, which determined the emergence of the term "*Chlamidozoon trachomatis*" (from the Greek *chlamys*—cloak, mantle), indicating the presence of a matrix around the accumulation of a group of microbial bodies. The designation "zoa" from the Greek τα ζώα—animals also appeared in the name, thus for the first time indicating a connection between chlamydia diseases in animals and humans.

For many years, there have been disputes about the true nature of chlamydia. Before the advent of structural and molecular genetic analysis methods, a final decision on their taxonomy and classification position remained difficult. Their eponymous names were in honour of the researchers who studied them: "miyagavanella," "halprovia," "bedsonia," "colesia," "reikeia," "pararickettsia," "neorickettsia," "coquetsia," etc. Initially, chlamydia were considered viruses due to their small size, ability to pass through filters with a diameter of 0.45 μm and a two-phase cycle of intracellular development. However, due to the presence of both DNA and RNA, the ability to synthesize proteins, lipids and nucleic acids, as well as sensitivity to antibiotics, they were finally classified as bacteria only in 1966.

The order *Chlamydiales*, according to modern systematics, is a taxonomic group that includes microorganisms with similar antigenic, morphological and biochemical characteristics. Initially, it was believed that this type of microorganisms includes only one family, that is *Chlamydiaceae*, but based on genetic analysis in 2018, eight other related families were added to the order: *Clavichlamydiaceae, Criblamydiaceae, Piscichlamydiaceae, Parachlamydiaceae, Rhabdochlamydiaceae, Simkaniaceae, Waddliaceae and Parilichlamydiaceae*. They contain both recognized genera and species, as well as as-yet-unrecognized candidates that are still under consideration. They are called chlamydia-like organisms (CLOs) or "environmental chlamydiae," because many of them were originally isolated from the environment [13].

However, these organisms are emerging pathogens as many: *Parachlamydia* sp., *Simkania* sp. and *Waddlia* sp., are associated with human disease, and others organisms, such as *Piscichlamydia* sp. and *Parilichlamydia* sp., aree associated with animal diseases. Their strictly intracellular nature and the requirement for cell culture have been key factors in characterizing the biology and pathogenicity of CLOs. Further research, as new isolation and diagnostic techniques are developed, is likely to help define the true pathogenic potential of CLOs. CLOs are increasingly being identified in mammals and also in birds, particularly poultry, but also in wild birds, seabirds and parrots. Many of these organisms are thought to cause disease in their respective hosts, which may have zoonotic significance.

The best-studied family *Chlamydiaceae*, which, according to recent data [14, 15], includes known human pathogens as well as animal pathogens (some of which have zoonotic potential), includes the genus *Chlamydia* and the recently added genus *Chlamydiifrater* (Table 1.1).

Currently, the genus *Chlamydia* includes 17 officially recognized species and 3 candidate species (Ca.).

Genus *Chlamydiifrater* includes two new species: *Chlamydiifrater phoenicopteri* and *Chlamydiifrater volucris*, both of which were isolated from wild flamingos (Phoenicopterus roseus) [16].

Amongst the species belonging to the genus *Chlamydia* [17], the best studied is *C. trachomatis*, which occurs predominantly in humans and causes trachoma and is the most common aetiology of bacterial sexually transmitted infections (STIs) worldwide [18]. The remaining *Chlamydia* species have documented zoonotic potential, namely, *C.* psittaci, C. abortus, C. caviae and C. felis. The organisms have varying degrees of host specificity: some *Chlamydia* species have been

Table 1.1 Species of representatives of the Chlamydiaceae family and natural "hosts"

Genus	Species	Host species
Chlamydia	*Chlamydia trachomatis*	Human
	Chlamydia pneumoniae	Humans, koalas, other marsupials, horses
	Chlamydia psittaci	Birds, horses
	Chlamydia avium	Pigeons
	Chlamydia buteonis	Hawks
	Chlamydia gallinacean	Birds: Order of gallinaceae
	Chlamydia ibidis	Ibises: Pelican-like birds
	Chlamydia abortus	Ruminants, pigs
	Chlamydia pecorum	Ruminants animals, pigs, koala
	Chlamydia spp.	Pigs
	Chlamydia felis	Cats
	Chlamydia caviae	Guinea pigs
	Chlamydia muridarum	Mice, hamsters
	Chlamydia crocodile	Reptiles, amphibians
	Chlamydia poikilothermis	Snakes
	Chlamydia serpentis	Snakes
	Chlamydia vaughanii	Fish
	Candidatus species (Ca.): Ca. *Chlamydia corallus,* Ca. *Chlamydia sanzinia,* Ca. *Chlamydia testudines*	Snakes Turtles
Chlamydiarrhea	*Chlamydiifrater phoenicopterid*	Flamingo
	Chlamydia volucris	

reported in only one host species, whilst others have been reported in multiple wild and domestic animal, as well as humans [15, 19–21].

In scientific papers, guidelines and encyclopaedias, the genus *Chlamydophila* is still unreasonably attributed to the family *Chlamydiaceae* [22]. According to the outdated views, 3 species belonged to the genus *Chlamydia (C. trachomatis, C. suis, C. muridarum*), the rest were transferred to the genus *Chlamydophila.* However, such a classification did not overstand the test of time: several groups of authoritative researchers addressed letters and articles to the editors of IJSEM with objections to such a reclassification. As a result, without receiving approval, in 2015, the recommendations of KD Everett et al. were rejected.

Currently, the LPSN (List of Prokaryotic names with Standing in Nomenclature), which is the most authoritative database on biological taxonomy and nomenclature of prokaryotes, positions the taxonomic status *of Chlamydophila* as "heterotypic synonym" instead of the legitimate "correct name," which automatically excludes this name from scientific and practical use [23].

1.2 Brief Characteristics of the Chlamydiaceae Family

1.2.1 Genus *Chlamydia*

1.2.1.1 *Chlamydia trachomatis*

The pathogen, previously traditionally considered an anthroponotic pathogen, can cause genital and generalized forms of the disease in both humans and animals, and cross-infections may occur. This type of *Chlamydia* is the cause of trachoma, mainly in people living in developing countries, and the cause of conjunctivitis and pneumonia in newborns [24–26].

Currently, numerous serovars *of C. trachomatis* have been described, each of which is associated with certain diseases: serovars A-C are the causative agents of trachoma; serovars D-K are the causative agents of urogenital chlamydia; sexually transmitted diseases of other localizations (paratrachoma, pharyngitis, proctitis, pelvic peritonitis, perihepatitis, arthritis); pathologies of newborns, and serovars L1-L3 are the causative agents of venereal lymphogranuloma. Although *C. trachomatis strains* share high nucleotide sequence similarity, the bacterial and host factors governing tissue and cell tropism remain largely unknown [27].

1.2.1.2 *Chlamydia pneumonia*

Species *Chlamydia pneumonia* was initially considered a human-specific microorganism, but has recently been isolated from horses, koalas, and other animals, including amphibians and reptiles. Genetic analysis has shown that the pathogen has crossed over from animals to *Homo sapiens* at least twice in the past.

Genetic and biological differences have made it possible to identify biovars within the species *C. pneumoniae*. It includes three biovars—*Human* and *Koala* (isolated from the koala—*Phascolarctos cinereus* and other Australian marsupials, as well as frogs and reptiles) and *Equine* (from horses). The strains TW-183, AR39, B21, CWL029, J138, LPCoLN have been identified.

In humans, *C. pneumonia* is considered one of the main pathogens of the respiratory tract, causing pharyngitis and other acute respiratory infections, bronchitis, sinusitis and pneumonia. According to numerous studies, seropositivity in adults for *C. pneumoniae* currently ranges from 60% to 80%. Most studies focus on assessing the role of this pathogen as a cause of persistent infections in chronic human diseases. They were based on the assumptions that this pathogen may be associated with bronchial asthma, lung cancer, sarcoidosis, COPD, reactive arthritis, cardiovascular and neurological diseases in humans, including Alzheimer's disease, multiple sclerosis, etc. [28–30].

Despite the simultaneous circulation of *C. pneumonia* in both humans and animals, human and animal isolates are heterogeneous biovars, and the possibility of its anthropozoonotic transmission has not been definitively established.

1.2.1.3 *Chlamydia psittaci*

C. psittaci as a model organism in studies of J.W. Moulder, A. Matsumoto, G.P. Manire, T.P. Hatch, P.B. Wyrick in the 1960s and 1970s laid the foundation for modern chlamydia research.

The first scientific article about chlamydial infection was devoted to an outbreak of psittacosis in humans (Ritter, 1879). Between 1890 and 1930, numerous serious outbreaks of psittacosis in humans occurred in Europe and North and South America (Hegler 1930; Meyer and Eddie 1935), all associated with the keeping, sale and purchase of parrots and other exotic birds. The establishment of the National Institutes of Health was prompted by an outbreak of psittacosis in the United States in 1930 (Lepore, 2009). Large outbreaks have since become rare as disease control has become more effective due to improved knowledge of aetiology and epidemiology, better diagnostic tools and the use of antimicrobial agents in therapy.

C. psittaci is a widespread zoonotic chlamydial species, with 464 bird species (the primary host) from 30 different orders susceptible. *C. psittaci* infection is particularly common in captive parrots and cockatoos (order *Psittaciformes),* where prevalence ranges from 16% to 81%, and in captive turtle doves and pigeons (order *Columbiformes*), where prevalence ranges from 13% to 95%. *C. psittaci* is also common in poultry and is considered endemic in the turkey industry. Additional orders of wild birds that have been infected include *Lariformes* (gulls) and *Anseriformes* (ducks and geese). The bacteria are spread between birds primarily by airborne transmission through inhalation of aerosols from eye or nasal secretions and dust from the feathers and faeces of infected individuals. Vertical broadcast pathogen [31].

However, the initial belief that *C. psittaci* primarily infects birds has been disproved, as the pathogen has been found in domestic animals such as cattle, sheep, pigs, horses, goats, and cats, as well as in wildlife and rodents. Strains of *C. psittaci* transmitted to humans from animals are less pathogenic.

C. psittaci is genetically variable, and genotypes have been designated based on outer membrane protein A (ompA) sequences. Several dozen *C. psittaci genotypes have been identified* (M56, Mat 116, WC, 6BC, etc.), which are also considered pathogenic for humans and capable of zoonotic transmission.

The antigenic properties of *C. psittaci* are determined by the presence of a heat-stable genus-specific lipopolysaccharide antigen, common with other *Chlamydia*, and species-specific proteins of the outer membrane. The microorganism has high virulence, disease caused by *C. psittaci* in humans is characterized by lung damage, development of endocarditis, serous meningitis, encephalitis and renal failure. Infection occurs through inhalation of aerosol and secretions during contact with sick animals, their carcasses or tissues. Infected faeces and feathers are considered to play a key role in zoonotic transmission [36].

1.2.1.4 *Chlamydia gallinacean, Chlamydia avium, Chlamydia ibidis, Chlamydia buteonis*

Until recently, avian chlamydia, called psittacosis or ornithosis, was thought to be caused only by *C. psittaci.* However, since 2009, cases of infection of birds with proposed new species of *Chlamydia* have been isolated and described in some European and Asian countries in chickens and urban pigeons: *Chlamydia gallinacean, Chlamydia ibidis, Chlamydia avium, chlamydia buteonis*. Thus, the World Organisation for Animal Health (WOAH) expanded the definition of avian chlamydiosis including parallel with *C. psittaci* also other *Chlamydia species*.

The species *C. gallinacea* has been found in poultry, guinea fowl, turkeys and ducks without showing signs of disease. It is believed that *C. gallinacea is* an endemic chlamydial species for chickens (*Gallus gallus domesticus*) with the ability to persist in their body for a long time, since experimentally infected chickens do not show any clinical pathology, although the isolated strain of *C. gallinacea* contained a plasmid. This chlamydia was subsequently isolated from chickens in various European countries, Argentina, Australia and China.

In South Korea, *C. gallinacea* was found in woodcocks *(Scolopax rusticola),* but based on genetic analyses, the Korean strain of *C. gallinacea* differed from the European and Chinese isolates.

The zoonotic potential of *C. gallinacea* was suggested following an outbreak of SARS in French slaughterhouse workers. A recent study in China detected *C. psittaci* and *C. gallinacea* DNA in whole blood, milk, faeces and vaginal swabs from clinically healthy dairy and beef cattle. The serovars obtained were identical to those found in birds in the same region, indicating possible transmission from poultry to ruminants, suggesting that *C. gallinacea* is an avian pathogen with potential to infect humans and other animals.

C. avium has been detected in pigeons and parrots (*Psittacula krameri*) in some European countries, but the zoonotic potential *of C. avium* is not yet known. Initial isolates *of C. avium* were obtained from cloacal, faeces and visceral swabs of birds with both asymptomatic forms and cases of clinical pathology and diarrhoea.

Other recently described chlamydial species in birds include *C. buteonis*, isolated from the red-shouldered hawk (*Buteo lineatus*), and *C. ibidis*, isolated from the sacred ibis (*Threskiornis aethiopicus*) and crested ibis (*Nipponia nippon).* To date, the virulence characteristics of *C. ibidis*, its geographic origin, pathogenicity in poultry, wild birds, or other animals, and zoonotic potential are unknown.

Several species of chlamydia, primarily associated with humans and other mammalian hosts, have also been identified in wild birds, including *C. trachomatis, C. abortus, C. pecorum, C. suis* and *C. muridarum*. C. *gallinacea* and *C. avium* are always found in bird flocks simultaneously with *C. psittaci*, but the ecology of the new chlamydial species requires further detailing [32, 37–40].

1.2.1.5 *Chlamydia abortus*

Initially, before the advent of molecular biology methods, chlamydiae of the species *C. abortus* were classified as *C. psittaci serovar* 1 of ruminants [41]. *C. abortus* bacteria are one of the main etiologic factors of chlamydial infectious abortions in small cattle (sheep and goats) and in cattle in many countries of the world. Strains *LLG*, S 26/3 have been identified.

The pathogen has also been associated with chlamydial abortions in horses, rabbits, guinea pigs, mice and pigs. Additionally, pregnant women working with animals infected with *C. abortus* are at risk of infection, as *C. abortus* is also a zoonotic agent capable of causing abortion in humans [42].

1.2.1.6 *Chlamydia pecorum*

Initially, *C. pecorum* was found in ruminants, pigs and koalas (marsupials). *Chlamydia* of this species is associated with a wide range of diseases. Thus, in koalas, *C. pecorum* causes conjunctivitis, infertility and diseases of the urogenital tract. In small and large cattle, horses and pigs, *C. pecorum* is associated with infections of the urogenital system, asymptomatic intestinal infections, abortions, conjunctivitis, mastitis, encephalomyelitis, enteritis, pneumonia, polyarthritis, pleurisy, pericarditis.

Strains E58, DBDeUG, IPTaLE, MC/MarsBar, P787, PV3056/3, VR629, W73 have been identified [43–47].

1.2.1.7 *Chlamydia suis*

Until 1999, *C. suis strains* were referred to as *C. trachomatis* due to sequence homology of the ompA gene. Currently, the pig is considered as the only known natural host of *C. suis*.

Strain MD56 has been identified. *C. suis* strains expressing a stable tetracycline resistance phenotype due to the presence of the tet resistance gene in the chromosome have been isolated from farms in the United States, Italy and Belgium. *C. suis* bacteria are characterized by a higher degree of genetic diversity compared to other *Chlamydia* species [48–50].

1.2.1.8 *Chlamydia felis*

C. felis includes isolates released from cats. This species is capable of causing a clinical form of infection in domestic cats, characterized by acute and chronic conjunctivitis. In addition, *C. felis* can reach the genital tract, causing the development of chronic salpingitis and oviduct infections. It also can be isolated from owners of domestic cats, but its pathogenicity for humans has not been fully determined. However, the possibility of developing follicular conjunctivitis in humans, functional liver disorders, endocarditis and glomerulonephritis upon infection has been established. This species of *Chlamydia* has also been isolated from HIV-positive patients with chronic conjunctivitis, and it was indistinguishable from *Chlamydia* isolated from cats. The first report of zoonotic transmission was associated with the development of acute follicular keratoconjunctivitis in a cat whose owner had a recent history of rhinitis and conjunctivitis.

This type of *Chlamydia* is represented by almost completely genetically identical isolates. However, they differ in extrachromosomal plasmids and pathogenic characteristics. Strain Fe/C-56 has been identified [51, 52].

1.2.1.9 *Chlamydia caviae*

Previously also considered as *C. psittaci,* it is now an independent species of *Chlamydia.* Most often, *C. caviae* causes conjunctivitis, rhinitis and urogenital inflammatory diseases, including abortions in guinea pigs, similar to the symptoms of infections caused by *C. trachomatis* in humans. The infection can be transmitted sexually or perinatally (prenatally—transplacentally, intranatally—during childbirth, or postnatally—during care of newborn individuals), most often by infecting newborn guinea pigs when passing through the birth canal of a sow infected with *C. caviae.* In laboratory conditions, as a result of infection with *C. caviae* strains, it was possible to cause experimental chlamydial infection in mice, hamsters and rabbits, but it is believed that in nature, these bacteria are capable of infecting only guinea pigs. Although *C. caviae* is considered a non-pathogenic microorganism for humans, and cases of pneumonia in adult patients caused by this pathogen have been reported after contact with guinea pigs, *C. caviae is* a good model for studying urogenital chlamydia in humans.

Although sexual transmission of *Chlamydia* infection by this species has so far been proven only for guinea pigs and humans, *C. caviae* can occasionally cause chlamydia in other animal species, particularly horses and rabbits [53–55].

1.2.1.10 *Chlamydia muridarum*

Chlamydia of this species were previously considered a subspecies of *C. trachomatis,* which is now recognized as a separate.

C. muridarum is considered non-pathogenic to humans, being the causative agent of chlamydia in hamsters and mice, as well as other rodents of the Muridae family. Bacteria of this species were first isolated in 1942 from the lungs of Swiss albino mice.

Identified strains MopnTet14, str. Nigg CM 972, str. Nigg 2 MCR, str. Nigg3 CMUT3-13, str. Nigg3 CMUT3-42, str. Nigg3 CMUT3-5, str. Weiss.

Currently, *C. muridarum* strains are actively used to model experimental chlamydial infections, including urogenital chlamydia and lymphogranuloma venereum in humans, demonstrating hydrosalpinx, cervical and vaginal infections in female mice and urethritis in males [56–60].

1.2.1.11 *Chlamydia crocodile*

In crocodiles (*Crocodylus niloticus* and *C. porosus*) *Chlamydia* was discovered in South Africa and Papua—New Guinea. In Thailand, the first outbreak of chlamydia in *Siamese crocodiles (C. siamensis)* was reported in 2012. Molecular evidence based on 16S ribosomal RNA (rRNA), 16S/23S rRNA gene and the major outer membrane protein (ompA) gene indicated that this outbreak was caused by a new species of *Chlamydia*, which was named *C. crocodili.* Clinical signs in infected crocodiles may be absent or may include kyphoscoliosis in juveniles, conjunctivitis, pharyngitis, ascites, depression, anorexia and death [61–66].

1.2.1.12 *Chlamydia poikilothermis, Chlamydia serpentine*

Recent reports indicate that snakes may harbour a significant number of diverse and unusual new species of chlamydia. In study of E. Staub et al. two new species of *Chlamydia* have been described: *Chlamydia serpentis* and *Chlamydia poikilothermis*, isolated from cloacal and choanal swabs of PCR-positive captive snakes from different Swiss snake collections. Whole-genome sequencing of the isolates confirmed the new species status [67–69].

1.2.1.13 *Chlamydia vaughanii*

Bacteria from the order *Chlamydiales*—chlamydial-like organisms—have been found in the aquatic environment as endosymbionts of amoebae and marine worms. They have also been reported as pathogens in fish, causing respiratory infections in the form of epithelial cystis of the gills. The common characteristic of these bacteria is the ability to infect fish epithelial cells, the prevalence of developmental forms characteristic of *Chlamydiales*, and to induce an immune response in the form of macrophage infiltration, as well as the impossibility of culturing them in vitro. These CLOs are the most common bacteria in the aquatic environment, which pose a real threat to the life and health of fish, and indirectly, perhaps, to the health of mammals, including humans [70, 71].

1.2.2 Candidatus Species (Ca.): Ca. *Chlamydia corallus*, Ca. *Chlamydia sanzinia*, Ca. *Chlamydia testudines*

Whole-genome sequencing of genomic DNA obtained from the choana of the clinically asymptomatic Madagascar tree boa (*Sanzinia madagascariensis volontany*) has identified a new species, Candidatus *Chlamydia sanzinia,* and similarly, Candidatus *Chlamydia corallus,* from the choana of the Amazonian emerald tree boa (*Corallus batesii*). These two new genomes show that both species fall in a phylogenetic clade with *C. pneumoniae* and *C. pecorum*. However, the availability of sample material and the lack of suitable culture systems in vitro are challenges for further characterization of new strains of Candidatus species [72, 73].

Some reports have described pathological conditions in turtles caused by *Chlamydiae* [74–76].

In particular, land and sea turtles are usually asymptomatic carriers of these bacteria, but ocular and respiratory symptoms, as well as fatal systemic infections, have been observed in some cases [77–79]. Otherwise, data on chlamydial infections in sea turtles are very scarce.

An outbreak of severe chlamydiosis has been discovered and studied in green sea turtles (*Chelonia mydas*) bred in captivity on a farm located in the British West Indies [80]. The affected turtles were weak, lethargic and unable to dive. Several animals died, and autopsies revealed lesions consistent with systemic infection. The liver, spleen and heart were the organs with the most severe changes, similar to lesions commonly seen in mammals and birds affected by *Chlamydia*. The causative agent is identified as *Chlamydia* sp. was detected in the lesions using Machiavelli staining, electron microscopy and detection of chlamydial antigen using monoclonal antibodies to *Chlamydia*, but the chlamydial species was not identified due to the inadequacy of the methods available over the years of study [80, 81]. Further analysis using PCR and sequencing of DNA extracted from the samples identified *C. abortus, C. pneumoniae* and *Neochlamydia* sp. *C. pneumoniae* was 100% similar to the human genotype. These results indicated that sea turtles may be carriers of pathogens capable of infecting other animals and humans [73, 81–86].

1.2.3 Genus *Chlamydiifrater*

During a routine examination of 15 apparently healthy captive flamingos at a zoo in 2011, an atypical strain of *Chlamydiaceae* was detected in cloacal swab samples using real-time PCR. Sequence analysis of the 16 S rRNA gene revealed high similarity to an uncultured clone 122 of the *Chlamydiales* bacterium, which had previously been found in gulls. As more samples were collected during annual flamingo banding campaigns in southern France from 2012 to 2015, Chlamydiaceae-specific DNA was detected by PCR in 30.9% of wild birds. Of these samples, three strains were successfully grown in cell culture. Ultrastructural analysis, comparison of 16S and 23S rRNA gene sequences, whole-genome analysis based on hybrid sequences of the new strains and subsequent calculation of taxonomic parameters showed that the relationship of the "flamingo" isolates to known representatives of the *Chlamydiaceae family* was sufficiently distant to indicate that these three strains belong to two separate species within the new genus. Based on these data, it was proposed to separate Chlamydiifrater gen. nov. as a new genus, and *Chlamydiifrater phoenicoptery* sp. *nov.* and *Chlamydiifrater volucris* sp. *nov.* as two new species of this genus [87].

1.2.4 Chlamydial-Like Organisms (CLOs)

Until recently, members of the family *Chlamydiaceae* were considered important pathogens of humans and animals with well-defined taxonomic diversity and host ranges. This paradigm has been challenged by molecular techniques that have revealed a greatly expanded taxonomic diversity encompassing other families of bacteria, *Chlamydia-related organisms* (CLOs), within the order *Chlamydiales* and an expanded host range for certain Chlamydial species, such as *C. psittaci* and *C. pneumoniae*, raising new questions about the role of cross-host transmission in the epidemiology of these pathogens. Moreover, these novel host studies have not only revealed expanded host ranges for existing species but have also identified new Chlamydial species, such as in reptiles and birds (Table 2).

Since 2014, new candidate chlamydia-like bacteria have been isolated from reptiles, amphibians, birds, fish and protozoa. They play a role in abortion in ruminants and women (families *Waddliaceae* and *Parachlamydiaceae)* and in epitheliocystitis and gill disease in fish (families *Simkaniaceae*, *Parilichlamydiaceae*, *Piscichlamydiaceae* and *Clavochlamydiaceae*).

Waddlia chondrophila and *Parachlamydia canthamoebae* have been isolated from the placentas of women with adverse pregnancy outcomes. *Waddlia chondrophila* was initially isolated from an aborted cow in the United States in 1986 and was initially classified as a rickettsia. Subsequently, in Germany, *W. chondrophila* was isolated from a stillborn foetus of a calf from a cow infected with *Neospora caninum*. The main pathological changes in that case were lymphohistocytic meningoencephalitis with fibrinous exudate and focal leukoencephalomalacia of the foetal brain with acute purulent pneumonia and bronchiolitis, whilst the aborted cow had multifocal purulent necrotizing placentitis with vasculitis. In studies by Swiss microbiologists, this bacterium was isolated in every hundredth case of late abortion in cattle.

Recently, this organism was detected in vaginal washes and placental tissues from cows in Tunisia with simultaneous infection with *Listeria monocytogenes*. However, in experimental infection, only one of nine heifers infected intravenously with *W. chondrophila* on day 105–110 of pregnancy showed inflammatory changes in the foetal membranes without abortion. For this reason, *W. chondrophila* is still considered an opportunistic organism, and its abortifacient role has not yet been confirmed.

Parachlamydia species have been associated with abortions in cattle and, to a lesser extent, small ruminants in Switzerland, England, Scotland, Ireland, Hungary and Tunisia. Infection has been associated with necrotizing or purulent placentitis, sometimes with the development of vasculitis. Non-suppurative interstitial pneumonia has also been reported in the foetal lungs. Parachlamydia antigen has been demonstrated in the cytoplasm of placental trophoblasts at sites of intense infiltration by polymorphonuclear neutrophils. Isolation of parachlamydia has often been accompanied by isolation of other abortifacients such as *Neospora caninum*, *Coxiella burnetii*, *C. abortus*, *Brucella abortus*, *Campylobacter* and infectious bovine rhinotracheitis virus (IBR). Chlamydia-like bacteria (*P.acanthamoebae*, uncultured chlamydia and *Rhabdochlamydia* species) have also been associated with pneumonia in cattle in Scotland. Parachlamydiae caused mild respiratory disease in calves when experimentally inoculated into the lungs. Clinical signs were largely dose dependent and were accompanied by macroscopic lung lesions. Severe interstitial pneumonia developed when mice were experimentally infected with *P. acanthamoebae* via the nasal and intratracheal routes.

The modes of transmission of chlamydia-like bacteria are unknown, but water sources may play a significant role. The zoonotic potential of these bacteria is very likely and may be expressed by termination of pregnancy and miscarriage in women, as well as pneumonia and bronchiolitis in children. Diagnosis of abortion in practical conditions does not include testing for chlamydia-like bacteria, so the prevalence of such infections in the animal kingdom and amongst people is not precisely determined [88–90].

Bacteria *Chlamydiales*, belonging to family *Rhabdochlamydiaceae*, were discovered in arthropods, in numerous numbers in cockroaches *Blatta orientalis* and ground isopods *Porcellio scaber* (Corsaro et al., 2007, Kostanjsek et al., 2004). Thus, arthropods represent a possible important reservoir for Chlamydiales bacteria that needs to be investigated [91].

In summary, it is worth noting that many bacteria of the order *Chlamydiales* are pathogens or emerging pathogens for both humans and animals, but their true diversity is largely underestimated and their ecology is not yet understood. Given their potential threat to human health, it is important to expand our knowledge of the diversity of chlamydiae and to determine the host range that these bacteria colonize [92–94].

References

1. Collingro A, et al. Chlamydiae in the environment. Trends Microbiol. 2020;28(11):877–88.
2. Kamneva OK, et al. Analysis of genome content evolution in PVC bacterial super-phylum: assessment of candidate genes associated with cellular organization and lifestyle. Genome Biol Evol. 2012;4(12):1375–90.
3. Horn M, et al. Illuminating the evolutionary history of chlamydiae. Science. 2004;304(5671):728–30.
4. Ishida K, et al. Amoebal endosymbiont Neochlamydia genome sequence illuminates the bacterial role in the defense of the host amoebae against legionella pneumophila. PLoS One. 2014;9(4):e95166.
5. Arthofer P, et al. Defensive symbiosis against giant viruses in amoebae. Proc Natl Acad Sci USA. 2022;119(36):e2205856119.
6. Dharamshi JE, et al. Gene gain facilitated endosymbiotic evolution of Chlamydiae. Nat Microbiol. 2023;8(1):40–54.
7. Borges AH, et al. Chlamydia trachomatis vaccine development—a view on the current challenges and how to move forward. Expert Rev Vaccines. 2022;21(11):1555–67.
8. Sevigny JL, et al. Marker genes as predictors of shared genomic function. BMC Genomics. 2019;20(1):268.
9. Johnson JS, al. Evaluation of 16S rRNA gene sequencing for species and strain-level microbiome analysis. Nat Commun. 2019;10(1):5029.
10. Gong W, et al. Estimation of 18S gene copy number in marine eukaryotic plankton using a next-generation sequencing approach. Front Mar Sci. 2019;6:1–5.
11. Wang Y, et al. Four superoxide dismutase (isozymes) genes of Bacillus cereus. Ann Microbiol. 2011;61:355–60.
12. Englesberg E, et al. Some enzymatic changes accompanying the shift from Anaerobiosis to Aerobiosis in Pasteurella Pestis1. J Bacteriol. 1954;68(2):178–85.
13. Bayramova F, et al. Insight into the biology of chlamydia-related bacteria. Microbes Infect. 2018;20(7–8):432–40.
14. Oren A, Göker M. Validation list no. 211. List of new names and new combinations previously effective, but not validly, published. Int J Syst Evol Microbiol. 2023;73:5845.
15. Cheong, et al. Chlamydiaceae: diseases in primary hosts and zoonosis. Microorganisms. 2019;7(5):146. https://doi.org/10.3390/microorganisms7050146.
16. Vorimore F, et al. Isolation of a new chlamydia species from the feral sacred Ibis (Threskiornis aethiopicus): c chlamydia ibidis. PLoS One. 2013;8:e74823.
17. Luu LDW, et al. Genome organization and genomics in chlamydia: whole genome sequencing increases understanding of chlamydial virulence, evolution, and phylogeny. Front Cell Infect Microbiol. 2023:13. https://doi.org/10.3389/fcimb.2023.1178736.
18. Jordan S, et al. Chlamydia trachomatis infections. In: Tan M, Hegeman JH, Sütterlin C, editors. Chlamydia biology: from genome to disease. Norfolk: Caister Academic Press; 2020. p. 1–30.
19. Sachse K, et al. Recent advances in epidemiology, pathology and immunology of veterinary chlamydiae. In: Tan M, Hegeman JH, Sütterlin C, editors. Chlamydia biology: from genome to disease. Norfolk: Caister Academic Press; 2020. p. 403–28.
20. Borel N, et al. Zoonotic transmission of chlamydia spp.: known for 140 years, but still underestimated. In: Sing A, editor. Zoonoses: infections affecting humans and animals. Cham: Springer; 2022. p. 1–28.
21. Albini S, et al. Update zum Zoonosepotential von Chlamydien. Schweiz Arch Tierheilkd. 2023;165(3):165.
22. Everett KD. Chlamydia and Chlamydiales: more than meets the eye. Vet Microbiol. 2000;75(2):109–26. https://www.ncbi.nlm.nih.gov/Taxonomy/Browser/wwwtax.cgi.
23. Schoch CL, et al. NCBI Taxonomy: a comprehensive update on curation, resources and tools. Database (Oxford). 2020;2020:baaa062. PubMed: 32761142 PMC: PMC7408187.
24. Malhotra M, et al. Genital chlamydia trachomatis: an update. Indian J Med Res. 2013;138(3):303–16.
25. Grygiel-Górniak B, et al. Chlamydia trachomatis-an emerging old entity? Rev Microorganisms. 2023;11(5):1283.
26. Mohammadpour M, et al. Trachoma: past, present and future. J Curr Ophthalmol. 2016;28(4):165–9.
27. Faris R, et al. Chlamydia trachomatis serovars drive differential production of proinflammatory cytokines and chemokines depending on the type of cell infected. Front Cell Infect Microbiol. 2019;9:399.
28. Hahn DL, et al. Chlamydia pneumoniae as a respiratory pathogen. Front Biosci. 2002;1(7):e66–76.
29. Roulis E, et al. Chlamydia pneumoniae: modern insights into an ancient pathogen. Trends Microbiol. 2013;21(3):120–8.
30. Porritt RA, et al. Chlamydia pneumoniae infection and inflammatory diseases. For Immunopathol Dis Ther. 2016;7(3–4):237–54.
31. Kaleta EF, Taday EM. Avian host range of Chlamydophila spp. based on isolation, antigen detection and serology. Avian Pathol. 2003;32(5):435–61.
32. Krawiec M, Piasecki T, Wieliczko A. Prevalence of chlamydia psittaci and other chlamydia species in wild birds in Poland. Vector Borne Zoonotic Dis. 2015;15(11):652–5.
33. Stokes HS, Martens JM, Walder K, et al. Species, sex and geographic variation in chlamydial prevalence in abundant wild Australian parrots. Sci Rep. 2020;10(1):20478.
34. Ornithosis KAP. Leningrad: medicine. Leningrad Department; 1973. p. 216p.

35. Knittler MR, Sachse K. Chlamydia psittaci: update on an underestimated zoonotic agent. Rev Pathog Dis. 2015;73(1):1–15.
36. Beeckman DSA, Vanrompay DCG. Zoonotic Chlamydophila psittaci infections from a clinical perspective. Clin Microbiol Infect. 2009;15(1):11–7.
37. Sachse K, Laroucau K, Riege K, et al. Evidence for the existence of two new members of the family Chlamydiaceae and proposal of chlamydia avium sp. nov. and chlamydia gallinacea sp. nov. Syst Appl Microbiol. 2014;37(2):79–88.
38. Laroucau K, Vorimore F, Aaziz R, et al. Chlamydia buteonis, a new chlamydia species isolated from a red-shouldered hawk. Syst Appl Microbiol. 2019;42:125997.
39. Vorimore F, Hsia R-C, Huot-Creasy H. Isolation of a new chlamydia species from the feral sacred ibis (Threskiornis aethiopicus): chlamydia ibidis. PLoS One. 2013;8(9):e74823.
40. Li Z, Liu P, Hou J. Detection of chlamydia psittaci and chlamydia ibidis in the endangered crested ibis (Nipponia nippon). Epidemiol Infect. 2020;8(148):e1.
41. Schautteet K, Vanrompay D. Chlamydiaceae infections in pigs. Review. Vet Res. 2011;42(1):29.
42. Essig A, Longbottom D. Chlamydia abortus: new aspects of infectious abortion in sheep and potential risk for pregnant women. Bacteriology. 2015;2:22–34.
43. Mojica S, Creasy HH, Daugherty S. Genome sequence of the obligate intracellular animal pathogen chlamydia pecorum E58. J Bacteriol. 2011;193(14):3690.
44. Rohner L, Marti H, Torgerson P, et al. Prevalence and molecular characterization of C. pecorum detected in Swiss fattening pigs. Vet Microbiol. 2021;256:109062.
45. Hagenbuch F, Loehrer S, Marti H, et al. Investigation of chlamydia pecorum in livestock from Switzerland reveals a high degree of diversity in bovine strains. Vet Microbiol. 2024;292:110057.
46. Marsh J, Kollipara A, Timms P, Polkinghorne A. Novel molecular markers of Chlamydia pecorum genetic diversity in the koala (Phascolarctos cinereus). BMC Microbiol. 2011;11(1):77.
47. Mohamad KY, Rodolakis A. Recent advances in the understanding of Chlamydophila pecorum infections, sixteen years after it was named as the fourth species of the Chlamydiaceae family. Vet Res. 2009;41(3):27.
48. Kieckens E, Van den Broeck L, Gils MV, et al. Co-occurrence of chlamydia suis DNA and chlamydia suis-specific antibodies in the human eye. Vector Borne Zoonotic Dis. 2018;18(12):677–82.
49. De Puysseleyr L, De Puysseleyr K, Braeckman L, et al. Assessment of chlamydia suis infection in pig farmers. Transbound Emerg Dis. 2017;64(3):826–33.
50. De Puysseleyr K, De Puysseleyr L, Dhondt H, et al. Evaluation of the presence and zoonotic transmission of chlamydia suis in a pig slaughterhouse. BMC Infect Dis. 2014;14:560.
51. Azuma Y, Hirakawa H, Yamashita A, et al. Genome sequence of the cat pathogen, Chlamydophila felis. Comparative study. DNA Res. 2006;13(1):15–23.
52. Hartley JC, Stevenson S, Robinson AJ, et al. Conjunctivitis due to Chlamydophila felis (chlamydia psittaci feline pneumonitis agent) acquired from a cat: case report with molecular characterization of isolates from the patient and cat. J Infect. 2001;43(1):7–11. https://doi.org/10.1053/jinf.2001.0845.
53. Ciuria S, Brouwer MSM, de Gier MM, et al. Chlamydia caviae in Swiss and Dutch Guinea pigs—occurrence and genetic diversity. Pathogens. 2021;10(10):1230.
54. Shomer N, Holcombe H, Harkness J. Biology and diseases of Guinea pigs. In: Laboratory animal medicine. Academic; 2015. p. 247–83.
55. Cheong HC, Lee CYQ, Cheok YY, et al. Chlamydiaceae: diseases in primary hosts and zoonosis. Microorganisms. 2019;7(5):146.
56. Pal S, de la Maza LM. Mechanism of T cell mediated protection in newborn mice against a chlamydia infection. Microbes Infect. 2013;15(8–9):607–14.
57. Pal S, Tifrea DF, de la Maza LM. Characterization of the horizontal and vertical sexual transmission of chlamydia genital infections in a new mouse model. Infect Immun. 2019;87(7):e00834–18.
58. St Jean SC, Arbona RJR, Mishkin N, et al. Chlamydia muridarum infection causes bronchointerstitial pneumonia in NOD.Cg-PrkdcscidIl2rgtm1Wjl/SzJ (NSG) mice. Vet Pathol. 2023;61(1):145–56.
59. Mishkin N, Miranda IC, Carrasco SE, et al. Chlamydia muridarum associated pulmonary and urogenital disease and pathology in a Colony of Enzootically infected Il12rb2 deficient and Stat1 knockout mice. Comp Med. 2024;74(2):121–9.
60. Whary MT, Baumgarth N, Fox JG, Barthold SW. Chapter 3: Biology and diseases of mice. In: Laboratory animal medicine. 3rd ed. Academic; 2015. p. 43–149.
61. Huchzermeyer FW, Gerdes GH, Foggin CM, Huchzermeyer KD, Limper LC. Hepatitis in farmed hatchling Nile crocodiles (Crocodylus niloticus) due to chlamydial infection. JS Afr Vet Assoc. 1994;65(1):20–2.
62. Huchzermeyer FW, Langelet E, Putterill JF. An outbreak of chlamydiosis in farmed Indopacific crocodiles (Crocodylus porosus). JS Afr Vet Assoc. 2008;79(2):99–100.
63. Sariya L, Kladmanee K, Bhusri B, Thaijongrak P, Tonchiangsai K, Chaichoun K, et al. Molecular evidence for genetic distinctions between Chlamydiaceae detected in Siamese crocodiles (Crocodylus siamensis) and known Chlamydiaceae species. Jpn J Vet Res. 2015;63(1):5–14.
64. Thongkamkoon P, Tohmee N, Morris EK, Inamnuay L, Lombardini ED. Combined fatal systemic chlamydia sp. and Aeromonas sobria infection in juvenile Siamese crocodiles (Crocodylus siamensis). Vet Pathol. 2018;55(5):736–40.
65. Shilton CM, Jerrett IV, Davis S, Walsh S, Benedict S, Isberg SR, et al. Diagnostic investigation of new disease syndromes in farmed Australian saltwater crocodiles (Crocodylus porosus) reveals associations with herpesviral infection. J Vet Diagn Invest. 2016;28(3):279–90.

66. Chaiwattanarungruengpaisan S, Thongdee M, Anuntakarun S, et al. A new species of chlamydia isolated from Siamese crocodiles (Crocodylus siamensis). PLoS One. 2021;16(5):e0252081.
67. Staub E, Marti H, Biondi R, et al. Novel chlamydia species isolated from snakes are temperature-sensitive and exhibit decreased susceptibility to azithromycin. Sci Rep. 2021;11(1):18244.
68. Laroucau K, Aaziz R, Lécu A, et al. A cluster of chlamydia serpentis cases in captive snakes. Vet Microbiol. 2020;240:108499.
69. Taylor-Brown A, Vaughan L, Greub G, et al. Twenty years of research into chlamydia-like organisms: a revolution in our understanding of the biology and pathogenicity of members of the phylum Chlamydiae. Pathog Dis. 2015;73:1–15.
70. Pawlikowska-Warych M, Deptuła W. Characteristics of chlamydia-like organisms pathogenic to fish. J Appl Genet. 2015;57:135–41.
71. Collingro A, Köstlbacher S, Mussmann M, et al. Unexpected genomic features in widespread intracellular bacteria: evidence for motility of marine chlamydiae. ISME J. 2017;11(10):2334–44. https://doi.org/10.1038/ismej.2017.95.
72. Taylor-Brown A, Bachmann NL, Borel N, Polkinghorne A. Culture-independent genomic characteriation of Candidatus chlamydia sanzinia, a novel uncultivated bacterium infecting snakes. BMC Genomics. 2016;17:710.
73. Taylor-Brown A, Spang L, Borel N, Polkinghorne A. Culture-independent metagenomics supports discovery of uncultivable bacteria within the genus chlamydia. Sci Rep. 2017;7(1):10661. https://doi.org/10.1038/s41598-017-10757-5.
74. Vanrompay D, De Meurichy W, Ducatelle R, Haesebrouck F. Pneumonia in Moorish tortoises (Testudo graeca) associated with avian serovar a chlamydia psittaci. Vet Rec. 1994;135:284–5.
75. Frutos MC, Monetti MS, Re VE, Cuffini CG. Molecular evidence of Chlamydophila pneumoniae infection in reptiles in Argentina. Rev Argent Microbiol. 2014;46:45–8.
76. Kabeya H, Sato S, Maruyama S. Prevalence and characterization of chlamydia DNA in zoo animals in Japan. Microbiol Immunol. 2015;59:507–15.
77. Hotzel H, Blahak S, Diller R, Sachse K. Evidence of infection in tortoises by chlamydia-like organisms that are genetically distinct from known Chlamydiaceae species. Vet Res Commun. 2005;29(Suppl S1):71–80.
78. Mitura A, Niemczuk K, Zaręba K, Zając M, Laroucau K, Szymańska-Czerwińska M. Free-living and captive turtles and tortoises as carriers of new chlamydia spp. PLoS One. 2017;12:e0185407.
79. Laroucau K, Ortega N, Vorimore F, Aaziz R, Mitura A, Szymanska-Czerwinska M, Cicerol M, Salinas J, Sachse K, Caro MR. Detection of a novel chlamydia species in captive spur-thighed tortoises (Testudo graeca) in southeastern Spain and proposal of Candidatus chlamydia testudinis. Syst Appl Microbiol. 2020;43:126071.
80. Homer BL, Jacobson ER, Schumacher J, Scherba G. Chlamydiosis in mariculture-reared green sea turtles (Chelonia mydas). Vet Pathol. 1994;31:1–7.
81. Bodetti TJ, Jacobson E, Wan C, Hafner L, Pospischil A, Rose K, Timms P. Molecular evidence to support the expansion of the host range of Chlamydophila pneumoniae to include reptiles as well as humans, horses, koalas and amphibians. Syst Appl Microbiol. 2002;25:146–52.
82. Aitken ID, Longbottom D. Chlamydial abortion. In: Aitken ID, editor. Diseases of sheep. Oxford: Blackwell Publishing; 2007. p. 105–12.
83. Pichon N, Guindre L, Laroucau K, Cantaloube M, Nallatamby A, Parreau S. Chlamydia abortus in pregnant woman with acute respiratory distress syndrome. Emerg Infect Dis. 2020;26:628–9.
84. Oren A, Garrity GM, Parker CT, et al. Lists of names of prokaryotic Candidatus taxa free. Int J Syst Evol Microbiol. 2020;70(7):5607–12.
85. Laroucau K, Ortega N, Vorimore F, et al. Detection of a novel chlamydia species in captive spur-thighed tortoises (Testudo graeca) in southeastern Spain and proposal of Candidatus chlamydia testudines. Syst Appl Microbiol. 2020;43(2):126071.
86. Ebani VV. Bacterial infections in sea turtles. Vet Sci. 2023;10(5):333.
87. Vorimore F, Hölzer M, Liebler-Tenorio EM. Evidence for the existence of a new genus Chlamydiifrater gen. nov. inside the family Chlamydiaceae with two new species isolated from flamingo (Phoenicopterus roseus): Chlamydiifrater phoenicopteri sp. nov. and Chlamydiifrater volucris sp. nov. Syst Appl Microbiol. 2021;44(4):126200.
88. Szymańska-Czerwińska M, Zaręba-Marchewka K, Niemczuk K. New insight on chlamydiae. J Vet Res. 2023;67(4):559–65.
89. Fedorova VA, Lyapina AM, Khizhnyakova MA, et al. Chlamydia of animals and humans. Moscow: Federal State Unitary Enterprise Academic Scientific Publishing, Production, Printing and Book Distribution Center "Nauka"; 2019. 135 p
90. Caspe SG, Hill H. Chlamydiosis in Animals. Animals (Basel). 2024;14(21):3130.
91. Croxatto A, Rieille N, Kernif T. Presence of Chlamydiales DNA in ticks and fleas suggests that ticks are carriers of Chlamydiae. Ticks Tick Borne Dis. 2014;5(4):359–65.
92. Stride MC, Polkinghome A, Nowak BF. Chlamydial infections of fish: diverse pathogens and emerging causes of disease in aquaculture species. Vet Microbiol. 2014;171(1–2):258–66.
93. Borel N, Polkinghorne A, Pospischil A. A review on chlamydial diseases in animals: still a challenge for pathologists? Vet Pathol. 2018;55(3):374–90.
94. Corsaro D, Greub G. Pathogenic potential of novel Chlamydiae and diagnostic approaches to infections due to these obligate intracellular bacteria. Clin Microbiol Rev. 2006;19(2):283–97.

Pathogenesis of Chlamydiosis 2

2.1 Structural and Functional Characteristics, Virulence Factors of *Chlamydia* spp.

Chlamydiae are prokaryotic, Gram-negative, obligate, intracellular parasites that function as "large viruses" (0.2–1.5 μm in size). Chlamydiae, like viruses, depend on host cells for energy metabolism. However, they are true bacteria and differ from viruses in many ways.

Chlamydia usually exist as immobile, spherical (cocci) microorganisms. They do not form spores or capsules and do not have flagella.

Like all bacteria, *Chlamydia* have DNA and RNA. They reproduce by binary fission and complete their two-phase development cycle within 40–60 h, whilst viruses undergo lytic and lysogenic phases in their life cycle. *Chlamydia* reproduce only in the cytoplasmic vesicles of living cells of their host. Chlamydia have a type of cells containing peptide glycan (probably represented by muramic acid). DNA appears as a heterogeneous mass inside the cytoplasm without a nuclear membrane. The size of the *Chlamydia* genome is $4–6 \times 10^8$ daltons, and the content of guanine and cytosine is 41–44%. Ribosomes appear as diffuse structures in the cytoplasm (they are absent in viruses). The cytoplasmic membrane is located under the cell wall and contains a large number of lipids, especially phospholipids.

Chlamydia virulence factors facilitate penetration into human tissues and enable the microorganism to hide from the immune system and use the host cell mechanisms to its advantage. These include

- Cell wall structure.
- Type III secretion systems.
- Chlamydial proteins present in the cytosol of infected cells (CPAF, HtrA, CT621 and CT622, CT311, CT795, glycogen synthase (GlgA) *of C. trachomatis,* outer membrane protein B *of C. trachomatis*.
- *Chlamydia*-induced antiapoptotic activity of infected host cells.
- Chlamydial cryptic plasmid.
- CT135 protein.
- Suppression of the NF-κB inflammatory pathway.
- Translocated actin-recruiting protein (TarP).
- Polymorphic proteins of the outer membrane of *Chlamydia* (Pmps). Studying the mechanisms of pathogenicity can lead to the development of new methods of combating this dangerous pathogen [1–20].

Chlamydia have some unique properties that distinguish them from other Gram-negative bacteria:

- Energy parasitism— microbiologists call Chlamydia "energy parasites," because they

V. Zinserling et al., *Chlamydia Infections*, https://doi.org/10.1007/978-3-031-99642-9_2

do not have an ATP-producing system, but they can obtain ATP from host cells.

- They have many metabolically active enzymes.
- FtsZ gene—*Chlamydia* lacks the FtsZ gene, which is necessary for all bacteria and archaea to form a septum during cell division.

Chlamydiae have a very complex growth and reproduction cycle, during which they pass through different phases. Growth, reproduction and maturation of chlamydiae in cell culture usually take 48 h. Their life cycle passes between two morphologically different forms or cell types: EB—elementary bodies or chlamydiospores; RB—reticular or initial bodies. In host tissues, under conditions unfavourable for *Chlamydia*, their life cycle naturally undergoes changes.

2.2 Interaction of *Chlamydia* with Host Cells

A unique feature of the life cycle of *Chlamydia* (alternation of morphological forms) underlies the pathogenesis of these bacteria.

The complex of pathogen–host interactions includes the introduction of *Chlamydia* into the cell, the disruption of intracellular processes of the host cell, the appropriation of host nutrients and evasion of the host immune response [21].

Chlamydia are capable of parasitizing almost all cells of the body, but they have the greatest tropism into columnar epithelium.

The main role in the initiation of *Chlamydia* transformation belongs to membrane structures. At the first stage, ligand–receptor interaction occurs between infectious (extracellular) or elementary bodies (EBs) and the host cell. All membrane proteins are involved in the adhesion process. Polymorphism of membrane proteins is associated with tissue tropism and presumably with the severity of the disease [22]. Then, effectors are "injected" into the host cell and the bacteria invade. During internalization, a vacuole (endosome) called a chlamydial inclusion is formed around the bacterium, in which EBs are transformed into reticular bodies (RBs) through intermediate bodies (IBs). Several EBs can simultaneously adhere to the host cell membrane, leading to the formation of multiple intracellular inclusions. Some types of *Chlamydia* (in particular, *C. trachomatis*) are characterized by the fusion of inclusions into one large vacuole [23]. Depending on the organ and tissue localization of the chlamydial infection focus, as well as the severity of the local and general immune response, the implementation of the intracellular cycle of *Chlamydia* development can occur in three main ways.

In exceptional cases, complete destruction of *Chlamydia* occurs in the host's phagolysosomal system.

In most cases, the productive phase of the *Chlamydia* life cycle begins. Metabolically active RBs quickly modify the vacuole membrane by producing and introducing bacterial proteins (early effectors) into it, which prevents inclusion degradation and facilitates its transport towards the microtubule-organizing centre (MTOC). Active binary divisions of microorganisms (8–12 cycles) occur inside the endosome. Reaching the nutrient-rich zone around the Golgi complex, intermediate forms of *Chlamydia* transform the vacuole membrane so that it becomes permeable to nutrients by producing "intermediate" effectors. Thus, metabolism is disrupted in the host cell and ATP (and other energy carriers) deficiency occurs, which leads to disruption of the cell membrane permeability. In this case, arachidonates (prostaglandins, thromboxane, leukotriene) are released, and lysosome activity is disrupted. At the end of the life cycle, RBs are asynchronously transformed into new-generation EBs via TBs synthesizing late effectors. By lysis or exocytosis, EBs leave the host cell and penetrate new cells. If *Chlamydia* exits by lysis, the host cell dies [24]. In general, the development cycle lasts 48–72 h [25].

In cases of metabolite deficiency in the host cell, inadequately implemented host defence mechanisms and irrational antibiotic therapy, *Chlamydia* persistence usually develops. Morphologically, this is manifested in the transformation of RB into aberrant bodies (ABs), which are in a state of proliferative and metabolic dormancy (hypobiosis) [24]. In this case, *Chlamydia* loses the ability to form colonies on laboratory nutrient media and acquire broad antibiotic resistance. The pathogenetic significance of AB lies, firstly, in the long-term survival of *Chlamydia* in the macroorganism without losing its pathogenic potential; secondly, in the formation of pronounced immunopathological reactions. These properties largely determine the development of chronic chlamydial infection. When the effect of stress factors ceases, the reverse transformation of AB into RT occurs [24].

In addition to the direct damaging effect of the microorganism, a significant role is played by the toxic activity inherent in all *Chlamydia*, associated with an endotoxin-like component and with toxic substances of the inflammatory type. Ultimately, oedema and hyperaemia of the mucous membrane develop in the area of the primary focus, the integrity of the epithelial layer is disrupted with partial desquamation of the epithelium; leukocyte and then lymphoid subepithelial infiltration occurs. In order to reduce the presentation of *Chlamydia* antigen fragments on the membrane surface and prevent their conjugation with ubiquitin and further activation along the corresponding proteolysis pathway, *Chlamydia* enzymes promote increased expression of the host cell's own antigens on the membrane surface. Thus, the activation of polymorphonuclear leukocytes is prevented, and the immune response of the macroorganism is paralyzed [26–28]. The consequence of these processes is the development of functional disorders of the affected organ.

Chlamydial infection is extremely rarely limited localization in the primary focus. Thus, with urogenital *Chlamydia*, the spread of microorganisms occurs in one of three ways:

- Transcanalicularly or via spermatozoa [29]—into the overlying genitourinary organs.
- Lymphogenously through the iliac lymph nodes into the spleen, and then into the gastrointestinal tract [30].
- Haematogenous route through transport within macrophages and neutrophils or independently of them —to distant organs [31].

The concept of the pathogenesis of chlamydial infection was formed by the mid-1990s on the basis of an analysis of scientific information on the clinical picture and epidemiology of diseases caused by *Chlamydia*, on morphofunctional disorders in patients and infected people, as well as on the basis of experimental modelling on animals.

The role of immunopathological mechanisms, in particular, the role of cytokines and heat shock proteins, as well as the genetic predisposition of the macroorganism to a particular disease in response to infection, have long determined the understanding of the pathogenesis of *Chlamydia*. However, in recent years, the development of gene manipulation approaches has expanded our understanding of molecular pathogenesis.

This section presents the general patterns of pathogenesis of diseases caused by various representatives of *Chlamydiales*.

Chlamydia causes many diseases with chronic inflammatory processes in all organs and systems of the human body and affects its reproductive function.

In recent decades, the pathogenesis of chlamydial lesions of the urogenital tract, nervous, cardiovascular, musculoskeletal and bronchopulmonary systems has been actively studied. Means and methods for treating patients with chlamydial infection continue to be developed, based on an understanding of the interaction of the pathogen and the macroorganism. *Chlamydia*, as intracellular obligate energy parasites, exhibit tropism for various types of epithelium, including squamous epithelium of the membranes of the brain and eyeball, fibrocytes, histiocytes, glial and muscle cells, neurons, monocytes, macrophages, etc. [32].

Chlamydial infection has a suppressive effect on the complement system [33], which is manifested in a decrease in the concentration of complement components C3a and C5a. This leads to inhibition of the chemotaxis of polymorphonuclear leukocytes at the site of inflammation and the release of mediators from mast and other cells [34].

Considering the existence of *Chlamydia* in the form of intra- and extracellular forms, it is necessary to distinguish two targets for the immune reactions of the macroorganism: EB, released from infected cells during replicative infection, and infected cells with RB located in them, expressing pathogen antigens on their surface. The cascade of immune reactions in chlamydial infection is caused by antigenic determinants—lipopolysaccharides (LPS), cell wall proteins (MOMP, OMP-2, OMP-3). Cell wall proteins and LPS have not only antigenic properties, but also are pronounced toxins. OMP-2 exhibits the properties of both endotoxin and exotoxin, which is partially secreted by the microbial cell into the external environment. In addition, OMP-2 has a superantigenic effect, which promotes non-specific activation of T-lymphocytes with subsequent formation of a large amount of interleukin-2 (IL-2) and tumour necrosis factor-α (TNFα). LPS, being a universal factor of *Chlamydia* pathogenicity, acts as an endotoxin, the target of which are cells of many human organs, including blood cells (granulocytes, monocytes). *Chlamydia* LPS, unlike cell wall proteins, is a weak antigen, and in small quantities, it stimulates the immune system, whilst in large quantities, on the contrary, it suppresses it. Being a superantigen, LPS causes non-specific stimulation of T- and B-lymphocytes and, as a consequence, the synthesis of a large number of cytokines, including IL-2 and TNFα, as well as polyclonal production of immunoglobulins [35].

The synthesis of antibodies of all classes to chlamydial antigens begins at the stage of elementary bodies, upon exit from the host cell.

EB and their individual antigen components are attacked by serum chlamydial antibodies in collaboration with phagocytes and complement, with the exception of secretory IgA and IgM, which perform their neutralizing functions independently. Five days after the primary colonization of *Chlamydia* and the release of the first EB, IgM antibodies appear, which are produced first to LPS, and then to MOMP. The main amount of IgM is in the vascular bed; in the secretions of the mucous membranes, IgM is found mainly in the form of secretory Ig M, which has neutralizing activity and is a powerful activator of complement. The presence of IgM antibodies indicates the activity of the process or the presence of infection, but the IgM titre can also increase with reactivation, reinfection or superinfection. The half-life of IgM antibodies is 5 days: they do not penetrate the placenta, can be synthesized in the foetus and belong to the newborn's own antibodies. Within 10–14 days after infection, IgA antibodies to the main protein MOMP and OMP-2 are synthesized in the blood serum; a decrease in the titre by the 2nd–4th month is an indicator of successful treatment. The half-life of IgA is 5–8 days. Secretory IgA is a powerful neutralizer and inhibits the adhesion of viruses and bacteria; in addition, it enhances the phagocytic activity of macrophages and polymorphonuclear cells in the blood and, to a lesser extent than IgM, activates complement components. Increased IgA titres are observed in primary *Chlamydia* and reinfection; titres increase to a lesser extent during exacerbation of the chronic process. Antichlamydial IgG is detected in the blood serum by the end of the third week after the appearance of the first EB. IgG is produced for chlamydial LPS and MOMP, the half-life is 23 days. IgG can also be detected in the secretion of mucous membranes in cases of increased permeability of the epithelial layer under inflammatory conditions, but without a secretory component. IgG enhances phagocytosis and complement-dependent lysis, and has a pronounced neutralizing effect. Diagnostically significant IgG titres are detected in chronic *Chlamydia*, and their significant increase occurs during an exacerbation of the process. Due to the weak antigen load in a local sluggish process, the development of serum antibodies in diagnostic titres occurs only in 60–70% of individuals with urogenital diseases [36]. In inflammatory pathology of the nose, paranasal sinuses and pharynx, diagnostically significant titres of antichlamydial immunoglobulins are detected even less often. Thus, according to the studies of Markina A.N. et al. (2021), only 33% (95%, CI 18–41%) of patients with verified chlamydial infection had serum chlamydial antibodies of isotype G to *C. pneumoniae* and *C. trachomatis*. Serum antichlamydial immunoglobulins of isotype A and M were detected in isolated cases [37, 38].

To eliminate *Chlamydia*-infected cells containing RB, the cellular link of immunity is activated with the involvement of T-helper lymphocytes of the first type (Th1).

The latter, with the help of activated macrophages, form a granuloma with subsequent digestion of chlamydial antigens.

The key role in the anti-chlamydial immune response belongs to cytokines, which are products of Th1 and activated macrophages. However, the intracellular existence of *Chlamydia* significantly limits the availability of their antigen substances and, accordingly, reduces the immunogenicity of the pathogen, and, consequently, the sanitizing effect of cytokines.

As a result of the immune response in the form of T-lymphocyte activation, the production of a cytokine profile begins, in particular, the anti-inflammatory cytokine IFNγ (interferon gamma), which activates macrophages, neutrophils, dendritic cells, increases cell resistance to intracellular microorganisms, stimulates the synthesis of IL-1, IL-2 and immunoglobulins [39]. High levels of IFNγ completely inhibit the growth of *Chlamydia*, low levels induce the development of morphologically abnormal intracellular forms.

Unfortunately, stable specific immunity to chlamydial infection is not developed. The insufficiency of the immune response is explained by the phenomenon of incomplete phagocytosis, which is manifested by a decrease in the bactericidal activity of neutrophils (according to the nitroblue tetrazolium reduction test), against the background of an increase in their number, tension in the phagocytic link and an inadequate response of the immune system to this infection.

Chronic chlamydiosis of any organs and systems causes more or less pronounced secondary immunodeficiency states of a combined type: decreased cellular immunity, phagocytic activity, increased concentration of circulating immune complexes, impaired interferon status and complement activity. When analysing immunograms of patients with chlamydial infection of the respiratory tract, compared with reference values, suppression of the T-cell link of immunity with activation of B-lymphocytes was revealed in almost half of the examined individuals. In addition, a third of patients showed changes in leukograms: relative and absolute eosinophilic leukocytosis. Our data also confirm this fact [39]. All of the above indicates the systemic impact of chlamydial infection of the respiratory tract, leading to an imbalance of homeostatic mechanisms in the human body.

The fundamental mechanism in the pathogenesis of chlamydial infection is the ability to persist, that is, the presence of the pathogen in the human body in a transformed form - the L-form.

The metabolic activity of *Chlamydia* in conditions of persistence is significantly reduced, growth is delayed and the transition from RB to EB is slowed down. Predisposing factors for the onset of *Chlamydia* persistence are inadequate etiotropic therapy, insufficient cellular and humoral immune response of the macroorganism [40]. In the case of *Chlamydia* persistence, a significant decrease or complete cessation of the production of MOMP is determined, which is the main immunogen of *Chlamydia*, imparting a high degree of specificity to the antibody and cellular immune responses of the macroorganism. The synthesis of LPS of the chlamydial cell wall is also reduced, but to a lesser extent than MOMP. However, along with this, persistent *Chlamydia* continues to synthesize and actively release heat shock protein (HSP-2), which is the dominant protein in most pathogenic microorganisms. It is the antigens of this protein that play the main role in the pathogenesis of persistent chlamydial infection. In humans, heat shock proteins are a family of various intracellular proteins involved in protein assembly and transport, and regulation of ATP activity. These proteins are related to stress cellular response proteins. Since chlamydial OMP-2 is characterized by a high degree (50%) of homology with the amino acid composition of human heat shock proteins, there is a high probability of developing autoimmune processes in a *Chlamydia*-infected macroorganism.

Chlamydial OMP-2 is a pronounced immunogen, which leads to increased production of various cytokines (IL-1, IL-2, TNFβ, IFNα, IFNβ, IFNγ) by immunocompetent cells and macrophages, suppressing active reproduction of RB, but not destroying these forms of *Chlamydia*, which ultimately contributes to the formation of persistence. Thus, in a persistent state, chlamydial infection is less immunogenic, and the immune response is less specific than in the productive variant of the course, since the response of the macroorganism is formed only to OMP-2 and LPS. Detection of high titres of antibodies to chlamydial OMP-2 is a marker of persistent chlamydial infection. The development of *Chlamydia* persistence is based on the combined action of a complex of cytokines that block the synthesis of MOMP and cause a deficiency of a number of metabolites necessary for differentiation of RB into EB. With minimal microbicidal effect on *Chlamydia*, biologically active cytokines lead to damage to the body's own cells with subsequent development of cicatricial-sclerotic changes in the mucous membrane. Cytokines IL-2, TNFβ, TNFα and IFNγ are producers of T-lymphocytes (Th0, Th1). IFNγ-stimulated macrophages synthesize IL-1, TNFα, IFNα, IFNβ and other biologically active substances. TNFβ and IL-1 promote fibroblast proliferation, leading to fibrous changes in the mucous membrane and submucosal layer. TNFα helps block the reproduction of intracellular RB by enhancing the expression of cell membrane proteins. Activated macrophages produce reactive oxygen species and free radicals, which, however, are not capable of causing significant harm to *Chlamydia*, since the cell wall strength is provided by antioxidant disulfide bonds between structural proteins. In addition, it is reinforced by a polysaccharide microcapsule resistant to superoxide radical oxidation. Therefore, *Chlamydia* are resistant to the products of the "respiratory explosion," and epithelial cells and other target cells of the host are damaged, which leads to scarring and sclerotic changes in the mucous membrane. If a high concentration of IFNγ inhibits the reproduction of *Chlamydia*, activates the lysis of the pathogen in macrophages and other phagocytic cells, then a low concentration promotes the development of L-like transformation of RB with subsequent transition to persistence. This is due to the fact that IFNγ enhances the expression of cell membrane antigens (MHC I, MHC II proteins, Fc receptors, ICAM-1, etc.). As a result, the adhesive capacity of the membranes of epithelial cells and fibroblasts increases, which significantly facilitates the penetration of *Chlamydia* into the cell [41]. In addition, low doses of IFNγ cause a decrease in the concentration of intracellular tryptophan, a metabolite necessary for the construction of MOMP, which also contributes to the development of persistence. An important role in the formation of atypical forms of *Chlamydia* belongs to the deficiency of metabolites such as Ca+ antagonists and cysteine. Thus, the effect of transforming factors leads to the formation of atypical forms of *Chlamydia*. As a result of the combined action of various cytokines of T-lymphocytes and macrophages, the synthesis of which is induced by chlamydial OMP-2, a "vicious circle" arises, leading to sluggish granulomatous inflammation with a proliferative-sclerosing component and the preservation of L-forms of *Chlamydia* with a minimal level of metabolism in the lesion. Persistence of *Chlamydia* leads to an extension of the inflammatory process with a tendency to the occurrence of cicatricial changes in tissues. The state of persistence is an unstable process, and when unfavourable factors disappear, the persistent form can easily switch to a cytocidal existence and manifestation of infection [42]. Depending on the species properties, different routes of infection are typical for representatives of the Chlamydiaceae family. For chlamydophilic infection, the aerosol route of infection is more typical, but given the tropism of this microorganism to blood cells, hematogenous and lymphogenous routes are possible. The mechanism of transmission of infection caused by *C. trachomatis* is contact, the most typical for it are sexual, contact-household, water, intrauterine, intra- and neonatal routes. There is evidence of the introduction of this pathogen to the mucous membrane of the upper respiratory tract through the lacrimal-nasal canal during chlamydial infection of the eyes. Damage to the respiratory tract by *Chlamydia* is also possible as a result of orogenital sexual contacts: *C. trachomatis* was isolated from the throat of 1.3% of homosexual men, and among heterosexuals: from 3.7% of men and 3.2% of women who practiced fellatio and cunnilingus. Susceptibility to chlamydial infection reaches 100%, it is especially high in individuals with immunodeficiency states. Depending on the massiveness of the infection, the presence of concomitant pathology and the state of the immune system, when *Chlamydia* affects the epithelial cells of the mucous membrane of the nose and throat, various ways of interaction of the pathogen with the macroorganism can be realized: spontaneous recovery, reproductive (cytocidal) and nonproductive variants of infection development. Spontaneous recovery is due to the destruction of *Chlamydia* in phagolysosomes under conditions of full implementation of the antimicrobial potential of infected epithelial cells and resistance factors of the macroorganism. Patterns and features of pathogenesis, as well as the frequency of spontaneous recoveries in chlamydial infection in otorhinolaringology have not yet been fully studied.

The pathogenesis of the cytocidal variant of urogenital *Chlamydia* development is described in sufficient detail in the literature. Considering the common biological characteristics of *C. pneumoniae* and *C. trachomatis* and the clinical and morphological manifestations of this infection, the pathogenesis of chlamydial lesions of the upper respiratory tract can be presented as follows. For the disease to occur, infectious particles (IPs) of *Chlamydia* must enter the epithelial cell and multiply in the phagosome, that is colonization of the pathogen must occur. In the process of fixation (adhesion) of EB to the plasma membrane of the epithelial cell, on the one hand, LPS and proteins of the cell wall of the microorganism participate; on the other hand, membrane receptor proteins of the target cell, complementary to the proteins of *Chlamydia*, too participate. Electrostatic and hydrophobic–hydrophilic interactions play an important role in adhesion. The phagosome membrane, formed from the protrusion of the plasma membrane of the epithelial cell, is not damaged by the lysosomal enzymes of the host cell due to the action of antilysosomal enzymes of *Chlamydia* and the presence of protective surface structures in the pathogen.

Chlamydia, during their replicative development cycle, use energy compounds, nucleotides, amino acids and cofactors of the host cell and alter the permeability of the plasma membrane, which disrupts the metabolism of the target cell, leading to its death. An important role in the destructive "effect" of *Chlamydia* is played by the stretching and rupture of the walls of phagosomes and the plasma membrane by numerous progenies of RB, which, with active reproduction, can occupy most of the cell [43]. As a result of the release of hydrolytic enzymes and toxic products of autolysis of destroyed epithelial cells, toxic substances of the *Chlamydia* themselves are released into the surrounding tissues, damage to the surrounding tissues occurs, and the integrity of the epithelial layer is disrupted. At the site of the primary focus, due to the activation of nonspecific and specific humoral cellular defence factors, oedema, hyperaemia, leukocyte and lymphocytic subepithelial infiltration occur, aimed at eliminating flotogenic principles and reparation of damaged tissues. The inflammatory process continues until all damaging factors are completely removed, including the pathogen itself and its fragments, or until a granulomatous fibrous tissue barrier is formed, limiting the lesion, or until *Chlamydia* transitions from the active form to the passive (L-form). The listed outcomes of the inflammatory reaction to the chlamydial pathogen determine the variants of the course of respiratory *Chlamydia*: an acute process with spontaneous recovery or recovery after the use of etiotropic, pathogenetic and symptomatic therapy, chronicity and persistence. The chronicity of infection is facilitated by ischemia in the lesion due to the action of arachidonates (thromboxanes, leukotrienes and prostaglandins), as well as paralysis of the cilia of the ciliated epithelium caused by *Chlamydia*. An important role in the pathogenesis of *Chlamydia* is played by local generalization of infection per continuitatem, that is sequential damage to the epithelial layer. In half of the cases of respiratory chlamydiosis, microbial associations of *Chlamydia* with other pathogenic and opportunistic microorganisms are observed, that is there is a mixed infection and polyetiology of inflammatory pathology. The spectrum of aetiologic agents of inflammatory diseases of the upper respiratory tract associated with chlamydial infection is quite extensive, and it is not always possible to reliably determine the species composition of its structure. The presence of a mixed infection promotes optimal adaptation of all aetiologic agents that make up the microbial association and enhances the pathogenic properties of each of them, promoting better resistance to antimicrobial factors. In addition, numerous studies have shown that different types of *Chlamydia* can act as pathogens simultaneously.

Thus, the inflammatory process of chlamydial aetiology most often proceeds asymptomatically, with a tendency to chronicity and generalization and requires timely diagnosis of intracellular bacterial infection and an adequate set of therapeutic measures and dispensary observation.

2.3 Functional State of the Immune System in Patients with Various Forms of Chronic Urogenital Chlamydial Infection

Considering that chronic urogenital chlamydial infection in most cases (70–80%) occurs as a mixed infection, we considered it appropriate to study immunological disorders in patients with localized and widespread forms of urogenital chlamydia, occurring according to the mixed STI variant. For this purpose, 228 patients with localized form of *Chlamydia* infection (LFHI) were examined. Of these, taking into account the structure of etiological factors, 5 experimental groups were formed: No. 1 (n = 48)—a group with monochlamydia; No. 2 (n = 34)—the disease had chlamydial-trichomonas aetiology; No. 3 (n = 92)—urogenital infection was caused by *Chlamydia*, mycoplasma and trichimonas; No. 4 (n = 26)—the disease was caused by an association of *Chlamydia* + ureaplasma + trichomonas; No. 5 (n = 28)—the infection was mixed (*Chlamydia* + trichomonas + bacteroids). Immunological disorders were determined using 50 different indicators that allowed us to assess the quantitative and functional state of various immune systems.

Depending on the nature of microbial associations, certain immune disorders were observed in patients with CI. Common features for all patients were that, regardless of the aetiology of the disease, most of the indicators differed from those in the control group (healthy), with the exception of the total number of leukocytes, lymphocytes, serum IL-2 levels, as well as its spontaneous production. In patients with monochlamydia, most indicators, compared with those in patients of other experimental groups, changed insignificantly compared with the control group. Thus, against the background of moderate signs of T-suppression, their cytokine status indicators also changed to a lesser extent than in patients with mixed infection. Against the background of insignificant activation of spontaneous IL-1 production, its induced production was reliably lower than in healthy individuals and lower than in other patients with mixed STIs.

At the same time, unlike most experimental groups, these patients had an insignificant increase in the content of this cytokine in the blood serum. In cases where *Chlamydia* was associated with other STI pathogens, the indices of induced production significantly increased compared to the control and similar indices in patients with monochlamydia. Spontaneous production of IL-1 increased in patients with mixed infection, but significantly differed from healthy subjects with the following microbial associations: *Chlamydia* + trichomonas + ureaplasma and *Chlamydia* + trichomonas + bacteroids. Spontaneous production of IL-2 in these patients was not activated, although its induced production significantly decreased only in patients whose infection was caused by such associations as *Chlamydia* + trichomonas + ureaplasma and *Chlamydia* + trichomonas + bacteroids. The spontaneous production of IL-6 and its content in the blood serum of patients (except for experimental group No. 6) of all groups did not differ from the control level. At the same time, the induced production of IL-6 was minimal in patients with monochlamydia and was significantly higher compared to the control. Almost similar features were characteristic of the indices of such a cytokine as TNF. The content of IL-8 in the blood serum was minimal in all patients, and its spontaneous production, although increased, was significantly higher in patients of experimental groups 3 and 5, whose mixed infection was caused by the association of *Chlamydia* with trichomonads, as well as mycoplasmas and bacteroids, respectively. Induced production of IL-8 in patients with monochlamydia remained at a normal level; however, in cases of associations of *Chlamydia* with other pathogens of STIs, it significantly increased compared to the control level, as well as the level in patients with monochlamydia. The parameters characterizing the migration, adhesive, phagocytic and bactericidal activity of neutrophils were in most cases significantly lower in these patients compared to the control. Their moderate decrease was observed only in monochlamydia, whilst in mixed infection with *Chlamydia*, they were in most cases significantly lower, in contrast to the parameters in patients with monochlamydial infection. The parameters characterizing the activation of the complement system moderately decreased in patients of all experimental groups. At the same time, only in patients with monochlamydia was a significant decrease in such a component as C1inh observed.

Thus, based on the analysis of the obtained research results, the following conclusion can be made. Patients with LFHI develop moderately expressed immunological disorders, which were minimal in patients with monochlamydia. In mixed infection with *Chlamydia*, they are more pronounced and indicate the immunosuppressive effect of trichomonads, mycoplasmas, ureaplasmas and pathogenic forms of bacteroids. This is supported by a more pronounced dysfunction of the immune system in patients with mixed infection, consisting in a significant decrease in CD4 and a reliable decrease in CD4/CD8 ($p < 0.05$). Pathognomonic for mixed STIs with *Chlamydia* was a constantly detected reliable increase ($p < 0.05$) in the number of cells carrying a membrane receptor to IL-2 (CD25). However, no significant differences were found in the serum content of the main cytokines and their spontaneous production. The associative nature of HI significantly increased the induced production of IL-1, IL-6, IL-8 and TNF against the background of a decrease in most indicators of migration, adhesive, phagocytic and bactericidal activity of neutrophils. The complement system was slightly activated in the examined patients. This is evidenced by a slight decrease in some of its components. In mixed infection with *Chlamydia*, only component such as C1inh reliably differed from the same indicator in patients with monochlamydia.

Based on the obtained research results, the following conclusions can be drawn.

In patients with chronic prostatitis and prostatovesiculitis, significant disturbances in the local cytokine status in the genitourinary tract are observed, which is manifested in an increase in the production of IL-8 against the background of a decrease in the content of IL-1 α.

A higher increase in the concentration of IL-8 and a significant decrease in IL-1 α in the ejaculate may indicate that patients are developing a more extensive local inflammatory process (prostatovesiculitis).

Persistent high levels of IL-8 and low concentrations of IL-1 α in the ejaculate of patients after completion of combination therapy may serve as additional markers of persistent chlamydial infection in the prostate gland.

2.4 Results of Correlation Analysis of Immunological Parameters in Patients with Localized and Widespread Forms of Urogenital Chlamydiosis

A regression analysis was conducted to identify the mathematical relationship between the most informative indicators of cellular immunity. The results of this analysis are presented in Fig. 2.1.

The presented graphs show that there is a specific mathematical relationship between the percentage of CD3 and CD4; CD3 and CD8; CD4 and CD20; CD20 and CD25; HLA II and CD20; CD20 and CD16; CD25 and HLA II; CD25 and

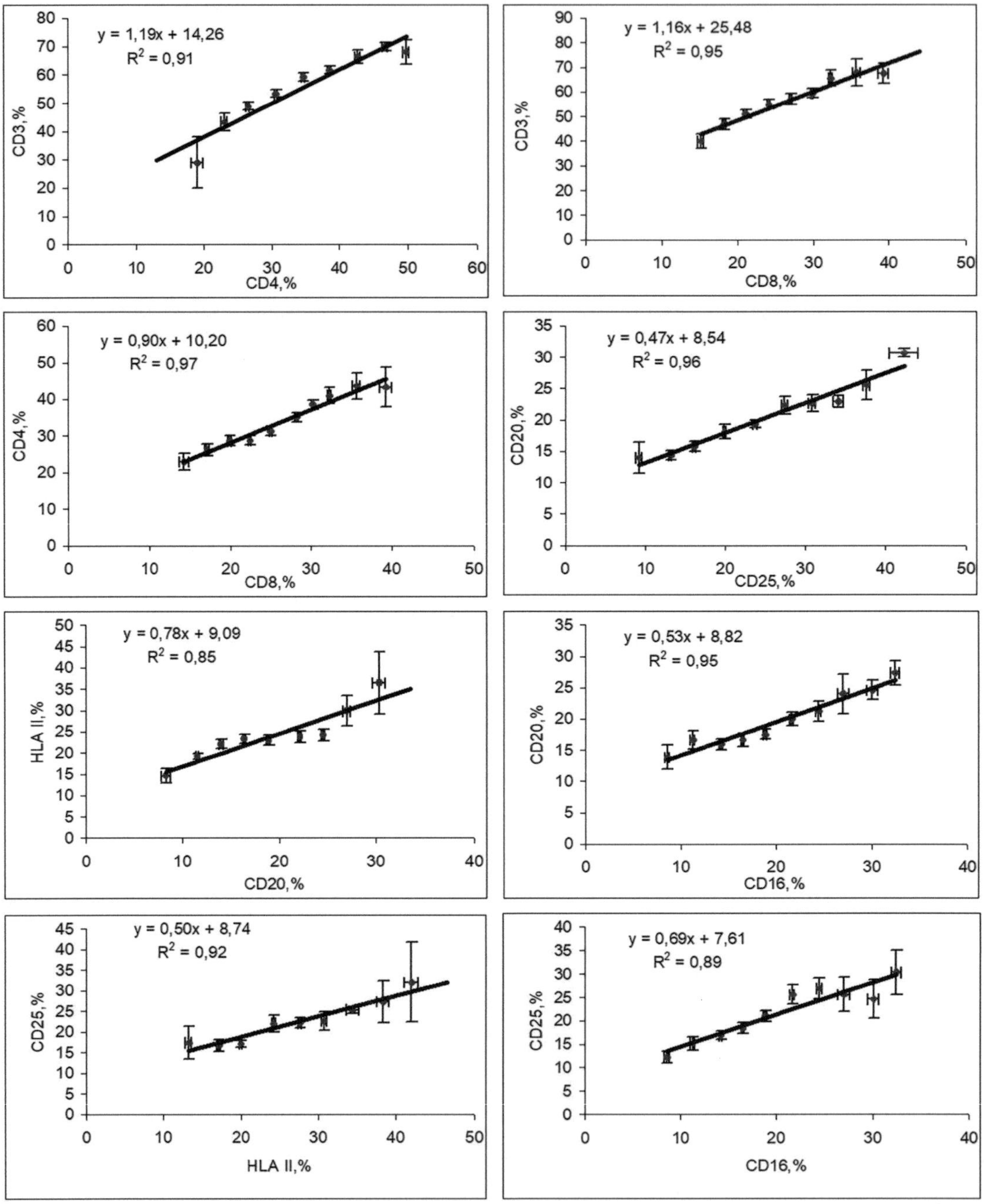

Fig. 2.1 The nature of the regression relationship between the indicators of cellular immunity in patients with urogenital chlamydia (analytical expression on the graphs is the linear regression equation)

CD16 in the blood of patients with chlamydial infection. The analysis of the results of correlation and regression analyses of immunological parameters in patients with chronic urogenital chlamydia allowed us to identify a number of interesting features that characterize the functional state of various links of the immune system in this group of patients. First of all, it should be noted that there are strong and moderate correlations between most immunological parameters in such patients; on the one hand, with the amount of antichlamydial antibodies in the blood serum, and on the other hand, with the severity of dysbiotic conditions in the normal intestinal flora. The obtained data indicate that there is probably a certain relationship between the state of the intestinal microbiocenosis and the functional state of such immune links as the T-link, the neutrophil-macrophage link and the complement system.

The general assessment of the features of the correlation dependence between antibody titres and the degree of intestinal dysbacteriosis, on the one hand, and immunological indices, on the other hand, showed that it is somewhat different in patients with LFHI and WFHI. Thus, in patients with LFHI, moderate and weak correlations between antibody titres and immunological indices prevailed, whilst strong and moderate correlations were more often determined between them and intestinal dysbacteriosis. In patients with RFHI, the correlation dependence between antibody formation and immunological indices (compared to those in patients with localized forms) decreased, whilst between dysbacteriosis and the same indices, it increased. This was probably due to the increased dysfunctional state of the immune system against the background of the development of more pronounced intestinal dysbacteriosis and immunodeficiency in this category of patients.

The obtained results indicate that patients with WFHI need rational immuno- and bacteriotherapy to a greater extent than patients with LFHI. We also came to this conclusion after studying the results of correlation and regression analyses of the parameters characterizing the state of the cellular link of immunity. Thus, it turned out that in patients with LFHI, strong correlation links between different lymphocyte subpopulations prevailed. In patients with common forms of *Chlamydia*, weak and moderate correlation links between these parameters prevailed. The results of correlation and regression analyses revealed the most pronounced correlation dependence between such parameters of cellular immunity as CD3 and CD4; CD3 and CD8; CD4 and CD20; CD20 and CD25; HLA II and CD20; CD20 and CD16; CD25 and HLA II; CD25 and CD16. The obtained results of the study of correlations between these indicators allowed them to be expressed in the form of mathematical formulas, which will probably have practical significance for the correct assessment of the functional state of cellular immunity in patients with urogenital chlamydia. The obtained research results have not only scientific but also practical significance, since they allow developing a targeted ("topical") programme of immunotherapy for patients with LFHI and WFHI.

The results of immunological studies conducted in patients with LFHI and WFHI allowed us to draw the following conclusions. Most patients are diagnosed with immunological disorders indicating the development of predominantly T-suppression against the background of a decrease in the immunoregulatory index, a decrease in the proliferative activity of lymphocytes and a violation of the functional activity of neutrophils. The data on the study of cytokine status indicators in these patients are of interest. It turned out that both in patients with LFHI and in patients with common forms of *Chlamydia*, spontaneous and induced production of IL-1 increases against the background of insignificant induced production of IL-2, an increase in spontaneous and induced production of IL-6, TNF, IL-8. It was found that the cytokine status indicators in patients with WFHI indicated a more significant (the differences were reliable) activation of cytokine production than in patients with LFHI. At the same time, the indices of spontaneous and induced migration activity of leukocytes were reduced, and the indices of O2-dependent antimicrobial system of neutrophils were significantly lower than in healthy individuals. Activation of the complement system is observed mainly in patients with WFCI, which confirmed the systemic nature of the inflammatory process. The results of the correlation analysis showed that this group of patients (especially in patients with WFCI) develop moderate disturbances of the functional relationships between the immunological indices of cellular immunity and cytokine status. The results of the correlation analysis also revealed disturbances in the correlation links between the immunological indices and such general criteria for assessing antichlamydial resistance as the activity of formation of antichlamydial antibodies and such an important indicator of general colonization resistance as intestinal dysbacteriosis.

Thus, the analysis of the obtained research results allowed us to draw the following conclusions.

- In patients with LFHI, immunological disorders develop to a lesser extent, whilst in patients with WFHI, they develop to a greater extent. In individuals with WFHI, they indicate the development of systemic inflammation.
- Considering that patients with LFHI are diagnosed with moderate signs of T-suppression against the background of significant disturbances in the cytokine status and the absence of signs of activation of the complement system, they are indicated for immunotherapy that restores these disturbances.
- Considering that patients with WFHI develop deeper immune changes against the background of disruptions in correlation links between both cellular immunity indicators and between different parts of the immune system, and disruptions are also formed between immune system indicators and colonization resistance (intestinal dysbacteriosis), they are more likely to benefit from replacement (cytokine) immunotherapy.

Of extreme importance in understanding the immunopathogenesis of chlamydial infection is the ability of *Chlamydia* itself to exist in the human body in the form of other main forms: reticular bodies (intracellular form) and elementary bodies (extracellular form). Considering that intracellular (reticular) forms of the pathogen produce antilysosomal enzymes that suppress antimicrobial systems both inside epithelial cells and inside neutrophils and macrophages. Therefore, intracellular digestion of *Chlamydia* inside phagocytes does not ensure their complete destruction. Therefore, conditions arise for intracellular circulation of the pathogen in the blood in the lymph, which leads to the generalization of the infectious process and the emergence of extraurogenital foci of infection.

Chlamydial infection has a suppressive effect on the complement system, which is manifested in a decrease in the concentration of complement components C3a and C5a. Ultimately, this leads to a decrease in neutrophil chemotaxis in the inflammation site and the release of leukocytes in the inflammation site and the release of mediators from mast and other cells. Given the 2-phase biological cycle of *Chlamydia* in the human body, there are 2 targets for immune responses of the macroorganism. The cascade of immune responses in chlamydial infection is caused by antigenic determinants—lipopolysaccharides (LPS), cell wall proteins (MOMP, OMP-2, OMP-3). Cell wall proteins and LPS have not only antigenic properties, but are also pronounced toxins. OMP2 exhibits the properties of both endotoxin and exotoxin, which are partially secreted by the microbial cell into the external environment. In this case, OMP2 has a superantigen effect, which enhances the nonspecific activation of T lymphocytes with the subsequent formation of a large amount of interleukin-2 (IL-2) and tumour necrosis factor-a (TNF-a). LPS acts as an endotoxin, the target for action of which are cells of many human organs, including blood cells (neutrophils, monocytes). Being a superantigen, LPS causes nonspecific stimulation of T and B lymphocytes, resulting in increased synthesis of a large number of cytokines, including IL-2 and TNF-a, as well as polyclonal production of immunoglobulins. The synthesis of antichlamydial antibodies begins at the stage of the appearance of elementary bodies when they exit cells infected with *Chlamydia*. These serum chlamydial antibodies, in collaboration with phagocytes and complement, perform their neutralizing functions independently: 5–7 days after the primary infection with *Chlamydia* and the release of the first elementary bodies from the cells, IgM antibodies appear. They are first produced to LPS, and then to MOMP. They are mainly found in the bloodstream, in the secretions of the mucous membranes in the form of secretory IgM, which is a powerful complement activator. Its presence indicates the activity of the process or a fresh infection.

And 10–14 days after infection, IgA antibodies begin to be synthesized in the blood serum. The half-life of IgA is 5–8 days. These antibodies are a strong neutralizer and inhibitor of adhesion of viruses and bacteria. They also enhance the phagocytic function of neutrophils and macrophages. An increase in IgA titres is observed with fresh primary chlamydial infection, as well as with reinfection, and to a lesser extent, titres increase with exacerbation of the chronic process.

In chronic persistent form of chlamydial infection, a weak antigen load is formed with a local sluggish inflammatory process. In this category of patients, the production of serum antibodies in diagnostic titres occurs only in, and 60–70% of individuals.

As a result of the launch of the immune response in the form of activation of T-lymphocytes, an increase in the production of the cytokine cascade is observed, including cytokines such as INF-gamma, which enhances the phagocytic activity of neutrophils and macrophages, as well as dendritic cells.

High levels of INF-gamma can inhibit the growth of *Chlamydia*, whilst low levels can induce the development of morphologically abnormal intracellular forms of *Chlamydia*.

It has been established that patients with chlamydial infection do not develop persistent specific immunity to this infection. This is explained by the phenomenon of incompleteness of phagocytes as a result of depression of their antimicrobial systems, which is manifested by a significant decrease in the bactericidal activity of neutrophils.

In cases of development of systemic (generalized) form of chlamydial infection with damage of various organs and systems in such patient's standard immune response to the existing inflammatory infectious process is not formed. In such cases, secondary immunodeficiency state of combined type is formed in patients: decrease of cellular immunity (T suppression); suppression of phagocytic activity and completeness of phagocytosis of neutrophils and macrophages due to suppression of their antimicrobial systems; increase of production of circulating immune complexes; disruption of interferon production; activation of complement.

The results of our studies also confirm these data. All the above information indicates the systemic influence of chlamydial infection on the immune system of such a category of patients, which ultimately leads to a pronounced imbalance of all links of the immune system, as well as most haemostatic mechanisms of the human body.

Depletion of the immune system function in patients with chlamydial infection contributes to the formation of a persistent chronic form of this pathology. This process is also facilitated by ineffective etiotropic therapy, as well as the presence of insufficient cellular and humoral immunity in the patient.

In such cases, *Chlamydia* reduce or completely stop the production of MOMP, which is the main immunogen of *Chlamydia*. At the same time, the production of LPS of the chlamydial cell wall is suppressed. But at the same time, persistent *Chlamydia* continue to synthesize heat shock protein (OMP-2). The antigen of this protein plays a major role in the pathogenesis of persistent chlamydial infection. In humans, these proteins are a family of various intracellular proteins involved in the assembly and transport of proteins and the regulation of ATP activity. These proteins are related to the proteins of the stress cellular response.

Detection of high titres of antibodies to chlamydial OMP-2 is an objective marker of persistent chlamydial infection. With minimal microbicidal effect on *Chlamydia*, biologically active cytokines lead to damage to the body's own cells with subsequent development of cicatricial-sclerotic changes in infected tissues.

In subsequent years, data appeared that, using immunohistological methods, signs of granulomatous inflammation were revealed in inflammatory foci in infected tissues of chlamydial aetiology.

Chlamydia, in the process of implementing their replicative development cycle, use energy compounds, nucleotides, amino acids, cofactors of host cells and disrupt the permeability of the plasma membrane.

Ultimately, this leads to metabolic disturbances in the target cell and even to its death. An important role in the destructive effect of *Chlamydia* is played by the stretching and rupture of the walls of phagosomes and the plasma membrane by a significant number of accumulated reticular bodies.

Ultimately, this leads to the release of hydrolytic enzymes and toxic substances of autolysis of destroyed epithelial cells, toxic substances of the *Chlamydia* themselves into the surrounding tissues, which leads to damage to the surrounding tissues, disruption of the integrity of the epithelial membrane. As a result of the activation of non-specific and specific defence factors, oedema, hyperaemia, leukocyte and lymphocyte subepithelial infiltration are formed in the inflammation focus, aimed at eliminating destructive principles and reparation of damaged tissues. In this case, the chronic inflammatory process continues until all damaging factors are completely removed, including the pathogen itself and its fragments, or until a granulomatous fibrous-sclerotic substrate is formed, which, as a barrier, will limit the inflammation focus and thus will contribute to the transition of the active form of infection to a persistent one.

Thus, the above-listed variants of the outcomes of the inflammatory reaction to tissues infected with *Chlamydia* determine the variants of the course of chlamydial infection with complete sanitation of the body from the pathogen (complete self-healing) or recovery after the use of complex etiotropic, pathogenetic and symptomatic therapy, as well as chronicization of the process or the transition of chlamydial infection to a persistent form. It should be noted that the chronicization of the inflammatory process can be facilitated by ischaemia in the lesion due to the action of arachidonates (thromboxanes, leukotrienes and prostaglandins). Both local and general generalization of the infection play an important role in the pathogenesis of *Chlamydia*, which ultimately leads to the sequential defeat of new tissues and organs by *Chlamydia*.

Most patients with chlamydial infection are diagnosed with mixed chlamydial infection, caused by the association of *Chlamydia* with opportunistic pathogens and opportunistic microorganisms (see also Chap. 8). In such cases, a mixed infection is observed, which determines the polyetiology of this inflammatory process.

References

1. Xaplanteri P, Rodis N, Potsios C. Virulence factors of chlamydia spp. involving human infections. In: Sarier M, editor. Chlamydia—secret enemy from past to present, Infectious diseases. Intechopen; 2023. p. 406. https://www.intechopen.com/books/12417.
2. Conrad T, Yang Z, Ojcius D, Zhong G. A path forward for the chlamydial virulence factor CPAF. Microbes Infect. 2013;15(14–15):1026–32.
3. Krüll M, Suttorp N. Pathogenesis of Chlamydophila pneumoniae infections—epidemiology, immunity, cell biology, virulence factors. In: Community-acquired pneumonia. Birkhäuser advances in infectious diseases. Basel: Birkhäuser; 2007.
4. Qi M, Lei L, Gong S, Liu Q, DeLisa MP, Zhong G. Chlamydia trachomatis secretion of an immunodominant hypothetical protein (CT795) into host cell cytoplasm. J Bacteriol. 2011;193(10):2498–509.
5. O'Connell CM, Ferone ME. Chlamydia trachomatis genital infections. Microbial Cell. 2016;3(9):390–403.
6. Heijne M, Jelocnik M, Umanets A, et al. Genetic and phenotypic analysis of the pathogenic potential of two novel chlamydia gallinacea strains compared to chlamydia psittaci. Sci Rep. 2021;11:16516.
7. Hudson AP. A major advance in elucidating the biology/pathobiology of chlamydia trachomatis. Infect Immun. 2013;81(3):622–4.
8. Byrne GI. Chlamydia trachomatis strains and virulence: rethinking links to infection prevalence and disease severity. J Infect Dis. 2010;201(S2):S 126-S133.
9. Beder T, Saluz HP. Virulence-related comparative transcriptomics of infectious and non-infectious chlamydial particles. BMC Genom. 2018;19:575.
10. Gong S, Lei L, Chang X, Belland R, Zhong G. Chlamydia trachomatis secretion of hypothetical protein CT622 into host cell cytoplasm via a secretion pathway that can be inhibited by the type III secretion system inhibitor compound 1. Microbiology (Reading). 2011;157(Pt 4):1134–44.

11. Wu X, Lei L, Gong S, et al. The chlamydial periplasmic stress response serine protease cHtrA is secreted into host cell cytosol. BMC Microbiol. 2011;11:87.
12. Lei L, Dong X, Li Z, Zhong G. Identification of a novel nuclear localization signal sequence in chlamydia trachomatis-secreted hypothetical protein CT311. PLoS One. 2013;8(5):e64529.
13. Lu C, Lei L, Peng B, et al. Chlamydia trachomatis GlgA is secreted into host cell cytoplasm. PLoS One. 2013;8(7):e68764.
14. Song L, Carlson JH, Whitmire WM, et al. Chlamydia trachomatis plasmid-encoded Pgp4 is a transcriptional regulator of virulence-associated genes. Infect Immun. 2013;81(3):636–44.
15. Qi M, Gong S, Lei L, et al. A chlamydia trachomatis OmcB C-terminal fragment is released into the host cell cytoplasm and is immunogenic in humans. Infect Immun. 2011;79(2193):e2203.
16. Hou S, Sun X, Dong X, et al. Chlamydial plasmid-encoded virulence factor Pgp3 interacts with human cathelicidin peptide LL-37 to modulate immune response. Microbes Infect. 2019;21(1):50–5.
17. Chen Q, Li Y, Yan X, et al. Chlamydia psittaci plasmid-encoded CPSIT_P7 elicits inflammatory response in human monocytes via TLR4/mal/MyD88/NF-κB signaling pathway. Front Microbiol. 2020;11:578009.
18. Mojica SA, Hovis KM, Frieman MB, et al. SINC, a type III secreted protein of chlamydia psittaci, targets the inner nuclear membrane of infected cells and uninfected neighbors. Mol Biol Cell. 2015;26(10):1918–34.
19. Whitewood AJ, Singh AK, Brown DG, Goult BT. Chlamydial virulence factor TarP mimics Talin to disrupt the Talin-vinculin complex. FEBS Lett. 2018;592(10):1751–60.
20. Vasilevsky S, Stojanov M, Greub G, Baud D. Chlamydial polymorphic membrane proteins: regulation, function and potential vaccine candidates. Virulence. 2016;7(1):11–22.
21. Luu LDW, Kasimov V, Phillips S, Myers GSA, Jelocnik M. Genome organization and genomics in chlamydia: whole genome sequencing increases understanding of chlamydial virulence, evolution, and phylogeny. Front Cell Infect Microbiol. 2023;13:1178736. https://doi.org/10.3389/fcimb.2023.1178736. PMID: 37287464; PMCID: PMC10242142
22. Abdelsamed, et al. Genetic variation in Chlamydia trachomatis and their hosts: impact on disease severity and tissue tropism. Future Microbiol. 8:1129–46. https://doi.org/10.2217/fmb.13.80.
23. Richards TS, Knowlton AE, Grieshaber SS. Chlamydia trachomatis homotypic inclusion fusion is promoted by host microtubule trafficking. BMC Microbiol. 2013;13:185. https://doi.org/10.1186/1471-2180-13-185.
24. Gitsels A, Sanders N, Vanrompay D. Chlamydial infection from outside to inside. Front Microbiol. 2019;10:2329. https://doi.org/10.3389/fmicb.2019.02329.
25. Elwell C, Mirrashidi K, Engel J. Chlamydia cell biology and pathogenesis. Nat Rev Microbiol. 2016;14(6):385–400.
26. Cram ED, Simmons RS, Palmer AL, Hildebrand WH, Rockey DD, Dolan BP. Enhanced direct major histocompatibility complex class I self-antigen presentation induced by chlamydia infection. Infect Immun. 2016;84:480–90. https://doi.org/10.1128/IAI.01254-15.
27. Pickering H, Teng A, Faal N, Joof H, Makalo P, Cassama E, et al. Genome-wide profiling of humoral immunity and pathogen genes under selection identifies immune evasion tactics of chlamydia trachomatis during ocular infection. Sci Rep. 2017;7:9634. https://doi.org/10.1038/s41598-017-09193-2.
28. Rajeeve K, Das S, Prusty BK, Rudel T. Chlamydia trachomatis paralyses neutrophils to evade the host innate immune response. Nat Microbiol. 2018;3:824–35. https://doi.org/10.1038/s41564-018-0182-y.
29. Makarounis K, Leventopoulos M, Georgoulias G, Nikolopoulos D, Zeginiadou T, Xountasi M, Kotrotsos P, Nosi E, Gennimata V, Venieratos D, Protogerou V, Tsilivakos V. Detection of chlamydia trachomatis inside spermatozoa using flow cytometry: effects of antibiotic treatment (before and after) on sperm count parameters. J Microbiol Methods. 2022;203:106604. https://doi.org/10.1016/j.mimet.2022.106604. Epub 2022 Oct 28. PMID: 36330892
30. Howe SE, Shillova N, Konjufca V. Dissemination of chlamydia from the reproductive tract to the gastro-intestinal tract occurs in stages and relies on chlamydia transport by host cells. PLoS Pathog. 2019;15(12):e1008207. https://doi.org/10.1371/iournal.ppat.1008207.
31. Zigangirova NA, Rumyantseva YP, Morgunova EY. Detection of C. trachomatis in the serum of the patients with urogenital chlamydiosis. BioMed Res Int. 2013;2013:489489, 7 pages. https://doi.org/10.1155/2013/489489.
32. Mandel CG, et al. Metabolism and physiology of pathogenic bacterial obligate intracellular parasites. Front Cell Infect Microbiol. 2024;14:1284701. https://doi.org/10.3389/fcimb.2024.1284701.
33. Tığlı GA. Immune response to Chlamydia. In: Sarier M, editor. Chlamydia—secret enemy from past to present [Internet], Infectious diseases. IntechOpen; 2023. https://doi.org/10.5772/intechopen.106108.
34. Chifiriuc MC, Socolov D, Moshin V, et al. Host immune response to chlamydia infection. In: Mares M, editor. Chlamydia [Internet]. Intech; 2012. https://doi.org/10.5772/1153.
35. Puy H, Fuentes V, Eb F, Orfila J. Biochemical characteristics and antigenic structures of chlamydia. Ann Biol Clin. 1989;47(8):485–91.

36. Puolakkainen M. Laboratory diagnosis of persistent human chlamydial infection. Front Cell Infect Microbiol. 2013;3:99.
37. Bragina EE, Orlova OE, Dmitriev GA. Some features of the life cycle of chlamydia. Atypical forms of existence: a review of the literature. Sexually Transmitted Diseases. 1998;1:3–9.
38. Poikonen K, Lajunen T, Silvennoinen-Kassinen S, Paldanius M, Leinonen M, Saikku P. Susceptibility of human monocytemacrophages to Chlamydia pneumoniae infection in vitro is highly variable and associated with levels of soluble CD14 and C. pneumoniae IgA and human HSP-IgG antibodies in serum. Scand J Immunol. 2008;67:279–84.
39. Sidorchuk S.N. Clinical and immunological features of pneumo-chlamydia in young people, 2004.
40. Jury B, Fleming C, Huston WM, LDW L. Molecular pathogenesis of Chlamydia trachomatis. Front Cell Infect Microbiol. 2023;13:1281823.
41. Brockett MR, Liechti GW. Persistence alters the interaction between chlamydia trachomatis and its host cell. Infect Immun. 2021;89(8):e0068520.
42. Beattie VL, Morrison RP, Byrne DI. Chlamydia persistence: from cell cultures.
43. Luu LDW, Kasimov V, Phillips S. Genome organization and genomics in Chlamydia: whole genome sequencing increases understanding of chlamydial virulence, evolution, and phylogeny.

3 Epidemiology of Chlamydial Infections

The role of *Chlamydia* as an aetiologic factor in many spontaneous infections of humans and various animal species has been determined relatively recently. Urogenital chlamydia was recognized as an STI in the 1970s and became subject to registration in 1988 (in the Russian Federation since 1993). Beginning in 1990, new cases were regularly registered in STI statistics. After 1995, the number of reported cases began to increase sharply. More and more couples began to seek treatment for infertility. It became a disease that was turning into a direct threat to the life on earth. Gradually, thanks to new research, many diseases were identified in which the role of *Chlamydia* is still questionable and requires study.

Currently, chlamydial infection is a diverse group of diseases caused by representatives of *Chlamydiales*. Its importance in human infectious pathology is determined by a long persistent course, gradually developing multifocal lesions of systems and organs and their medical and social consequences [1–3].

3.1 Infections Due to *Chlamydia trachomatis*

3.1.1 Urogenital Chlamydiosis

Urogenital chlamydiosis (UGC), caused by *C. trachomatis*, remains the most common bacterial sexually transmitted infection (STI). It remains a major public health problem, particularly in low- and middle-income, resource-limited countries.

Because chlamydial infections are asymptomatic in 80% of women and 50% of men, infections often stay undetected, untreated and unreported.

C. trachomatis infection occurs through oral, vaginal or anal sexual contact. Therefore, clinical manifestations reflect its practice.

Oral-genital and oral-anal sex are considered as one of the mechanisms of transmission of *C. trachomatis* in humans. The role of oral transmission of the pathogen through cunnilingus, fellatio and analingus as an important aspect of the epidemiology of UGH requires further study.

Most extragenital infections in women are asymptomatic: 100% of cases of pharyngeal chlamydiosis, 36–100% of cases of rectal chlamydiosis. Cases of rectal chlamydiosis without previous anal sex have been reported in a significant number of women. Extragenital infections are more common in men who have sex with men (MSM). The prevalence of rectal chlamydiosis in MSM (ranged from 2.1% to 23% (mean 8.9%), pharyngeal chlamydiosis—from 0% to 3.6% (mean 1.7%). The prevalence of extragenital infections amongst MSM (HIV-positive heterosexual men) in the studies reviewed ranged from 0% to 11.8% for rectal chlamydiosis (mean 7.7%), from 0% to 22.0% for pharyngeal chlamydiosis (mean 1.6%).

Chlamydiosis frequency is highest in people whose partners are already infected. Other risk

V. Zinserling et al., *Chlamydia Infections*, https://doi.org/10.1007/978-3-031-99642-9_3

factors include the following: frequent changes of sexual partners; unprotected sexual intercourse; non-traditional sexual intercourse; early onset of sexual activity; wearing an intrauterine device; other STI in the medical history.

If left untreated, chlamydial infection can lead to long-term irreversible outcomes including epididymitis, orchitis, cancer, ectopic pregnancy, infertility in both women and men, adverse pregnancy outcomes, neonatal deaths and congenital anomalies, and it can facilitate HIV transmission.

A common complication of genital chlamydia in women is pelvic inflammatory disease (PID), which includes any combination of endometritis, salpingitis, tubo-ovarian abscess and pelvic peritonitis. PID can lead to ectopic pregnancy, infertility and chronic pelvic pain [4–17].

The prevalence of UGH is estimated at 131 million cases annually [18].

The prevalence of chlamydial infection in the population varies depending on age, with the highest incidence observed in individuals under 25 years of age.

The incidence rates of UGH have remained largely unchanged over the past few years, even in countries with screening programmes (e.g. the UK) and active STI testing, treatment, partner notification and post-treatment retesting (Sweden, the Netherlands, etc.).

In 2023, there were 230,199 confirmed cases of *Chlamydia* reported in the 27 EU/EEA countries, for an overall notification rate of 70.4 cases per 100,000 population. When the rate is analysed over time amongst countries providing data, this represents an increase in the overall notification rate of 3% compared to 2022 and 13% compared to 2014.

After reaching record high notification rates in 2022, the increase in chlamydiosis notification rates slowed in 2023 amongst both women and men. Notification rates continued to be highest amongst women aged 20–24 years in 2023, although there was a 2% decrease in the rate for this population compared with 2022. In 2023, transmission between MSM accounted for 20% of chlamydia cases, a 4% increase compared with 2022. National chlamydia case notification rates ranged from 0.1 to 626 cases per 100,000 population. Differences in chlamydia testing policies, case finding and reporting strategies are thought to have a greater impact on reported chlamydia numbers than actual differences in epidemiology [19–21].

In the United States, according to the CDC, more than 1.6 million cases of chlamydiosis were diagnosed and registered in 2023 (stable trends are observed in dynamics, change <1.0%) [22, 23].

Chlamydial infection amongst U.S. men and women aged 15–39 years was estimated to be 2.35% [24].

At the same time, a different picture is observed in the Russian Federation. Over the course of several years, a steady downward trend in the incidence of UGH has been recorded, which rather reflects incomplete registration than actual incidence and requires further comprehensive study and analysis [25, 26] .

According to federal statistical reporting in the Russian Federation, the incidence of *Chlamydia* infection in 2021 was 17.9 cases per 100,000 population.

Available data on the prevalence of UGH in Russia were obtained only from small high-risk population groups, such as young (16–24 years) female university students [27], men with acute urethritis [28] or young (15–19 years) adults [29–31].

3.1.2 Lymphogranuloma Venereum

Lymphogranuloma venereum (LGV) is a disease caused by invasive *C. trachomatis* serovars (L1, L2, or L3).

Unlike genovars A–K, which remain confined to the mucosa, genovar L strains are invasive and can disseminate through the underlying connective tissue and affect regional lymph nodes.

Mixed infections with genovar L plus D–K strains [32] and mutant strains with recombinant DNA from L plus D–K strains [33] have been described, the clinical significance of which is unknown.

Globally, LGV is thought to be responsible for 2–10% of genital ulcer diseases in regions such as Southeast Asia and Africa, although these figures are based on older studies [34]. In many high-income countries, LGV is endemic amongst MSM, primarily amongst those co-infected with HIV [35].

Neither the degree of infectivity nor the reservoir of the disease has been precisely defined. Transmission is mainly attributed to asymptomatic carriers [36].

Transmission in the MSM population may be partly explained by anogenital contact. Since the ratio of genital to anorectal LGV infections is 1 in 15 in some settings, 4 other modes of transmission are suspected [37].

Classic LGV is characterized by the development of a transient genital ulcer or papule, followed by the development of painful inguinal and/or femoral lymphadenopathy (usually unilateral). If left untreated, the infection can lead to long-term complications such as deep tissue abscesses, strictures, fissures and chronic pain.

Lymphogranuloma venereum is common in tropical and subtropical regions worldwide. It is endemic in parts of Africa, Asia, South America and the Caribbean and was previously thought to be rare in industrialized countries. However, since 2003, it has remained endemic amongst European MSM.

Outbreaks have also been reported in North America and Australia, primarily amongst MSM who are co-infected with human immunodeficiency disease (HIV).

In the United States, recognizing LGV outbreaks and understanding its epidemiology is difficult, because testing to confirm infection with *C. trachomatis* (serovars L1–L3) is not routinely performed due to the limited number of commercially available tests in the United States, and while urogenital chlamydia is a nationally notifiable disease, LGV as a distinct entity is not notifiable.

In those European countries that routinely use confirmatory testing for LGV and have robust surveillance and reporting systems for LGV (e.g. the UK, France and the Netherlands), the incidence of LGV has been shown to be steadily increasing. However, the availability of LGV diagnostic testing and case reporting varies across European countries.

LGV infections in heterosexuals in Europe are extremely rare and there is no evidence of transmission in the European heterosexual population. Most cases in Europe are caused by serovars/genovars *Chlamydia trachomatis* L2b and L2 [38, 39].

Confusion in the identification of new and emerging strains highlights the importance of strictly adhering to the nomenclature rules developed by the International Committee on Prokaryotic Taxonomy Subcommittee on Chlamydia Taxonomy [40].

It has been suggested that the LGV epidemic amongst MSM in Europe, caused by the L2b subspecies, may have been introduced to Europe from the United States towards the end of the previous century through a global, tightly interconnected network of sexual contacts amongst MSM [41, 42].

Endemic cases of LGV infection in heterosexuals in Europe are extremely rare, and there is no evidence of LGV transmission in the European heterosexual population [43–46].

Lymphogranuloma venereum is a relatively common cause of proctitis and proctocolitis in MSM, but it rarely causes genital or oropharyngeal infections. Rectal ulceration, bleeding, tenesmus, cramping and lower abdominal pain are the main clinical features, and long-term infection may lead to the development of perirectal abscesses, fissures and systemic symptoms such as fever, malaise, weight loss and fatigue. Today, in developed countries, LGV is predominantly associated with rectal infection, and the classic signs of inguinal lymphadenopathy are becoming less common [47–55].

Lymphogranuloma venereum can occur at any age; however, the highest incidence of LGV occurs in the sexually active population between the ages of and 40 years. Lymphogranuloma venereum probably affects both sexes equally, although it is more common in men, because the early manifestations of LGV are more obvious in them [56]. There is a significant association between HIV-infected patients and LGV [57]. Men usually develop the acute form of the disease, whereas women often develop complications in the later stages of the disease.

The prevalence of HIV amongst MSM with LGV ranges from 67% to 100% in 13 descriptive studies. There is a significant association between HIV and LGV (odds ratio 8.19, 95% CI 4.68–14.33) [35, 58]. Moreover, hepatitis C is associated with LGV in the current epidemic amongst MSM [59–67].

3.1.3 Trachoma

Trachoma, an eye disease caused by the bacterium *C. trachomatis* (serotypes A–C), is one of the oldest documented diseases in the world: Evidence suggests that it has been around for over 10,000 years. Traces of it can be found throughout history, from Ice Age skeletons and ancient manuscripts. But it was not until the twentieth century that the cause of the disease was discovered, which is now a public health problem in 38 countries, causing blindness or visual impairment in about 1.9 million people (about 1.4% of all blindness worldwide). Blindness due to trachoma is irreversible (see Sect. 5.2).

Trachoma is hyperendemic in many poor and rural areas of Africa, Central and South America, Asia, Australia and the Middle East.

As of April 2024, 103 million people live in trachoma-endemic areas and are at risk of blindness due to trachoma. Africa remains the most affected continent where the most intensive efforts to combat the disease are being undertaken. Elimination programmes in endemic countries are implemented using the WHO-recommended strategy (since 1993).

In 1996, WHO established the WHO Alliance for the Global Elimination of Trachoma by 2020. The alliance is a partnership that supports member states.

The World Health Assembly adopted resolution in 1998, aiming for the global elimination of trachoma as a public health problem with 2030 as the target date.

As of 21 October 2024, WHO has verified that 21 countries—Benin, Cambodia, China, Gambia, Islamic Republic of Iran, Lao People's Democratic Republic, Ghana, India, Iraq, Malawi, Mali, Mexico, Morocco, Myanmar, Nepal, Oman, Pakistan, Saudi Arabia, Togo, Vanuatu and Viet Nam—have eliminated trachoma as a public health problem.

The burden of trachoma on affected individuals and communities is enormous. The economic cost of lost productivity due to blindness and visual impairment is estimated at US$2.9–5.3 billion per year, rising to US$8 billion if trichiasis is included.

The infection is spread through personal contact (hands, clothing, bedding or hard surfaces) and by flies that have come into contact with secretions from the eyes or nose of an infected person. Repeated episodes of infection over many years can cause the eyelashes to retract and rub against the surface of the eye. This causes pain and can lead to permanent damage to the cornea.

In 2023, 130,746 people received surgery for advanced disease and 32.9 million people were treated with antibiotics. Global antibiotic coverage in 2023 was 29%.

The infection is transmitted by direct or indirect transfer of secretions from the eyes and nose of infected individuals, especially young children, who are the main reservoir of infection. These secretions can be spread by certain species of flies [68, 69].

3.2 Infections Caused by *Chlamydia pneumonia*

Pneumochlamydia (*C. pneumoniae infection*) is an anthropozoonotic infectious disease caused by *C. pneumoniae,* transmitted by airborne droplets, characterized by various forms of the infectious process: from an asymptomatic form, acute respiratory infection of mild course, interstitial damage to lung tissue to damage of the central nervous system, joints, organ eyes, frequent reinfection.

This infection also correlates with the development of other infectious and non-infectious diseases: bronchial asthma; infection after lung transplantation; cardiovascular diseases and atherosclerosis; Alzheimer's disease, multiple sclerosis, age-related macular degeneration, etc.

Persistent *C. pneumoniae* infection in organ transplant recipients (whether donor, primary, or reactivated) poses a serious health risk.

Pathogenic to human strain Human (formerly TWAR—Taiwan acute respiratory agent) was named by combining the letter designations of two primary isolates, TW-183 and AR-39, which were described as strains of *C. psittaci*. TW-183 was isolated from the conjunctiva of a patient in Taiwan. AR-39 was isolated in 1983 in the United States from the oropharynx of a patient with acute respiratory disease. A similar strain, IOL-207, was also obtained from the conjunctiva in Iran and isolated in cell culture in the United Kingdom. Upon further study, the new species of *Chlamydia* was named *C. pneumoniae* .

This microorganism is considered one of the most widespread species of *Chlamydia* in the biosphere.

The source of infection is a patient with a manifest form of pneumonia or recovering from an infection.

Pneumochlamydia is released into the external environment with nasopharyngeal secretions when coughing, sneezing, talking and is transmitted by airborne droplets.

Most people encounter *C. pneumoniae* throughout their lives: by age 20, 50% of people have antibodies, and by age 60–70, 80%. The incidence is highest amongst young people.

The disease occurs at any time of year. Outbreaks of community-acquired pneumonia and upper respiratory tract infections (pneumonic and nasopharyngeal forms) caused by this pathogen occur from time to time around the world. Outbreaks of pneumochlamydiosis most often occur in crowded settings, including college dormitories, detention or correctional facilities, hospitals, long-term care facilities, military training facilities, schools. Outbreaks can last a long time for several reasons. First, people without symptoms can spread the bacteria. This includes a 3–4-week incubation period. Second, because *C. pneumoniae* infections are usually mild, people usually do not require treatment, but they can be contagious for several weeks after symptoms begin.

Thus, studies based on patients with community-acquired pneumonia are likely to underestimate the true incidence of *C. pneumoniae* infection .

A large study of patients with community-acquired pneumonia requiring hospitalization in the United States showed that *C. pneumoniae* is a rare cause of infection in children and adults [70, 71].

C. pneumoniae infection cannot be fully accounted for as sporadic cases remain unreported. Pneumochlamydiosis is not a nationally notifiable disease. Surveillance systems to collect case information are lacking. However, outbreak studies and investigations provide useful information [72].

Despite the simultaneous circulation of *C. pneumoniae* in both humans and animals, human and animal isolates are heterogeneous biovars, and the possibility of its anthropozoonotic transmission has not been definitively established.

3.3 Infections by *Chlamydia psittaci*

Ornithosis (psittacosis, parrot fever; ornis, genitive case ornithos—bird; syn.: psittacosis, psittacosis, from the Greek psittakos—parrot) is a zoonotic infectious disease caused by *C. psittaci*, characterized by fever, intoxication, specific damage to the lungs, central nervous system and hepatosplenic syndrome (see more details in Sect. 5.4) .

Most reported cases of ornithosis in humans result from direct contact with birds (primarily parrots). Signs of illness in infected birds may include lethargy, respiratory distress, anorexia and conjunctivitis, although infection may be subclinical.

Infection usually occurs through inhalation of microorganisms that enter the air from dried faeces (secretions) of infected birds (airborne and airborne dust routes). Infection can occur during care, slaughter and processing of birds and animals that excrete the pathogen with faeces, urine, amniotic fluid, aborted foetuses and with secretions from the mucous membranes of the eyes and nasopharynx.

Feathers and contaminated with secretions dry excrements can be carried by air currents to a considerable distance from the source of infection. Alimentary infection is possible (when consuming contaminated food products).

There are known isolated infections from sick people.

There is evidence of spread of *C. psittaci* from wild birds to horses and subsequently to humans in Australia, with a highly virulent strain of *C. psittaci* associated with loss of reproductive function in horses and subsequent disease in humans.

In February 2024, Austria, Germany, Denmark, Sweden and the Netherlands notified the European Union Early Warning and Response System (EWRS) of an increase in ornithosis cases observed in 2023 and early 2024, and particularly noticeable from November 2023 to December 2023 onwards. Five fatal cases were reported.

Although ornithosis is a nationally notifiable disease, a number of factors may limit the completeness of reporting and thus affect our understanding of epidemiological risk factors and trends in incidence. The incidence of ornithosis is sporadic, but occupational and familial outbreaks occur (mean 8.3 cases per year, range 2–21 cases per year). The main age group of cases is people aged 40–65 years; however, it is unclear whether this is due to age differences in susceptibility or exposure to risk.

Since 2018, there have been fewer than 100 cases of psittacosis reported per year in the United States.

These statistics may not be an accurate reflection of the actual number of cases in humans due to limited research and imperfect diagnostic methods.

Epidemic outbreaks may occur at poultry farms, meat-processing plants, pet stores and zoos. The risk group includes livestock breeders, farmers, veterinarians, meat processing plant workers, taxidermists, hunters, etc. The main sources of infection in a family outbreak are decorative indoor birds and pigeons.

Since the identification of *C. psittaci* in birds, several new *Chlamydia* species have been described, and it is likely that some older reports of *C. psittaci* infections are actually infections with other *Chlamydia* species, particularly studies based on serologic data alone.

Globally, *C. psittaci* is

- Recognized as a significant zoonotic pathogen, with outbreaks frequently reported.
- Is thought to be the cause of approximately 1% of cases of community-acquired pneumonia (CAP) [73, 74].

3.4 Diseases Caused by *Chlamydia felis, Chlamydia abortus,* and *Chlamydia caviae*

There is evidence in the literature that *Chlamydia* lacks strict specificity in relation to its biological hosts. Thus, in recent years, with the development of molecular genetic methods, more and more reports have appeared that *Chlamydia* isolated from animals and birds, when entering the human body, can cause diseases with a variety of clinical presentations, from a mild form of acute respiratory disease and pneumonia to meningoencephalitis, from enteritis to abortion and severe generalized infection [75–85].

References

1. Cheong HC, Lee CYQ, Cheok YY, et al. Chlamydiaceae: diseases in primary hosts and zoonosis. Microorganisms. 2019;7(5):146.
2. Baud D, Regan L, Greub G. Emerging role of Chlamydia and Chlamydia-like organisms in adverse pregnancy outcomes. Curr Opin Infect Dis. 2008;21(1):70–6.
3. Borel N, Sachse K. (2023). Zoonotic transmission of chlamydia spp.: known for 140 years, but still underestimated. In: Sing A, editor. Zoonoses: infections affecting humans and animals. Cham: Springer; 2023. https://doi.org/10.1007/978-3-030-85877-3_53-1.
4. Dewart CM, Bernstein KT, De Groote NP, Romaguera R, Turner AN. Prevalence of rectal chlamydial and gonococcal infections: a systematic review. Sex Trans Dis. 2018;45:280–93.

5. Leenen. J., van Liere GAFS, Hoebe CJPA, Hogewoning AA, de Vries HJC, Dukers-Muijrers NHTM Preceding oropharyngeal Chlamydia trachomatis infection is not a risk factor for anorectal Chlamydia trachomatis infection in men who have sex with men (MSM) and women: Proceedings of the Fourteenth international symposium on human chlamydial infections. 2018, July 1–6; Zeist; The Netherlands. The Netherlands; 2018: 89–93.
6. Dukers-Muijrers NH, Schachter J, van Liere GAFS, Wolffs PFG, Hoebe CJPA. What is needed to guide testing for anorectal and pharyngeal chlamydia trachomatis and Neisseria gonorrhoeae in women and men? Evidence and opinion. BMC Infect Dis. 2015;15:533.
7. Barbeyrac B, Baita D, Touati A, Bebear C, Peuchant O. Does Chlamydia trachomatis anal infection occur with vaginal infection in women? In: Proceedings of the Fourteenth international symposium on human chlamydial infections. 2018, July 1–6. Zeist, The Netherlands; 2018. p. 95–7.
8. Rank R, Yeruva L. Hidden in plain sight: chlamydial gastrointestinal infection and its relevance to persistence in human genital infection. Infect Immun. 2014;82(4):1362–71. https://doi.org/10.1128/IAI.01244-13.
9. Moncada J, Schachter J. In vitro survival of Chlamydia trachomatis in a low pH environment. In: Proceedings of the Fourteenth international symposium on human chlamydial infections. 2018, July 1–6. Zeist, The Netherlands; 2018. p. 131–3.
10. Bavoil P, Marques PX, Brotman R, Ravel J. Does active oral sex contribute to female infertility. J Infect Dis. 2017;216(8):932–5.
11. Workowski KA, Bolan GA. Sexually transmitted diseases treatment guidelines 2015. MMWR Recomm Rep. 2015;64(33):1–137.
12. van Liere GAFS, Dukers-Muijrers NHTM, Hoebe CJPA. Oropharyngeal Chlamydia trachomatis testing and positivity at an STI clinic in the past 5 years; testing more and finding even more. In: Proceedings of the Fourteenth international symposium on human chlamydial infections. 2018, July 1–6. Zeist, The Netherlands; 2018. p. 173–7.
13. van Rooijen MS, van der Loeff MFS, Morré SA, van Dam AP, Speksnijder AGCL, de Vries HJC. Spontaneous pharyngeal chlamydia trachomatis RNA clearance. A cross-sectional study followed by a cohort study of untreated STI clinic patients in Amsterdam, The Netherlands. Sex Trans Infect. 2015;91(3):157–64.
14. Tjahyadi D, Ropii B, Tjandraprawira KD, et al. Female urogenital chlamydia: epidemiology, chlamydia on pregnancy, current diagnosis, and treatment. Ann Med Surg. 2022;75:103448.
15. Salari N, Olfat N, Ghasemi H. The global prevalence of Chlamydia trachomatis genital infection in pregnant women: a meta-analysis. Arch Gynecol Obstet. 2025;311(2):529–42.
16. Adachi KN, Nielsen-Saines K, Klausner JD. Chlamydia trachomatis screening and treatment in pregnancy to reduce adverse pregnancy and neonatal outcomes: a review. Front Public Health. 2021;9:531073.
17. Zhao P, Liang P, Wang J, et al. Chlamydia cases in women of reproductive age, 2006–2020: an analysis of surveillance data from Southern China. BMC Public Health. 2025;25(1):158.
18. World Health Organization (WHO). The global health observatory. https://www.who.int/data/gho/data/themes/topics/indicator-groups/indicator-group-details/GHO/chlamydia.
19. European Center for Disease Prevention and Control (ECDC). Chlamydia—Annual Epidemiological Report for 2023 https://www.ecdc.europa.eu/en/publications-data/chlamydia-annual-epidemiological-report-2023.
20. European Center for Disease Prevention and Control. A systematic review and meta-analysis of the prevalence of chlamydia, gonorrhoea, trichomoniasis and syphilis in Europe. Stockholm: ECDC; 2024.
21. Barbaric J, Kuchukhidze G, Seguy N, et al. Surveillance and epidemiology of syphilis, gonorrhoea and chlamydia in the non-European Union countries of the World Health Organization European region, 2015 to 2020. Euro Surveill. 2022;27(8):2100197.
22. National Overview of STIs in 2023. https://www.cdc.gov/sti-statistics/annual/summary.html.
23. Huai P, Li F, Chu T, et al. Prevalence of genital chlamydia trachomatis infection in the general population: a meta-analysis. BMC Infect Dis. 2020;20(1):589.
24. Kreisel KM, Weston EJ, St Cyr SB, Spicknall IH. Estimates of the prevalence and incidence of Chlamydia and gonorrhea among US men and women. Sex Transm Dis. 2021;48(4):222–31.
25. Kubanova AA, Kubanov AA, Melekhina LE. Dynamics of changes in intensive indicators of sexually transmitted infections in the assessment of the epidemiological process and health status of the population of The Russian Federation for 2006–2016. Bull Dermatol Venereol. 2018;91(1):27–37. (in Russian)
26. Abramov AA. Territorial distribution of urogenital chlamydia, gonorrhea and associated complications in The Russian Federation. Epidemiol Vaccine Prev. 2024;23(2):25–35. (in Russian)
27. Khryanin AA, Reshetnikov OV, Vlaspolder F. Comparison of APTIMA COMBO 2 assay with polymerase chain reaction Roche assay for detection of chlamydia trachomatis in endocervical swabs. Int J STD AIDS. 2007;18:871–2.
28. Taylor-Robinson D, Renton A, Jensen JS, et al. Association of Mycoplasma genitalium with acute non-gonococcal urethritis in Russian men: a comparison with gonococcal and chlamydial urethritis. Int J STD AIDS. 2009;20:234–7.

29. Shipitsyna E, Krasnoselskykh T, Zolotoverkhaya E, et al. Sexual behaviours , knowledge and attitudes regarding safe sex, and prevalence of non-viral sexually transmitted infections among attendees of youth clinics in St. Petersburg, Russia. J Eur Acad Dermatol. 2013;27:e75–84.
30. Smelov V, Thomas P, Ouburg S, Morré SA. Prevalence of genital Chlamydia trachomatis infections in Russia: systematic literature review and multicenter study. Rev Pathog Dis. 2017;75(7):ftx081.
31. Smelov V, Quint KD, Pleijster J. Chlamydia trachomatis serovar distributions in Russian men and women: a comparison with Dutch serovar distributions. Drugs Today. 2009;45(Suppl B):33–8.
32. Quint KD, van Doorn LJ, Kleter B, et al. A highly sensitive, multiplex broad-spectrum PCR-DNA-enzyme immunoassay and reverse hybridization assay for rapid detection and identification of chlamydia trachomatis serovars. J Mol Diagn. 2007;9:631–8.
33. Somboonna N, Wan R, Ojcius DM, et al. Hypervirulent chlamydia trachomatis clinical strain is a recombinant between lymphogranuloma venereum (L(2)) and D lineages. MBio. 2011;2:e00045-11.
34. de Vries HJC, Shiva Nagi Reddy B, Khandpur S. Lymphogranuloma venereum. In: Gupta S, Kumar B, editors. Sexually transmitted infections. 2nd ed. New Delhi: Elsevier; 2012. p. 506–21.
35. Ronn MM, Ward H. The association between lymphogranuloma venereum and HIV among men who have sex with men: systematic review and meta-analysis. BMC Infect Dis. 2011;11:70.
36. Saxon C, Hughes G, Ison C, Group ULC-F. Asymptomatic lymphogranuloma venereum in men who have sex with men, United Kingdom. Emerg Infect Dis. 2016;22:112–6.
37. de Vries HJ. The enigma of lymphogranuloma venereum spread in men who have sex with men: does ano -oral transmission play a role? Sex Transm Dis. 2016;43:420–2.
38. Vall -Mayans M, Caballero E, Sanz B. The emergence of lymphogranuloma venereum in Europe. Lancet. 2009;374:356.
39. de Vrieze NH, de Vries HJ. Lymphogranuloma venereum among men who have sex with men. An epidemiological and clinical review. Expert Rev Anti-Infect Ther. 2014;12:697–704.
40. Seth-Smith HM, Galan JC, Goldenberger D et al. Concern regarding the alleged spread of hypervirulent lymphogranuloma venereum chlamydia trachomatis strain in Europe. Eur Survey 2017; 22(15).
41. Spaargaren J, Schachter J, Moncada J, et al. Slow epidemic of lymphogranuloma venereum L2b strain. Emerg Infect Dis. 2005;11:1787–8.
42. Smelov V, Vrbanac A, van Ess EF, et al. Chlamydia trachomatis strain types have diversified regionally and globally with evidence for recombination across geographic divides. Front Microbiol. 2017;8:2195.
43. Peuchant O, Baldit C, Le Roy C, et al. First case of chlamydia trachomatis L2b proctitis in a woman. Clin Microbiol Infect. 2011;17:E21–3.
44. Verweij SP, Ouburg S, de Vries H, et al. The first case record of a female patient with bubonic lymphogranuloma venereum (LGV), serovariant L2b. Sex Transm Infect. 2012;88:346–7.
45. Heiligenberg M, Verweij SP, Speksnijder AG, Morre SA, de Vries HJ, van der Loeff MF S. No evidence for LGV transmission among heterosexuals in Amsterdam, The Netherlands. BMC Res Notes. 2014;7:355.
46. Touati A, Vernay-Vaisse C, Janier M, et al. Did L strains responsible for lymphogranuloma venereum proctitis spread among people with genital Chlamydia trachomatis infection in France in 2013? Sex Transm Dis. 2016;43:374–6.
47. de Vrieze NH, van Rooijen M, Schim van der Loeff MF, de Vrieze HJ. Anorectal and inguinal lymphogranuloma venereum among men who have sex with men in Amsterdam, The Netherlands: trends over time, symptomatology and concurrent infections. Sex Transm Infect. 2013;89:548–52.
48. de Vrieze NHN, Versteeg B, Bruisten SM, van Rooijen MS, van der Helm JJ, de Vries HJC. Low prevalence of urethral lymphogranuloma venereum infections among men who have sex with men: a prospective observational study, sexually transmitted infection clinic in Amsterdam, The Netherlands. Sex Transm Dis. 2017;44:547–50.
49. Desclaux A, Touati A, Neau D, et al. Extra-rectal lymphogranuloma venereum in France: a clinical and molecular study. Sex Transm Infect. 2018;94:3–8.
50. Peuchant O, Touati A, Sperandio C, et al. Changing pattern of chlamydia trachomatis strains in lymphogranuloma venereum outbreak, France, 2010–2015. Emerg Infect Dis. 2016;22:1945–7.
51. Touati A, Peuchant O, Henin N, Bebear C, de Barbeyrac B. The L2b real-time PCR targeting the pmpH gene of Chlamydia trachomatis used for the diagnosis of lymphogranuloma venereum is not specific to L2b strains. Clin Microbiol Infect. 2016;22:574.e7–9.
52. Harris SR, Clarke IN, Seth-Smith HM, et al. Whole-genome analysis of diverse chlamydia trachomatis strains identifies phylogenetic relationships masked by current clinical typing. Nat Genet. 2012;44(413–419):S1.
53. Borges V, Gomes JP. Deep comparative genomics among chlamydia trachomatis lymphogranuloma venereum isolates highlights genes potentially involved in pathoadaptation. Infect Genet Evol. 2015;32:74–88.
54. de Vries HJ, Schim van der Loeff MF, Bruisten SM. High-resolution typing of chlamydia trachomatis: epidemiological and clinical uses. Curr Opin Infect Dis. 2015;28:61–71.
55. Hadfield J, Harris SR, Seth-Smith HMB, et al. Comprehensive global genome dynamics of chlamydia trachomatis show ancient diversification followed by contemporary mixing and recent lineage expansion. Genome Res. 2017;27:1220–9.

56. Ceovic R, Gulin SJ. Lymphogranuloma venereum: diagnostic and treatment challenges. Infect Drug Resist. 2015;8:39–47.
57. Rönn MM, Ward H. The association between lymphogranuloma venereum and HIV among men who have sex with men: systematic review and meta-analysis. BMC Infect Dis. 2011 Mar;18(11):70.
58. de Barbeyrac B, Laurier-Nadalie C, Touati A et al. Observational study of anorectal chlamydia trachomatis infections in France through the lymphogranuloma venereum surveillance network, 2010–2015. Int J STD AIDS 2018.
59. Gotz HM, van Doornum G, Niesters HGM, den Hollander JG, Thio HB, de Zwart O. A cluster of acute hepatitis C virus infection among men who have sex with men–results from contact tracing and public health implications. AIDS. 2005;19:969–74.
60. van de Laar TJ, Van der Bij AK, Prins M, et al. Increase in HCV incidence among men who have sex with men in Amsterdam most likely caused by sexual transmission. J Infect Dis. 2007;196:230–8.
61. Vanhommerig JW, Lambers FA, Schinkel J, et al. Factors for sexual transmission of hepatitis C virus among human immunodeficiency virus-infected men who have sex with men: a case-control study. Open Forum Infect Dis. 2015;2:ofv115.
62. Stoner BP, Cohen SE. Lymphogranuloma Venereum 2015: clinical presentation, diagnosis, and treatment. Rev Clin Infect Dis. 2015;61(Suppl 8):S865–73.
63. Lymphogranuloma Venereum (LGV). Sexually transmitted infections treatment guidelines, 2021.
64. de Vries HJC, de Barbeyrac B, de Vrieze NHN. 2019 European guideline on the management of lymphogranuloma venereum. Practice guideline. J Eur Acad Dermatol Venereol. 2019;33(10):1821–8.
65. Papp JR, Schachter J., Gaydos CA, Van Der Pol B. Recommendations for the laboratory-based detection of chlamydia trachomatis and Neisseria gonorrhoeae 2014.
66. Oda G, Chung J, Lucero-Obusan C, Holodniy M. Clinically defined lymphogranuloma Venereum among US veterans with human immunodeficiency virus, 2016–2023. Microorganisms. 2024;12(7):1327.
67. https://www.std.uw.edu/go/comprehensive-study/chlamydial-infections/core-concept/all.
68. Toumasis P, Vrioni G, Tsinopoulos IT, et al. Insights into pathogenesis of trachoma. Microorganisms. 2024;12(8):1544.
69. Lynch KD, Apadinuwe SC, Lambert SB. A national survey integrating clinical, laboratory, and WASH data to determine the typology of trachoma in Nauru. PLoS Negl Trop Dis. 2022;16(4):e0010275.
70. Jain S, Self WH, Wunderink RG, Fakhran S, et al. Community-acquired pneumonia requiring hospitalization among US adults. N Engl J Med. 2015;373(5):415–27.
71. CDC Chlamydia pneumoniae Infection https://www.cdc.gov/cpneumoniae/index.html.
72. https://www.cdc.gov/cpneumoniae/php/surveillance/index.html.
73. Wang J, Wang B, Xiao J, et al. Chlamydia psittaci: a zoonotic pathogen causing avian chlamydiosis and psittacosis. Virulence. 2024;15(1):2428411. https://doi.org/10.1080/21505594.2024.2428411.
74. Knittler MR, Sachse K. Chlamydia psittaci: update on an underestimated zoonotic agent. Pathog Dis. 2015;73(1):1–15. https://doi.org/10.1093/femspd/ftu007. Epub 2014 Dec 4
75. Borel N, Ciuria S, Flury T, et al. Zoonotic potential of Guinea pigs: outbreak of cryptosporidiosis combined with chlamydiosis in a breeding Guinea pig herd. Schweiz Arch Tierheilkd. 2023;165(1):59–63. https://doi.org/10.17236/sat00383.
76. Chlamydia—Annual Epidemiological Report for 2022.
77. Chlamydia https://www.who.int/news-room/fact-sheets/detail/chlamydia.
78. https://www.ecdc.europa.eu/en/publications-data/chlamydia-annual-epidemiological-report-2022.
79. Li C, Ong J, Tang W, Wang C. Editorial: Chlamydia trachomatis infection: epidemiology, prevention, clinical, and basic science research. Front Public Health. 2023;11:1167690. https://doi.org/10.3389/fpubh.2023.1167690. eCollection 2023
80. Low N, Redmond S, Uusküla A, et al. Screening for genital chlamydia infection. Cochrane Database Syst Rev. 2016;2016(9):CD010866. https://doi.org/10.1002/14651858.CD010866.pub2.
81. Marra CA, Patrick DM, Reynolds R, Marra F. Chlamydia trachomatis in adolescents and adults. Clin Econ Implic. 1998;13:191–222.
82. Rowley J, Hoorn SV, Korenromp E, et al. Chlamydia, gonorrhoea , trichomoniasis and syphilis: global prevalence and incidence estimates. Bull World Health Organ. 2019;97(8):548–562P. https://doi.org/10.2471/BLT.18.228486.
83. Tang W, Mao J, Li KT, et al. Pregnancy and fertility-related adverse outcomes associated with Chlamydia trachomatis infection: a global systematic review and meta-analysis. Sex Transm Infect. 2020;96(5):322–9. https://doi.org/10.1136/sextrans-2019-053999. Epub 2019 Dec 13
84. World Health Organization. Sexually transmitted infections (STIs). https://www.who.int/news-room/fact-sheets/detail/sexually-transmitted-infections-(stis). 2022.
85. Global health strategies for HIV, viral hepatitis and sexually transmitted infections 2022–2030.

4 Laboratory, Instrumental and Morphological Diagnostics of Chlamydial Infections

4.1 Modern Aspects of Diagnostics of Diseases Caused by *C. trachomatis*

Laboratory diagnostics of urogenital chlamydial infection is a key moment in establishing a final diagnosis, which is due in most cases to the absence of pathognomonic symptoms in these diseases and the frequent combination of infection with other pathogens of STIs. Currently, there is no single algorithm and scheme for diagnostic examination of patients with suspected chlamydiosis. Today, there are dozens of manuals and guides on diagnostics and treatment of chlamydial infection, allowing one to get an idea of both the range of methods used in Russia and abroad, and the implementation of individual laboratory diagnostic procedures. However, most of them provide information on the principles and standard capabilities of various methodologies, but do not aim to systematically cover the most probable reasons for the decrease in the effectiveness of laboratory and, as a consequence, clinical diagnostics of chlamydiosis (including common forms of this infection), which is often encountered in the practical work of medical institutions and reduces the quality of medical care [1].

Thus, the main value of molecular genetic diagnostic methods for *Chlamydia* is undoubtedly their high sensitivity. A large number of studies have been conducted to assess the comparative sensitivity of various methods for detecting *Chlamydia* in clinical samples, a significant part of which confirms the need for the integrated use of PCR, direct immunofluorescence (DIF) and the culture method (CM). Significant advances in molecular genetic technologies have made it possible to detect various types of *Chlamydia*, including those not cultured on cell lines and culture embryos.

However, there are currently no laboratory diagnostic algorithms for both acute and chronic forms of chlamydial infection. These difficulties are due to the high dependence of laboratory diagnostic results on the following factors:

- Selection of the appropriate laboratory research method.
- Proper preparation of the patient for the examination.
- Correct collection by the doctor of material for examination from primary (urethra, cervical canal of the cervix, oropharynx, conjunctiva) and secondary (sputum, cerebrospinal fluid, blood leukocyte concentrate, synovial fluid, biopsies from lymph nodes and rectal mucosa, etc.) foci of chlamydial infection.
- Correct preliminary preparation of the collected material and timeliness of the study.
- Proper storage and delivery of material to the laboratory.
- Material and technical support for laboratory research.
- The level of qualification of the medical personnel conducting the study.

V. Zinserling et al., *Chlamydia Infections*, https://doi.org/10.1007/978-3-031-99612-9_4

The basic principles of diagnosing chlamydial infection are the same as for other bacterial pathologies. Test procedures include

- Direct visualization of the agent in clinical samples by staining (bacterioscopic method).
- Determination of specific chlamydial antigens in clinical samples.
- Direct isolation from the patient's tissues (bacteriological method).
- Serological tests that detect antibodies (demonstrating changing titres).
- Determination of specific chlamydial genes in clinical samples.

In this guide, we have summarized our (A.L. Poznyak, S.N. Sidorchuk, V.A. Zinserling) experience in diagnosing chlamydial infection).

4.2 Indications for Testing for Urogenital *Chlamydia*

The following are subject to mandatory examination for urogenital *Chlamydia*: patients with acute and chronic inflammation of the pelvic organs (cystitis, prostatitis), chronic inflammatory diseases of the genitourinary system (women—primarily with lesions of the cervix); menstrual cycle disorders such as metrorrhagia, patients with a history of infertility of unclear genesis for 2–3 years (both in women and men); patients with habitual miscarriage; pregnant women with a complicated obstetric history (non-viable pregnancy, spontaneous abortions, premature births, low birth weight babies, polyhydramnios) and with complicated pregnancy (threat of miscarriage, polyhydramnios, placentitis, etc.), newborns with diagnosed chlamydial infection in the mother, women planning to terminate a pregnancy, before therapeutic and diagnostic curettage of the mucous membranes of the cervix and body of the uterus, during other intrauterine interventions, when using intrauterine contraception, examination of ejaculate donors.

In addition, analysis for the presence of *C. trachomatis* is prescribed to clarify the aetiology of the disease in the following situations: detection of Chlamydia in HIV-infected individuals, patients with undifferentiated arthritis, chronic conjunctivitis, dry eye syndrome, fever of unknown genesis, with secondary immunodeficiency states, unexplained weight loss of more than 5 kg over 3–6 months, with changes in the general blood test (anaemia, thrombocytopenia, leukopenia or leukocytosis, increased ESR), changes in urine tests (leukocyturia, proteinuria), when it is necessary to clarify the nature of organ damage, the presence of simultaneous damage to many organs and systems, etc.; when monitoring the effectiveness of antibacterial treatment; for the purpose of screening population groups at increased risk of developing urogenital *Chlamydia* (individuals with increased sexual activity and frequent changes of sexual partners).

When studying the anamnestic data, the following is determined: the patient's suspected source of infection; the time elapsed from the moment of sexual contact with the suspected source of infection until the appearance of subjective symptoms; the results of examination of sexual partners; obstetric-gynaecological, urological and sexual anamnesis data; the presence of STIs in the anamnesis and at present; allergy anamnesis data; the presence of somatic diseases; data on the intake of medications, including antibacterial ones, over the past 3 months [2, 3].

4.3 Methodological Aspects of Laboratory Diagnostics of *Chlamydia*

The clinical material for testing for the presence of *Chlamydia* in samples may include scrapings of epithelial cells from the mucous membranes of the urethra, cervical canal, vagina, posterior pharyngeal wall, nose, conjunctiva, rectum, sputum, bronchoalveolar lavage, cerebrospinal fluid, blood leukocyte concentrate, synovial fluid, ejaculate, prostate secretion, the first portion of freely released morning urine in men and women, as well as vaginal discharge in women, biopsies of the conjunctiva, testicles, endometrium, lymph nodes and synovial membrane of the joints [4, 5].

Microscopic examination is used to verify the presence of an inflammatory process in the genitourinary organs. The diagnostic criteria confirming the presence of urethritis in men are as follows: detection of 5 or more leukocytes in the field of vision in smears from the urethra at a magnification of ×1000; detection of 10 or more leukocytes in the sediment of the first portion of urine. The diagnostic criterion confirming the presence of urethritis in women is: detection of 10 or more leukocytes in the field of vision in smears from the urethra at a magnification of ×1000. The diagnostic criterion confirming the presence of cervicitis in women is: detection of 20 or more leukocytes in the field of vision in smears from the cervical canal at a magnification of ×1000.

Laboratory diagnostics of urogenital *Chlamydia* includes a number of methodological approaches. The most common method is immunofluorescence, less commonly used is polymerase chain reaction, and only in some laboratories does the culture method of detecting *Chlamydia* is applied. Serological blood testing for the determination of immunoglobulins IgG, IgM, IgA to C. trachomatis is also available. Other methods for diagnosing urogenital chlamydial infection are rarely used. Comparison of methods and clinical materials showed the ambiguity of the tests used in clinical practice. The search for the most sensitive and specific tests, the creation of a research algorithm formed the basis of many years of work by various authors. The variety of methods for laboratory diagnostics of chlamydial infection and clinical material used for research pose the task of optimizing these methods for laboratories [6].

None of the listed methodological approaches ensure 100% reliability of the results obtained. Therefore, today, the integrated application of two methods based on different principles is considered as the "gold standard" [7].

Laboratory diagnostic situations arising in urogenital *Chlamydia* can be divided into two groups.

The first group includes cases when markers of the pathogen itself are detected in the material from various parts of the genital tract and extragenital localization, regardless of whether antibodies against *Chlamydia* are present in the blood. This group includes results obtained using immunofluorescence, polymerase chain reaction and cultural studies.

The second group consists of situations in which immunoglobulins to *C. trachomatis* of various classes are detected in the blood of patients, but markers of these microorganisms in the urogenital tract are not detected.

4.4 Diagnostic Value of the Results Obtained by Various Methods of Diagnosing Chlamydial Infection

4.4.1 Direct Immunofluorescence (DIF) Method

It is known that when using the DIF method, false-positive results are relatively often obtained. Obtaining false-positive results can be caused, first of all, by the low quality of diagnostic kits, the subjective nature of the interpretation of the data obtained and the use of test systems with polyclonal antibodies [8].

The provision that additional confirmation of positive results is required remains unchanged [1, 8].

The following diagnostic kits are used to perform DIF for the purpose of diagnosing *Chlamydia*: « Chlamyset Antigen » (Orion diagnostica, Finland), « DFA Micro—Tract » (Siva USA), « Chlamydia direct IF » (Bio—Merieux UK), " ChlaMonoScreen " (Niramedic, Russia), " ChlamiSlight " (Labdiagnostics, Russia), " ChlamiDif " (Diamed, Russia).

4.5 Molecular Biological Methods for Diagnosis *of C. trachomatis*

Currently, a significant number of test systems based on various molecular biological approaches are offered for detection of *Chlamydia* nucleic acids in biological material samples. In this regard, the choice of test systems for use in a specific laboratory is a rather difficult task. In this case, the decisive factors should not be such obvious parameters as cost and convenience in everyday work, but sensitivity and specificity. In the current situation, the requirements for in-laboratory validation of test systems are increasing sharply. Methods for detection of nucleic acids can be divided into two groups: associated and not associated with nucleic acid amplification. The main methods not associated with nucleic acid amplification include various versions of methods based on hybridization of target nucleic acids and complementary probes containing radioactive or other labels. The best example of such a method is the PACE® 2 CT test (Gen-Probe, Inc. San Diego, CA), approved by the FDA in 1988. The test is based on the hybridization of a DNA probe with a specific region of the 16S ribosomal RNA of *C. trachomatis*. In recent years, NAAT (nucleic acid amplification tests) have gradually replaced other diagnostic methods due to their high sensitivity, specificity, reproducibility and high throughput. Calculations by TJ Battle et al. showed that when using non-amplification methods for diagnosing chlamydial infection (culture method, direct immunofluorescence method, ELISA method with antigen detection), 20–40% of *C. trachomatis* infection cases are missed [9].

All amplification methods can be divided into three groups: based on signal, target and probe amplification.

When using signal amplification methods, there is no increase in the concentration of the target or probe during the reaction. A significant increase in the analytical sensitivity of the method is achieved by binding multiple labelled molecules to the target. One variant of this approach (hybrid capture assay (hybrid molecule capture method) is used in commercial test systems for detection of C. trachomatis—HC2® CT ID (Qiagen Germantown, MD). The method is based on hybridization in solution of target DNA and RNA probe. The resulting hybrid molecules are captured by immobilized antihybrid antibodies. Then, antihybrid antibodies labelled with alkaline phosphatase are attached to the immobilized hybrid molecules. The reaction is assessed by the intensity of luminescence; its high sensitivity is determined by the fact that many molecules of labelled antibodies are attached to one hybrid molecule (DNA + RNA).

When using probe amplification, the amplification product is represented only by the nucleotide sequences included in the probe. The best-known version of this method is the ligase chain reaction, implemented in the commercial product LCx Probe System (Abbot). However, in 2003 the manufacturer withdrew the test system from the market.

All methods related to this group of target amplification are based on the implementation of enzymatic reactions, during which one or more enzymes synthesize multiple copies of the target nucleic acid [3].

4.5.1 Classical PCR

Amplification of the target DNA is carried out in repeated cycles, each of which includes denaturation (formation of single-stranded molecules) of the target DNA at a temperature of more than 90 °C; annealing of each single-stranded DNA molecule of a complementary oligonucleotide primer when the temperature is lowered to 55–65 °C; completion (synthesis) of a double-stranded DNA molecule from each primer as a result of the enzymatic activity of thermostable DNA polymerase using deoxynucleoside triphosphates contained in the reaction mixture at a temperature of 72 °C.

At the end of the cycle, the target DNA fragments are doubled. When n cycles are performed, the number of target DNA fragments will be 2n. In practice, approximately 30 amplification cycles are performed to obtain amplification products (amplicons) in quantities sufficient for their detection by conventional analytical methods. Initially, during PCR, after each annealing of the primers, a new portion of DNA polymerase had to be added to the reaction mixture, since the previously added enzyme was inactivated at high temperatures during the denaturation stage. A high amplification reaction rate was achieved by using a thermostable DNA polymerase and by creating programmable thermal cyclers that ensure rapid and precise changes in the temperature of the reaction mixture.

Several methods are used to detect amplification products. The most common detection method is horizontal electrophoresis of the reaction mixture sample obtained after amplification in an agarose gel. The PCR result is considered positive when a DNA fragment is detected whose molecular weight corresponds to the molecular weight of the control sample amplicon. For this purpose, markers (DNA fragments of known molecular weight), positive and negative controls must be used during electrophoresis. The significant disadvantages of the method are: subjectivity of the operator's assessment of the electrophoresis results, low productivity, impossibility of automating the process, difficulty in quantitatively assessing the PCR products in each specific sample. The greatest danger is the possibility of producing a non-specific product similar in size to the product being detected during PCR. With the existing detection system, the operator may issue a false-positive result [10].

An alternative to electrophoretic methods for detecting PCR- amplified DNA are hybridization-fluorescence detection methods. In the course of this detection method, the amplified DNA hybridizes with both primers and fluorescently labelled oligonucleotides probes specific to the internal sequence of the analysed fragment. The resulting hybrid is automatically registered by a fluorescent or photometric reader. Thus, in the hybridization method of DNA detection, the specificity of the amplification reaction is ensured, firstly, by hybridization with primers, and secondly, by hybridization with specific probes.

The PCR method in its classical version was initially used to detect *C. trachomatis* DNA using test systems constructed in each laboratory independently (home-made). Currently, such test systems are being replaced by commercial test systems. In most test systems, the target is the cryptic plasmid or 23S rRNA of *C. trachomatis*.

PCR in its classic version is used in commercial test systems manufactured by Roche Molecular Diagnostics Pleasanton, CA (AMPLICOR® CT/NG Test for Chlamydia trachomatis and COBAS AMPLICOR® CT/ NG Test for Chlamydia trachomatis). The target in the indicated test systems is a cryptic plasmid. There are a number of domestic PCR test systems for detecting *Chlamydia trachomatis*, approved for medical use. Test systems based on the principle of classical PCR are the least convenient in everyday work (especially when performed manually), but are distinguished by their relatively low cost. To increase the sensitivity and specificity of classical PCR, its variant was developed, called nested PCR. In this case, two pairs of primers are used. After amplification using the first pair of primers, the obtained amplicons are used in the second round of PCR with the second pair of primers. The second pair of primers anneal on the internal regions of the amplicons, thus the product of the second round of amplification is shorter than the product of the first round. Increased sensitivity and specificity of nested PCR is achieved by increasing the total number of amplification cycles (15–30 in each round) and annealing the second pair of primers only on the fragments obtained in the first round. The nested PCR method is used mainly for research purposes and has not found wide application in commercial test systems.

From a practical point of view, multiplex PCR is very promising. In this variant, several pairs of primers specific to different targets are located in the same tube, which allows the detection of several targets simultaneously. Designing primers and optimizing conditions for multiplex PCR is somewhat more complicated than solving these problems for classical PCR, since it is necessary to exclude possible complementarity between different primers and ensure the same annealing temperature for them. Multiplex PCR is somewhat inferior in sensitivity to the usual reaction [1, 11].

4.5.2 Real Time PCR

One of the fundamental drawbacks that complicates the use of classical PCR in diagnostics is the extremely high sensitivity of this method, which increases the likelihood of false-positive results due to cross-contamination of the samples being tested. The likelihood of cross-contamination can be prevented by using real-time PCR due to the fact that the processes of amplification and detection of amplification products occur simultaneously in the same test tube. To detect amplification products, fairly complex technologies have been developed based on a set of enzymatic reactions that result in a fluorescent signal in the reaction mixture, the intensity of which is proportional to the amount of the formed amplification product. The specificity of the fluorescent signal can be achieved by using DNA probes complementary to the internal regions of the DNA fragment limited by primers. TaqMan probes and "molecular beacons" are the most widely used.

Real-time PCR can be used to determine the quantitative content of target DNA in a biological sample. The feasibility of quantitative detection of *C. trachomatis* in urogenital chlamydial infection has not yet been determined, but the determination of DNA concentration [12, 13].

Quantity of *C. trachomatis* is an important additional diagnostic measure. It probably allows assessing the activity of the infectious process depending on its nature, prevalence, combination with other pathogens of urogenital pathology, the presence of complicated forms of the disease (infertility, *Chlamydia*-induced arthropathy).

Real-time PCR requires special thermal cyclers with precision optics that allow monitoring the fluorescence intensity in the reaction mixture. Modern thermal cyclers for real-time PCR are equipped with channels for detecting fluorescence in several wavelength ranges (up to 5–6), which allows developing multiplex reaction formats.

4.5.3 Transcription-Based Amplification Methods

In addition to PCR, a method of DNA amplification, RNA amplification methods have begun to attract increasing attention. Transcription-based amplification methods are isothermal (target amplification occurs at a constant temperature), the target being the pathogen's RNA. The prototype of these methods is the process that occurs during the replication of retroviruses. At the initial stages of the reaction, with the participation of reverse transcriptase, complementary DNA is synthesized on the target RNA matrix, and then multiple copies of RNA are synthesized with the help of RNA polymerase. Currently, two variants of the amplification method in question are widespread, protected by patents of the manufacturing companies: transcription-based amplification (TMA—TranscriptionMediatedAmplification—Gen-Probe, Inc. San Diego, CA, and nucleic acid sequence-based amplification (NASBA—Nucleic Acid Sequence Based Amplification)—BioMerieux [14].

The differences between the above variants are related to the different origins of the enzymes used in the reactions and different methods of detecting the amplification products. The TMA test systems (manufactured by Gen-Probe) use reverse transcriptase with endogenous RNase activity and RNA polymerase of the T7 bacteriophage. Hybridization is used to detect the amplification product—single-stranded RNA. The test systems are produced for the detection of C. trachomatis (APTIMA CT®Assay) and for the simultaneous detection of C. trachomatis and N. gonorrhoeae (APTIMA Combo 2® Assay). The latter test system also uses preliminary enrichment of the target RNA on magnetic particles, which allows to overcome to a large extent the problem of the presence of amplification inhibitors in the clinical sample. The NASBA test systems (manufactured by BioMerieux) use the reverse transcriptase of the avian myeloblastosis virus, RNase H and RNA polymerase of the bacteriophage T7. Hybridization is also used to detect amplification products, but in a slightly different format than in the TMA test systems. Since the target for NASBA is the RNA molecules of ribosomes (ribosomal RNA) of microorganisms, this provides a number of advantages over PCR. Firstly, the number of ribosomes: one *Chlamydia* cell contains from several thousand to several tens of thousands. For comparison: even multi-copy DNA regions used as a target for PCR do not exceed two dozen per bacterial cell. Thus, NASBA can be used to detect pathogens even in cases where their number is too small and insufficient for detection by PCR. Secondly, while DNA is a fairly stable material and its detection does not yet mean the presence of viable microorganisms, RNA, on the contrary, is an extremely unstable material and degrades quite quickly when microorganisms die and are destroyed. This makes it possible not only to more accurately judge the presence of a current infection, but also to more accurately and reliably assess the results of the treatment. Finally, since the PCR method has a higher analytical sensitivity compared to other laboratory methods—microscopy, DIF, culture method—the use of these methods to confirm PCR results is not always correct. In this case, NASBA can be used as a confirmatory test for PCR results, especially in the absence of clinical signs of infection. Real-time amplification product detection technology (NASBA-Real-Time) using specific fluorescent probes further increases the specificity of the test and the objectivity of the laboratory test results. The main disadvantage of transcription-based test systems is their high cost and the need to use strictly defined equipment [15].

4.5.4 Amplification with Strand Displacement

The chain displacement amplification method is an isothermal method, conceptually it is very complex, but in technical implementation it is very simple. The method is the intellectual property of Becton Dickinson, the test systems are marketed under the name "BD ProbeTec ™ ET C. trachomatis and N. gonorrhoeae amplified DNA Assay » for the simultaneous detection of *C. trachomatis* and *N. gonorrhoeae*.

Despite the growing popularity of molecular biological methods for diagnosing urogenital chlamydial infection among doctors, they are also not perfect, since false-positive and false-negative results cannot be excluded.

4.6 Cultural Method

In the era of increasing resistance of most *Chlamydia* to antimicrobial drugs, resistance to them is of particular concern in the treatment of chlamydial infection, especially its chronic forms [16].

Recently, there have been reports of treatment failures associated with *C. trachomatis* strains that are resistant to several drugs. Therefore, in recent years, there has been an active study of *Chlamydia* sensitivity to antichlamydial drugs in cell cultures [1].

Many researchers have shown that the use of McCoy cells for susceptibility testing *of C. trachomatis* and Hep-2 cells for testing for *C. pneumoniae* gives the most reliable and consistent results.

For many years, the culture method (CM) has been the preferred method for diagnosing *C. trachomatis* infections, as it allows detecting viable microorganisms. However, this method is not standardized, resulting in discrepancies in data obtained from different diagnostic centres. At the same time, its high specificity allows recommending its use for diagnosing *C. trachomatis* in extragenital areas and, most importantly, as an assessment of treatment effectiveness. Most researchers have concluded that with a 100% specificity of the culture method, its sensitivity remains very low—from 40% to 60%. With the introduction of PCR into practice, cell culture sowing still remains the standard, but only for certain clinical situations. Technical difficulties and the long duration of this study make it less convenient, although the pathogen is most often detected by the culture method. Therefore, the use of this method, especially in complex cases, is certainly necessary.

For cultural studies, various types of cells with high sensitivity to *Chlamydia* are used: McCoy, Hela-229, L-229, BHK-221. Preference is given to mixed cell lines (KK lines LLC-MK520, BHK-21 and L59290). Given the existing difficulties in using this method for diagnosing persistent forms of chlamydial infection, we use a mixed transplantable cell culture

LLC + MK2 + L929 + BHK-21C, with previously reduced resistance.

The culture method has long been considered the gold standard, but it has proven to be ineffective in isolating aberrant or antibiotic-resistant *Chlamydia* species and in diagnosing latent persistent forms of chlamydial infection, leading to false-negative results. The sensitivity of the method is considered to be 40–60%, specificity is about 100%, although in general, the diagnostic efficiency does not exceed 70–85%, which does not meet modern requirements [16, 17].

However, an important advantage of the cultural method is the isolation of only live forms of the *Chlamydia* pathogen.

Currently, the method is not recommended for routine laboratory diagnostics [17].

The cultural method has recently begun to be used for diagnostics of persistent forms of chlamydial infection. For these purposes, multiple passages of *Chlamydia* on cell cultures are carried out in order to achieve the effect of "reversions" of persistent forms of *Chlamydia* with the formation of typical elementary and reticular bodies. But these multiple passages of the pathogen on cell culture must be carried out after using various methods that stimulate the reproduction of *Chlamydia* in cells. The widespread use of this method is hindered by its complexity, relative high cost, delayed receipt of results (not earlier than 72 hours) and the risk of infection of personnel. In addition, the diagnostic value of the cultural method is reduced when using clinical materials from patients with a chronic form of infection who have received multiple courses of antibacterial therapy. When using the cultural method, it is necessary to take into account that the probability of isolating *C. trachomatis* can be influenced by the following factors:

- Gender of the patients examined (the percentage of *Chlamydia* isolation is higher in women than in men).
- Patients taking antibiotics (it is advisable to carry out culture studies on individuals who have not taken antibiotics in the last month).
- Duration of the disease (the pathogen is isolated more often during a long course of the disease than during a short one).
- Method of collecting material (in case of urogenital *Chlamydia*, the best results are obtained by collecting clinical material using a Volkmann spoon, endourethral curette or cytological brush; in case of persistent form of the disease—by examining ejaculate).
- The time of delivery of the material to the laboratory (it should not exceed 1.5 h; it is permissible to store clinical material in a freezer at $-18–20^{0}$ C for up to 2 weeks; however, this reduces the isolation of the pathogen and extends the time of its cultivation).
- The cell culture line used (mixed continuous cell cultures, weakened beforehand with prednisolone, are best).
- Quality of the transport medium (to prevent the growth of contaminating microflora, it is advisable to add penicillin, streptomycin, kanamycin, amphotericin, to which *Chlamydia* has a high resistance).

In recent years, coherent optical methods of laboratory diagnostics have been used to improve the quality of diagnostics of *Chlamydia* cultured on chicken embryos (CE). The method allows observing changes in CE infected with *Chlamydia* no earlier than 4–5 days after infection. For early detection of changes in microcirculation in CE (both intact and infected with *Chlamydia*), installations were developed using the NI- Elvis station. The method is based on the use of a laser spectrum microscope when scanning samples of CE infected with *Chlamydia*.

4.7 Rapid Tests in the Diagnosis of Sexually Transmitted Infections

The development of rapid tests that allow for an aetiological diagnosis to be established within a few minutes or tens of minutes, preferably during a patient's appointment with a doctor, is one of the main areas of modern microbiological diagnostics, including STI diagnostics. Timely etiotropic treatment provides a better clinical effect, and limiting the use of empirical antibiotic therapy in the long term can help reduce the development of antibiotic resistance in microorganisms. In addition, it is necessary to take into account that a significant proportion of patients do not come for a follow-up appointment, so immediately initiated treatment can reduce the risk of complications in infected individuals, as well as the spread of infections.

To date, the vast majority of rapid tests for the diagnosis of STIs are based on immunological reactions (mainly immunochromatography and agglutination) to detect antigens or antibodies [18].

Modern immunological rapid tests have a fairly high specificity, but their sensitivity varies significantly (Table 4.1).

In general, rapid immunological tests have a fairly high sensitivity for detecting antibodies, due to their high content in the blood, but they are less sensitive when detecting antigens. Thus, most immunological rapid tests for the diagnosis of chlamydial and gonococcal infections have a sensitivity of 50–70%. It should be emphasized that the sensitivity indicators significantly depend on the reference test, in relation to which the diagnostic characteristics of the test being evaluated are determined. For example the sensitivity of one of the tests for detecting *Chlamydia* (Clearview Chlamydia test) was 95% when compared with the results of a cultural study [19], and only 32.8% when compared with the results of PCR [20].

Since only molecular biological methods can currently provide adequate diagnostics of many infections, including urogenital tract infections, rapid tests based on nucleic acid analysis methods have been developed in recent years by global diagnostic system manufacturers. In order for these methods to be used in a doctor's office, the reaction time must be reduced and the process fully automated. One solution to this problem is the use of microfluidic technologies. Microfluidics is an interdisciplinary science that describes the behaviour of small volumes and flows of liquids, and molecular diagnostics is one of the most important areas of its application. Bioanalytical systems based on microfluidics allow for the miniaturization and integration of processes that are traditionally performed on a full scale as a sequence of individual operations. Thus, using microfluidic technologies, immunological rapid tests based on miniaturized enzyme immunoassay for serological diagnosis of syphilis and HIV

Table 4.1 Modern commercial rapid tests for the diagnosis of sexually transmitted infections

Pathogen	Test	Duration of analysis	Test principle	Sensitivity (%)	Specificity (%)	Source
Chlamydia trachomatis	*Chlamydia* rapid test (diagnostics for the real world)	30 min	Immuno-chromatographic analysis	41.2–83.5	98.9	[16, 25, 39]
	BioStar OIA *Chlamydia* test (Inverness)	30 min	Optical immunoassay	59.4–73.8	98.4–100	[4, 15]
	Clearview Chlamydia test (Alere)	15 min	Immuno-chromatographic analysis	32.8–95	97.9–99.6	[37, 38, 46]
	QuickVue *Chlamydia* test (Quidel)	12 min	Immuno-chromatographic analysis	25–65	100	[35]
	GeneXpert CT/NG (Cepheid)	90 min	Nucleic acid amplification (real-time PCR)	97.4–98.7	99.4–99.9	[11]

have recently been developed, the sensitivity and specificity of which were comparable to those of traditional serological tests, while only 1 μl of whole blood was used for analysis [21].

Miniaturization of PCR systems can also provide significant advantages, including reduced analysis time, reduced reagent consumption, portability, and the ability to integrate multiple pre- and post-PCR processing modules into a self-contained system with full automation [22].

Multiplex testing, that is simultaneous testing for a range of microorganisms that may occur at a given anatomical site in a given clinical condition, is also a technological approach that can reduce the time to establish an etiologic diagnosis.

An example of the fusion of nucleic acid amplification (real-time PCR), microfluidic and multiplex technologies is the commercially available GeneXpert system (Cepheid), designed for the simultaneous diagnosis of chlamydial and gonococcal infections in the physician's office [23]. Manual operations are reduced to a minimum, namely, to the introduction of material from the patient into the cartridge. The test is easy to use, has high sensitivity (above 97%) and specificity (above 99%). However, it can hardly be called an ideal rapid test is lengthy (the duration of the analysis is about 90 minutes), expensive (requires expensive equipment).

Significant potential for the creation of rapid tests also lies in the use of electrochemical DNA biosensors [24, 25].

The method is based on the interaction between the microorganism's nucleic acid, amplified or non-amplified, and complementary oligonucleotide probes immobilized on microelectrodes (sensors), resulting in the generation of an electrochemical signal detected by the sensor. This approach is implemented in the diagnostic platform for rapid diagnostics of STIs developed by Atlas Genetics. This is a rapid test (analysis time is about 25 min), fully automated, based on PCR amplification followed by electrochemical detection of amplification products. The sensitivity and specificity of the test are very high—in preclinical trials they were 98.1% and 98%, respectively, for the detection of *C. trachomatis* [26], and 95.5% and 95.7%, respectively, for the detection of T. vaginalis [27]. This system is currently not commercially available.

A significant drawback of analytical PCR systems in the context of their use for rapid diagnostics is the need for complex and often expensive equipment. The solution to this problem could be facilitated by the introduction of isothermal amplification methods, when the amplification reaction occurs at a fixed temperature in a conventional thermal block.

The sample preparation for amplification consists of its simple dilution, and the stage of analysis of the amplification products is reduced to installing the tube with amplicons after the reaction in the cassette for subsequent colorimetric detection. The test has a sensitivity and specificity comparable to PCR, is easy to use, does not require tools and equipment (except for a microdispenser and a thermal block), which makes it potentially suitable for rapid diagnostics. It is believed that the development of rapid tests based on isothermal amplification methods is an important direction in the development of rapid diagnostics of infectious diseases [28].

Thus, modern rapid tests, mostly based on immunological reactions, are usually highly specific, but their sensitivity is not high enough, especially for tests for antigen detection. Recent advances in molecular diagnostic technologies (amplification, microfluidic, biosensor) open up opportunities for creating highly sensitive and highly specific, easy-to-use, affordable rapid tests for STI diagnostics.

4.8 Serological Tests (Enzyme-Linked Immunosorbent Assay, Indirect Immunofluorescence)

Serological methods are auxiliary in diagnostics of urogenital *Chlamydia*. Currently, using the serological method, it is possible to detect IgM, IgG and IgA to *C. trachomatis* in biological fluids (blood, ejaculate, synovial fluid, cerebrospinal fluid). A feature of UGC is significant individual variability in the onset of formation, severity and duration of the humoral immune response, which significantly complicates the interpretation of both positive and negative results of serological tests.

This is due to non-absolute species specificity chlamydial antigens (AG) of the outer membrane, low immunogenicity of individual strains *of C. trachomatis*, individual differences in the dynamics and strength of the immune response at different stages of infection. According to the presence or absence of antibodies to *Chlamydia*, serologically positive and negative patients are distinguished. It is believed that the results of tests for the presence of antichlamydial IgM in the blood does not coincide with the clinical picture. It is possible that the detection of antibodies of this class has greater practical significance in the examination of pregnant women; in male chlamydiosis, no patterns of IgM determination have been described. The detection of these immunoglobulins is diagnostically valuable only in the examination of people infected with *C. trachomatis* for the first time. Among the main reasons for the failure of species-specific IgM diagnostics of UGH should highlight the low level of synthesis of this class of antibodies to membrane proteins of *C. trachomatis* during primary infection and its short duration. The latter, taking into account the predominantly erased symptoms of primary chlamydial lesions of the genitourinary system and, accordingly, the prevalence of late seeking medical care, leaves minimal chances for registering species-specific IgM. A more pronounced immune response is formed to the genus-specific lipopolysaccharide, however, in this case, serum IgM to all representatives of the genus *Chlamydia* is registered in the ELISA, which makes it difficult to establish an evidentiary relationship between a positive result of such a serological analysis and an early stage of infection caused specifically by *C. trachomatis*. In addition to the high probability of obtaining a false-positive clinical conclusion about the presence of UGC based on a positive result of IgM testing in ELISA with LPS-AG, the use of such test systems also determines the risk of false-negative responses in the case of an actual primary infection with *C. trachomatis*. If the primary infection caused by *C. trachomatis* was previously preceded by episodes of infection with other representatives of the genus *Chlamydia*, repeated synthesis of IgM to genus-specific LPS will most likely not be initiated.

For IgG to *C. trachomatis*, diagnostic titres have been established. According to the observations of V.V. Mikhailichenko et al. (2000), the determination of antichlamydial IgG can be considered a screening test, but the IgG titre cannot be used to make a diagnosis. Detection of antichlamydial IgG in the blood, regardless of their titre, indicates only two facts: the patient had *Chlamydia* and was cured by the time of examination, or the patient has been suffering from *Chlamydia* for some time. The latter can only be proven by identifying the pathogen in the patient. If *Chlamydia* is not detected in PCR and culture, then even a high or, more importantly, increasing IgG titre (in the absence of IgA) is not always a basis for establishing a diagnosis of Chlamydia. An increase in titre by more than 4 times is rare, and a change in value by 2 times is within the error of the method. It is more difficult to interpret the situation in which a positive result of direct immunofluorescence, not confirmed by polymerase chain reaction and culture research, is combined with the detection of only antichlamydial IgG. In this case, it is advisable to choose the tactics of dynamic observation of the patient, during which the diagnosis will be specified.

Unlike IgG, detection of IgA to C. trachomatis in the blood allows diagnosis. It is known that detection of antichlamydial IgA is a sign of an acute inflammatory process caused by *Chlamydia*. The presence of IgA is always combined with the presence of IgG in the blood, although the value of their ratio may vary. The presence of IgA in the blood, even when it is not possible to detect the pathogen in PCR and the culture method, is regarded by many authors as a manifestation of an actively ongoing chlamydial process. This probably also applies to those cases when the IgA titre is below the diagnostic one. In such a situation, the possibility of a cross-reaction with low titres of antichlamydial immunoglobulins, clinical manifestations in the patient and his sexual partner, as well as social circumstances are taken into account. The minimum necessary measures include dynamic clinical and laboratory observation, which allows for the final exclusion of infection or timely initiation of antibacterial therapy. It is most appropriate to conduct simultaneous determination of IgA and IgG to species-specific AG of *C. trachomatis*, obtained, as a rule, on the basis of recombinant or synthetic outer membrane proteins (OMP) of the causative agent of UGH. The use of such ELISA test systems ensures the detection of chlamydial antibodies circulating in the blood serum and, at the same time, significantly reduces the risk of cross-interactions with antibodies to other representatives of *Chlamydia*, in particular to C. pneumoniae. In contrast, the use of ELISA test systems based on genus-specific lipopolysaccharide (LPS) of *Chlamydia* can significantly complicate the differential diagnosis of UGC with other *Chlamydia*, primarily with infection caused by *C. pneumoniae*, especially in the absence of symptoms of respiratory or urogenital tract infection.

At the same time, in connection with the considered shortcomings of IgM serodiagnostics of UGC, it is appropriate to assess the reliability and practical applicability of complex and detailed algorithms for assessing the results of determining various classes of chlamydial antibodies proposed in some manuals for doctors. They are based on existing ideas about the patterns of the typical immune response of the body to the presence of *C. trachomatis*, which consist in the fact that during primary infection, a sequential synthesis of specific AT classes M, A and G is initiated. It is also believed that during reinfection with the UGC pathogen or during UGC reactivation, it is possible to register mainly specific IgG and IgA with a minimal probability of detecting IgM. Based on the assessment of the variants of combinations of positive and negative results of serological studies for various classes of antibodies to C. trachomatis, it is proposed to conduct an in-depth interpretation and establishment of the form of UGC in a patient with primary or repeated infection, chronic course, relapse of UGC or persistence, as well as a history of infection. In addition to taking into account the features of the combination of positive and negative responses to IgM, IgG and IgA, the assessment of titers of these antibodies in positive sera serves as an objective basis for differential clinical diagnosis of UGC. However, the ranges of titres of antibodies of various classes recommended for serological identification of each of the listed clinical variants of UGC are determined with a fourfold or more range, and therefore they inevitably overlap and reduce the possibilities of serological differentiation of forms of acute and chronic chlamydial infection to a minimum. It is also necessary to take into account the multifactorial complexities of reliable IgM testing of UGC, consistent with the indications of the need for extremely cautious interpretation of serological test results, especially when IgM is detected. Obviously, the most frequently performed single test in practice provides satisfactory serological differential diagnostics of only two opposite conditions—"there is an infection" or "there is no infection, but there is residual seropositivity." The basis for the first conclusion is simultaneously positive test results for IgA and IgG or only for IgA in any titres, for the second—only for IgG. It should be noted that it is advisable for a practicing physician to operate with these generalized conclusions, since clarification of the variants of fresh or chronic chlamydial infection cannot be carried out without taking into account clinical and anamnestic data. On the other hand, the international classification of diseases ICD-10 suggests differentiating UGC only from the standpoint of topical diagnostics without specifying the stage of infection. The simplicity and rationality of this classification of UGH quite adequately reflect the real possibilities and complexities of objective clinical and laboratory diagnostics of chlamydial infection, preventing unfounded decisions and actions of the doctor, including the establishment and frequent attempts to treat difficult to prove persistent chlamydial infection [15].

Thus, when the antigen of the pathogen is detected in the material from various segments of the human genital tract using immunofluorescence, polymerase chain reaction and culture studies, regardless of whether antibodies against *Chlamydia* are present in the blood, it is necessary to make a diagnosis of "chlamydiosis". The absence of chlamydial antibodies in this situation indicates a possible seronegative variant of the infection. In cases where immunoglobulins to *C. trachomatis* are determined in the blood of patients, and markers of these microorganisms are not detected in the urogenital tract, there is no reason to make a diagnosis of "chlamydiosis". There is no doubt that serological methods are inferior in information content to PCR, CM and even DIF in fresh clinically expressed UGC and in any other variants of infection accompanied by the isolation of the pathogen or its molecular markers from parts of the genital tract accessible for taking scraping material. It is these patients that dermatovenerologists and urologists most often encounter. However, obstetricians and gynaecologists often have to establish or exclude the role of *C. trachomatis* in the development of tubal infertility and inflammatory diseases of the pelvic organs (PIDs). The reason for the ineffectiveness of diagnostics may also be the development of cicatricial changes in the foci of chronic infectious lesions. In such cases, the pathogen, its DNA or antigen are not always present in the material obtained from the lower sections of the genitourinary tract, and negative results of CM, PCR and DIF do not exclude the diagnosis of PID of chlamydial aetiology. In this case, the only way to obtain material for a reliable direct study is laparoscopy, which, however, is not widely used in routine practice even abroad due to the high cost of the procedure and possible difficulties in identifying mild inflammation in the fallopian tube. In this situation, the value of detecting chlamydial antibodies increases significantly, since the results of immunoserology are an inexpensive alternative to laboratory confirmation of clinical suspicions of chlamydial PID [29].

Despite a number of difficulties in interpreting the results of immunoserological studies conducted to diagnose UGC, test systems for detecting antibodies to C. trachomatis are widely used in healthcare practice.

4.8.1 Immunoblotting

Immunoblotting allows to reveal the humoral immune response of the macroorganism to individual chlamydial proteins. The technique of immunoblotting of *Chlamydia* was developed by Batteiger, Newhall and Jones in 1982. Subsequent studies showed that the main cross-reacting antigens *of Chlamydia trachomatis* and *Chlamydophylla psitaci* are LPS, proteins of 57–62 kDa and MOMP (Mondesire et al., 1989). Serum from many individuals, without any indication of current or past chlamydial infection, reacts (although weakly) with *C. trachomatis* MOMP in immunoblotting. Serum from patients with chlamydial infection reacts most strongly with proteins of 60–62 kDa. Moreover, the degree of expression of this reaction in convalescents is greater than in individuals with acute infection (Newhall et al., 1982; Cevenini et al., 1986). Women who developed salpingitis after an abortion were less likely to have IgA antibodies to 60–62 kDa proteins and IgG antibodies to 75 kDa proteins, compared to women who did not develop salpingitis after an abortion. The titres of these antibodies in patients were significantly lower than in healthy women. Thus, using immunoblotting, it was shown which antigens cause a protective humoral immune response in patients with *Chlamydia* (Brunham et al., 1987). The two most notable proteins of the 60–62 kDa chlamydial protein family are outer membrane protein 2 (Omp—2) and heat shock protein Hsp60. The serum of almost 100% of patients with ectopic pregnancy and pelvic inflammatory disease reacts with Omp2 and Hsp60, 81% and 31%, respectively (Wagar et al. 1990).

4.9 Determination of Serotypes and Molecular Biological Characteristics of C. *trachomatis*

The main problems associated with the diagnosis of inflammatory syndromes associated with *Chlamydia* in practical health care are caused, first of all, by insufficient information on the molecular organization of these microorganisms and their distinctive properties, as well as on the molecular mechanisms of the microorganism-host cell relationship. Serologically, the *C. tra-*

chomatis species is divided into 18 main serovars marked with letters of the English alphabet from A to L. Serovars D-K are detected in various clinical forms of urogenital pathology in humans. From 60% to 80% of all strains are serotypes D, E and F with minor variations in the world. The serotype can determine the infectivity of the pathogen, which is measured by the number of inclusions forming units (IFU) of *Chlamydia* in clinical samples. There are publications establishing the relationship between serotypes, molecular biological characteristics of *C. trachomatis* and various clinical manifestations of chlamydial infection. Comparative analysis of the serological variant of the pathogen with clinical manifestations showed that more frequent causes of inflammatory processes of the urogenital tract are serotypes D and K of *C. trachomatis*, causing the development of urethritis, adnexitis, endocervicitis and other pathologies.

4.10 Diagnosis of Urogenital *Chlamydia* Associated with Trichomonas Invasion

Based on our many years of experience in examining and treating patients with STIs, and literature data for widespread forms of chlamydial urogenital infection, the detection rate of *T. vaginalis* can reach 70–80%.

In most cases, atypical forms of trichomonads with altered metabolism and morphology are detected. New information has appeared on the intracellular absorption and the possibility of intracellular storage of *Chlamydia* by vaginal trichomonads in vitro, which, despite this, retained the ability to reproduce and did not lose their infectivity. These features contribute to the maintenance of a chronic inflammatory process in the genitourinary tract, which is manifested by moderate general infectious intoxication, subfebrile temperature, slightly expressed signs of a local inflammatory process in various parts of the genitourinary tract (urethritis, prostatitis, urethroprostatitis, cystitis, cervicitis, colpitis). These facts in most cases are the reasons for unsuccessful courses of therapy for patients with genitourinary chlamydiosis. When trichomonads are lysed (e.g. as a result of exposure to antiprotozoal drugs), *Chlamydia* are released from them and contribute to the maintenance of a chronic inflammatory process in the surrounding tissues. The ineffectiveness of treatment of urogenital trichomoniasis with antitrichomoniasis drugs from the nitroimidazole group is most often associated, according to a number of authors, with low zinc levels in the blood, low absorption of the drug, low concentration of the drug in the foci of inflammation or inactivation of the drug under the influence of vaginal microflora, as well as with the widespread distribution of resistant strains of T. vaginalis to antitrichomoniasis drugs from the nitroimidazole group. According to our data, the latter circumstance causes frequent relapses of chlamydial infection, coinciding with clinical and laboratory signs of relapses of urogenital trichomoniasis in 23.4% of patients.

It is important to note that in mixed infections, *Chlamydia* often remains undetected. The use of antibiotics in the treatment of concomitant infections leads to changes in the antigenic structure of the *Chlamydia* cell wall, complicating the diagnosis and, accordingly, the treatment of *Chlamydia*.

4.11 Diagnosis of Widespread Forms of Chlamydial Infection

Despite numerous publications on the study of various problems associated with urogenital chlamydial infection, course of this infection in young people and associated diseases needs further study [30].

Urogenital chlamydiosis is characterized by a wide variety of clinical manifestations. The introduction of new diagnostic methods has allowed not only to expand the spectrum of pathology caused by *C. trachomatis*, but also to verify that diagnostic options are possible not only for localized forms of this infection, but also with damage to the musculoskeletal system, central nervous system, respiratory tract, otorhinology organs, eye, cardiovascular system. However, there is no consensus among researchers on the nature of the development of these forms of chlamydial infection.

In order to study the distinctive clinical features of the course of localized (LFCI) and widespread forms (WFCI) of chronic urogenital chlamydial infection, we analysed the frequency of the main clinical syndromes in 650 patients. Of these, 298 had localized (urethritis, prostatitis) and 352 had widespread forms of chlamydial infection (urogenital *Chlamydia* complicated by neurochlamydiosis, *Chlamydia*-induced arthropathy, vasculitis, myocarditis, proctosigmoiditis).

The presented data show that the most typical syndromes in patients with urogenital chlamydiosis were general infectious intoxication syndrome (41.2%), asthenovegetative syndrome (40.9%), inguinal lymphadenitis (40.8%), and immunodeficiency syndrome (63.1%). It turned out that for patients with LFCI, the most typical, along with syndromes of damage to the genitourinary tract (urethritis, prostatitis), were general infectious intoxication (27.2%), inguinal lymphadenitis (31.2%), asthenovegetative syndrome (75.8%), and manifestations of immunodeficiency (32.9%). However, these syndromes were significantly more often diagnosed in patients with WFCI. In addition, this category of patients was characterized by such syndromes as intestinal dysbacteriosis (92.1%), chronic conjunctivitis (84.4%), arthralgic syndrome (33.2%), meningeal syndrome (27.6%), hepatosplenic syndrome (23.6%), allergic syndrome (32.6%), and anemia syndrome (12.2%). The most characteristic phenomenon for this form of infection was the detection chlamydemia (63.4%) [31].

Thus, the distinctive features we identified in the diagnosis of the main clinical syndromes in patients with LFCI and WFCI were probably due to the influence of *Chlamydia* on various organs and systems of infected individuals. The clinical distinctive features identified in this case should be used for differential clinical and laboratory diagnostics of these forms of urogenital chlamydial infection.

Taking into account the above, we considered it expedient to conduct a comprehensive diagnosis of chlamydial lesions using modern laboratory and clinical-instrumental research methods. For this purpose, the list of clinical material from patients with suspected extraurogenital foci of CI was significantly expanded. To substantiate the formation of WFCI in patients, we additionally used the methods of histochemical assessment of the morphofunctional state of the mucous membranes affected by *Chlamydia*, as well as the electron microscopy. To clarify the localization of foci of chronic infection, in these patients additionally were used ultrasound investigation of the pelvic organs and radioisotope scintigraphy. Analysis of the results of *C. trachomatis* diagnostics in various clinical materials from patients with LFCI and WFCI made it possible to identify a number of distinctive features. Thus, in patients with LFCI, *Chlamydia* were diagnosed only in the genitourinary tract. The frequency of their detection significantly increased after the use of biological provocation with betaleukin. The most informative clinical material in such patients was: prostate secretion, ejaculate and centrifugate of the first portion of urine. The use of biological provocation with betaleukin increased the frequency of detection of *Chlamydia* in scraping material from the urethra by 1.5–2 times. In patients with WFCI, *C. trachomatis* was detected both in the urogenital tract and beyond it: in the oropharynx, conjunctiva, paranasal sinuses, synovial fluid and peripheral blood. The use of biological provocation with betaleukin also reliably increased the frequency of detection of *Chlamydia* in various clinical materials. In patients with WFCI, occurring as a monoinfection, chlamydemia was diagnosed in 69.1% of cases, and in similar patients with mixed STIs involving *Chlamydia*—in 84.9%. At the same time, using the culture method, it was possible to isolate "viable" *Chlamydia* from peripheral blood in 47.1% of individuals with monochlamydia and in 30.1% of those with mixed STIs involving Chlamydia. The low percentage of "viable" *Chlamydia* detected in the blood of patients with mixed infection was probably due to their predominant intracellular localization in neutrophils and macrophages, as well as the antagonistic interaction of Chlamydia with mycoplasmas, ureaplasmas and bacteroids. The study of the morphofunctional state of the urethral mucosa in patients with LFCI and WFCI helped to identify symptoms that allow us to some extent to explain the mechanisms of interaction of *Chlamydia* with epithelial cells, as well as the formation of sclerotic areas in tissues. We suggested that the formation of extraurogenital foci of CI occurs on the background of irreversible sclerotic and alterative changes in the mucous membrane of the urogenital tract. Probably, these changes contribute to the translocation of *Chlamydia* through the altered mucous membrane into the blood and lymph. The use of transabdominal and transrectal ultrasound scanning of the pelvis in men with LFCI and WFCI allowed us to find out that 76.2% of patients with chronic prostatitis of chlamydial aetiology have ultrasound signs of various pathological processes in the prostate gland. At the same time, in patients with WFCI, these changes were diagnosed reliably more often. Probably, the detected ultrasound changes in the prostate gland were a consequence of sclerotic and alterative processes caused by *Chlamydia* on the glandular tissue. It cannot be ruled out that these pathological changes could also contribute to the translocation of *Chlamydia* into the blood and lymph. The use of electron microscopy also made it possible to identify changes in the morphofunctional state of the maxillary sinus mucosa and cerebrospinal fluid cells infected with *Chlamydia* in patients with a widespread form of urogenital chlamydiosis. The results obtained proved the presence of *Chlamydia* in these clinical materials, as well as their proliferation on the background of sclerotic and alterative changes in *Chlamydia*-infected tissues. The most convincing data on the formation of extraurogenital foci in patients with chronic urogenital chlamydiosis were obtained by radioisotope scintigraphy. This method made it possible to identify multiple sites of increased accumulation of autoleukocytes (AL) in both men and women with suspected WFCI. The results of using radioisotope scintigraphy made it possible to detect foci of chronic inflammation in patients with WFCI not only in the genitourinary organs, but also in the wall of the proctosigmoid intestine, in the oropharynx, heart, paranasal sinuses, pelvic lymph nodes, and large joints. Etiological decoding of the identified foci of chronic infection in those examined using modern laboratory methods (DIF, PCR, CM) made it possible to identify C. trachomatis in them, which proves their chlamydial nature [1, 32].

4.12 Diagnosis of Persistent Forms of Chlamydial Infection

Significant difficulties arise in diagnosis of the persistent form of infection, when obtaining material for direct detection of the pathogen is difficult or impossible. In the case of persistence of *C. trachomatis* using the culture method is also difficult. The use of cell culture requires multiple passages, since in persistent infection chlamydiae are not cultured due to the non-infectivity and non-productivity of persistent inclusions as a result of minimal metabolism in the pathogen cell itself. The direct immunofluorescence method is also uninformative for diagnosing persistent infection. In persistence, the production of MOMP and LPS is blocked, and detection of the antigen on the surface of elementary bodies (EB) of *C. trachomatis* using monoclonal antibodies is not possible. In addition, persistence usually implies a relatively low concentration of infectious bodies in epithelial cells, which, given the above-mentioned “quantitative census” for fluorescent bodies required for a positive result, makes the diagnosis even more problematic. Diagnosis of persistent chlamydiosis is difficult regardless of gender. In chronic chlamydial cervicitis in women complicated by lesions of the upper urogenital tract, the use of cell culture and direct immunofluorescence methods is also unacceptable for confirming the etiological diagnosis. The PCR method, due to its high sensitivity and controlled specificity, allows detecting persistent infections, but requires provocative measures in preparing patients before collecting material. Alternative methods for diagnosing persistent *Chlamydia* can be serological methods with the determination of antibodies against the pathogen and the dynamics of their titre. In particular, the level of chlamydial antibodies of the IgG class is

2–4 times higher in extragenital manifestations of chlamydial infection than in uncomplicated *Chlamydia* of the lower urogenital tract.

Thus, a peculiar situation has developed in the laboratory diagnostics of chlamydial infection: on the one hand, a significant number of test systems and diagnosticums are used, on the other hand, there are difficulties with interpretation of the results obtained. Unified clinical and laboratory algorithms for examining patients with inflammatory urogenital diseases are necessary, there is also need for simultaneous determination of concomitant opportunistic microflora. Reliable data on the presence (absence) of *C.trachomatis* can only be obtained based on the results of a comprehensive examination of patients. If urogenital *Chlamydia* is suspected, DIF with cell culture or PCR analysis is preferable. Serological tests (ELISA) are of auxiliary importance and for the diagnosis of *Chlamydia* must be used in combination with cell culture or PCR analysis. The absence of antibodies of both classes (or their low titres) with a positive PCR may indicate an inadequate immune response, long-term chronic course of *Chlamydia*, persistent infection, *Chlamydia*-induced arthropathy, sclerotic and fibrous lesions of the genitourinary organs.

In world practice, a huge experience has been accumulated, indicating the need to implement a comprehensive approach to clinical and laboratory examination of patients, since the use of diverse methodologies that complement and confirm each other increases the reliability of the diagnosis and eliminates technical errors. In our opinion, it is necessary to focus on the analysis of the practically achievable information obtained by individual methods or their combinations. Such an approach can contribute to the formation of a critical attitude of specialists to the results of laboratory diagnostic studies and their choice of the correct tactics for managing the patients being examined.

The reliability of laboratory data and the validity of clinical conclusions can be achieved only with a combination of high quality of selected laboratory diagnostic tools, sufficient qualifications of laboratory personnel and the necessary level of training of physicians capable of critically analysing the totality of laboratory and clinical-anamnestic data.

4.13 Laboratory and Instrumental Diagnosiss of Pneumochlamydia

In a blood test, the number of leukocytes is usually normal; there may be a moderate shift in the leukocyte formula to the left due to band elements, and a normal or moderately increased ESR. Urinalysis may reveal febrile albuminuria and cylindruria. Chest X-ray reveals interstitial pneumonia in most patients.

Specific laboratory diagnostics of pneumochlamydia is difficult due to the characteristics of the pathogen, the course of the infection, the low concentration of the pathogen in the inflammatory foci, the presence of cross-serological reactions with *C. trachomatis* and *C. psittaci* antigens; therefore, it is advisable to conduct a comprehensive examination using various methods.

Diagnosis is based on the results of serological tests detecting specific IgG, IgA and IgM. The pathogen antigen is determined using a direct immunofluorescence reaction (DIF) with monoclonal antibodies labelled with a fluorochrome .

To identify the pathogen, PCR is used, as well as the reaction of transcription amplification (NASBA—nucleic acid sequence-based amplification), which allows the diagnosis of *Chlamydia* RNA.

The material for the study is the patient's blood serum, scrapings from the mucous membrane of the mouth and nasopharynx, nasopharyngeal washes, sputum, bronchoalveolar lavage, tissues of affected vessels or organs, mononuclear cells of peripheral blood, in case of endocarditis—blood or fragments of heart valve tissue obtained during surgery.

4.14 Laboratory and Instrumental Diagnosis of Ornithosis

In a blood test, the total number of leukocytes is normal or slightly elevated (leukocytosis at the height of the disease is evidence of a secondary infection); lymphocytosis, monocytosis (absolute and relative), a significant (40–60 mm/h) increase in ESR, eosinophilia—during the recovery period.

Urine analysis shows no characteristic changes; signs of toxic kidney damage may appear (single erythrocytes, cylinders, traces of protein).

When examining sputum, an increased number of leukocytes (including monocytes), eosinophils and alveolar macrophages, alveolar epithelium, and sometimes erythrocytes are detected.

In patients with severe disease, neutrophil, D-dimer, lactate dehydrogenase, interleukin (IL)-2, IL-6, and IL-10 levels are significantly higher, while lymphocyte, CD3+ T cell, and CD4+ T cell counts, CD4+/CD8+ T cell ratio, and albumin levels are significantly lower than in patients with mild disease.

Radiographic changes in the lungs during the development of pneumonia are characterized by interstitial changes—increased pulmonary pattern, peribronchial or perivascular infiltration, which is manifested by a reticular pattern, band-like darkening along the vessels and bronchi with the most frequent localization of the process in the root areas and in the lower lobes of the lungs. Against this background, infiltrates of various sizes and shapes, single or multiple, may appear. Involvement of peribronchial lymph nodes, lymph nodes of the roots of the lungs, and exudative pleurisy are possible. Radiographic changes resolve within an average of 6 weeks.

Computed tomography of patients with severe disease demonstrates large areas of lung tissue consolidation; ground glass opacities are possible with an increased risk of multilobular lesions and pleural effusion.

If *meningitis* develops, pleocytosis in the CSF is moderate, usually does not exceed 300–500 cells in 1 μl, in the first days neutrophils predominate in it, then lymphocytes (up to 80–90%), the content of sugar and chlorides is normal, the protein level is slightly increased. Changes in the cerebrospinal fluid can persist for 3–4 weeks.

The diagnosis of ornithosis in humans is considered established upon laboratory confirmation using serological and molecular genetic methods.

Metagenomic next-generation sequencing (mNGS) enables rapid and accurate detection of potential pathogens, whether bacteria, fungi, viruses or parasites. It is increasingly used to diagnose infectious diseases, especially when traditional diagnostic methods have limitations. Studies have shown that mNGS is the most promising method for comprehensive diagnosis of infections, especially severe pneumonia.

The material for testing for ornithosis is blood serum, sputum, bronchoalveolar lavage, cerebrospinal fluid; autopsy material—blood, exudate, biopsies of organs and tissues (lungs, heart, etc.).

Paired sera are examined at an interval of 14 days; diagnostic antibody titers in the complete serum count, ELISA. Serological tests are retrospective, cross-reactions with other *Chlamydia* are possible, antibacterial therapy can delay or reduce the formation of antibodies. Thus, complement-fixing antibodies appear no earlier than the 4th–6th day of illness, and with early antibacterial therapy—on the 2nd–3rd week. Maximum antibody titres are recorded on the 4th–5th week with their subsequent rapid decrease [33–41].

4.15 Morphological Methods for Diagnosing *Chlamydia*

Morphological diagnostics of *Chlamydia* is used much less frequently than laboratory diagnostics. The literature provides only very brief descriptions of the structural changes that develop in humans and does not highlight diagnostically significant ones. The description of the histological signs of diseases caused by *Chlamydia* is presented in many veterinary research papers. A detailed description of the pathomorphological changes in anthroponotic *Chlamydia* is extremely rare in world literature. The author of the first and in many ways priority thematic works was A.V. Zinserling [39] Later, the Morphological characteristics of *Chlamydia* are given in a number of publications by V.A. Zinserling [40].

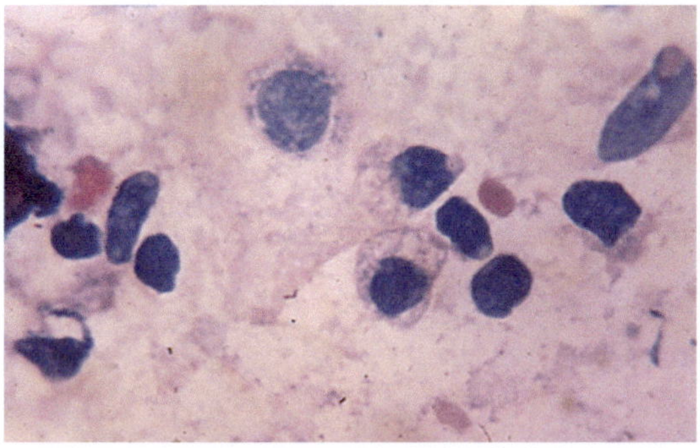

Fig. 4.1 Characteristic cytological changes in *Chlamydia* in a smear from the lungs. Haematoxylin-eosin staining. Magnification 1000

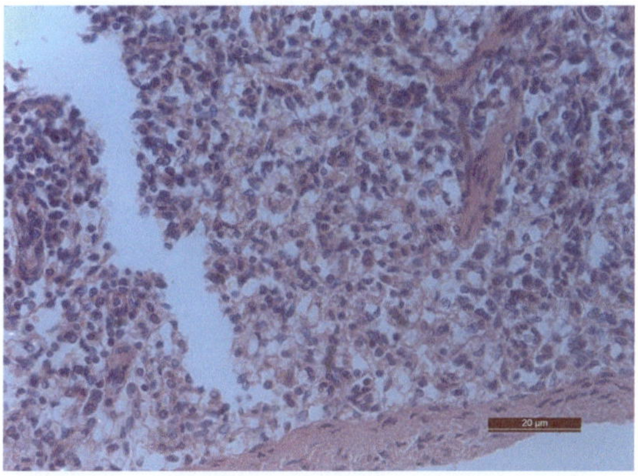

Fig. 4.2 Characteristic changes in the lungs in *Chlamydia*. In the lumen of the alveoli, macrophages with vacuolated cytoplasm. G-E staining. Magnification 640

For morphological diagnostics, both histological and cytological preparations can be used (Figs. 4.1 and 4.2).

The greatest diagnostic value when using haematoxylin-eosin screening staining is the detection of small vacuolization of various affected cells (epithelial, macrophages, nerve, etc.).

Of key importance is the detection of intracellular small elementary and larger extracellular reticular particles, which are detected much less frequently, only during an active infectious process. To detect these particles using light microscopy, additional staining methods must be used. We have the greatest positive experience using the PAS reaction (Fig. 4.3a) and various modifications of azure-eosin staining, including Machiavelli's (Fig. 4.3b).

Fundamentally characteristic extra- and intracellular inclusions can also be detected by electron microscopic examination (Fig. 4.4).

For final verification of the diagnosis, immunohistochemical studies are necessary due to the possibility of the appearance of similar structural changes in infectious processes of other aetiologies, primarily mycoplasmosis.

The inflammatory reaction can be of varying severity and is nonspecific; the predominance of neutrophilic leukocytes is uncharacteristic.

4.15.1 Immunohistochemical and Immunocytochemical Methods

This method is used mainly for scientific and expert purposes. Personal experience speaks of its reliability in the study of any materials (lungs, brain, placenta, internal organs in case of intrauterine *Chlamydia*) (see Chaps. 5 and 6). Information about its use in the literature is rather limited. Thus, with its help, *Chlamydia* were detected in cystitis, chronic endometritis and in the placenta of women with a history of habitual miscarriage. In 2016, Van Kruninjen with the help of detected Chlamydia trachomatis in the cytoplasm of macrophages of the submucosa and serous membrane of the colon and ileum in 5 of 19 patients with Crohn's disease [41].

Therefore, immunohistochemistry can be used as a cost-effective screening test in surgical pathology biopsy in high-risk patients [42].

Also, the immunohistochemistry method can be used to detect previously unrecognized infection in men with obstructive azoospermia [43].

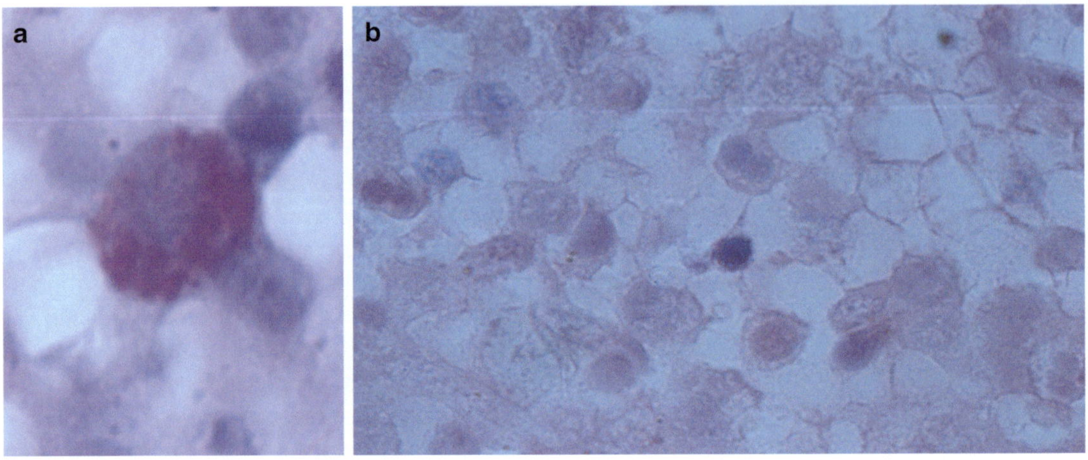

Fig. 4.3 Extra- and intracellular inclusions in the lungs in *Chlamydia*. (**a**) With PAS reaction Magnification 1000 (**b**) With azur-zosin staining Magnification 640

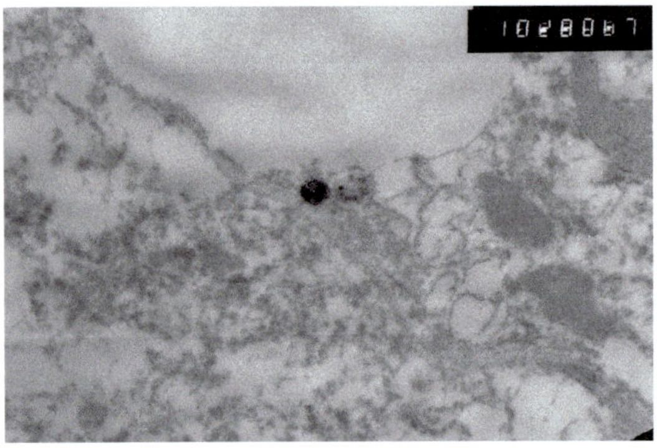

Fig. 4.4 Extra- and intracellular bodies of *Chlamydia* in the lungs under electron microscopy

References

1. Lobzin YV, Poznyak AL, Sidorchuk SN. Chlamydial infections: a guide for doctors. St. Petersburg: Foliant; 2010. p. 488p.
2. Gomberg MA, Soloviev AM. Modern tactics of treatment of patients with various forms of urogenital Chlamydia. Attend Physic. 2003;7:50–3.
3. Rodrigues R, Silva AR, Sousa C, Vale N. Addressing challenges in Chlamydia trachomatis detection: a comparative review of diagnostic methods. Medicina. 2024;60:1236.
4. Bryan ER, McLachlan RI, Rombauts L, Katz DJ, Yazdani A, Bogoevski K, Chang C, Giles ML, Carey AJ, Armitage CW, Trim LK, McLaughlin EA, Beagley KW. Detection of Chlamydia infection within human testicular biopsies. Hum Reprod. 2019;34(10):1891–8.
5. Papp JR, Schachter J, Gaydos CA, van der Pol B. Recommendations for the laboratory-based detection of Chlamydia trachomatis and Neisseria gonorrhoeae—2014. MMWR Recomm Rep. 2014;63:1–19.
6. Kopnina EO. Modern approaches to diagnostics of chlamydia: literature review. Lab Diagn Infect Dis. 2006;1(3):23–6.
7. Radzivil TT, Druzhinina TV, Pavlyuk AV, Koroleva IV. Efficiency of diagnostics of urogenital Chlamydia using various laboratory methods. "VectorBest News".—Koltsovo. 2005;4(38):3–5.
8. Papp JR, Schachter J, Gaydos CA, Van Der Pol B. Recommendations for the laboratory-based detection of Chlamydia trachomatis and Neisseria gonorrhoeae. Atlanta: Centers for Disease Control and Prevention (CDC), US Department of Health and Human Services; 2014.
9. Battle TJ, Golden MR, Suchland KL, et al. Evaluation of laboratory testing methods for Chlamydia trachomatis infection in the era of nucleic acid amplification. J Clin Microbiol. 2001;39:2924–7.
10. Sarır M, Duman I, Göktaş S, Demir M, Kukul E. Results of multiplex polymerase chain reaction assay to identify urethritis pathogens. J Urol Surg. 2017;4:18–22.
11. Johnson RE, Newhall WJ, Papp JR, Knapp JS, Black CM, Gift TL, Steece R, Markowitz LE, Devine OJ, Walsh CM, et al. Screening tests to detect Chlamydia trachomatis and Neisseria gonorrhoeae infections—2002. MMRW Recomm Rep. 2002;11:1–38.
12. Gharsallah H, Frikha-Gargouri O, Bom RJ, Hammami A, Bruisten SM. Comparison of reverse hybridization and ompA sequencing methods applied on Chlamydia trachomatis strains from Tunisia. Microbiologyopen. 2018;7(2):e00549. https://doi.org/10.1002/mbo3.549.
13. Mohseni M, Sung S, Takov V. Chlamydia. StatPearls Publishing: St. Petersburg; 2023.

14. Deiman B, van Aarle P, Sillekens P. Characteristics and applications of nucleic acid sequence-based amplification (NASBA). Mol Biotech. 2002;20:163–79.
15. Domeika M, Savicheva A, Sokolovskiy E, et al. Guidelines for the laboratory diagnosis of Chlamydia trachomatis infections in East European countries. J Eur Acad Dermatol Venereol. 2009;23(12):1353–63. https://doi.org/10.1111/j.1468-3083.2009.03328.
16. Shao L, Guo Y, Jiang Y, Liu Y, Wang M, You C, Liu Q. Sensitivity of the standard Chlamydia trachomatis culture method is improved after one additional in vitro passage. J Clin Lab Anal. 2016;30:697–701.
17. Meyer T. Diagnostic procedures to detect Chlamydia trachomatis infections. Microorganisms. 2016;4:25.
18. World Health Organization. Laboratory diagnosis of sexually transmitted infections, including human immunodeficiency virus. Geneva: World Health Organization; 2013.
19. Stratton NJ, Hirsch L, Harris F, de la Maza LM, Peterson EM. Evaluation of the rapid CLEARVIEW Chlamydia test for direct detection of chlamydiae from cervical specimens. J Clin Microbiol. 1991;29(7):1551–3.
20. Yin YP, Peeling RW, Chen XS, Gong KL, Zhou H, Gu WM, Zheng HP, Wang ZS, Yong G, Cao WL, Shi MQ, Wei WH, Dai XQ, Gao X, Chen Q, Mabey D. Clinic-based evaluation of clearview Chlamydia MF for detection of Chlamydia trachomatis in vaginal and cervical specimens from women at high risk in China. Sex Transm Infect. 2006;82:v33–7.
21. Chin CD, Laksanasopin T, Cheung YK, Steinmiller D, Linder V, Parsa H, Wang J, Moore H, Rouse R, Umviligihozo G, Karita E, Mwambarangwe L, Braunstein SL, van de Wijgert J, Sahabo R, Justman JE, El-Sadr W, Sia SK. Microfluidics-based diagnostics of infectious diseases in the developing world. Nat Med. 2011;17(8):1015–9.
22. Park S, Zhang Y, Lin S, Wang TH, Yang S. Advances in microfluidic PCR for point-of-care infectious disease diagnostics. Biotechnol Adv. 2011;29(6):830–9.
23. Gaydos CA, Van Der Pol B, Jett- Goheen M, CT/NG Study Group. Performance of the cepheid CT/NG Xpert rapid PCR test for the detection of Chlamydia trachomatis and Neisseria gonorrhoeae. J Clin Microbiol. 2013;51:1666–72.
24. Ferguson BS, Buchsbaum SF, Swensen JS, Hsieh K, Lou X, Soh HT. Integrated microfluidic electrochemical DNA sensor. J Clin Microbiol. 2006;44(2):561–70.
25. Hsieh K, Patterson AS, Ferguson BS, Plaxco KW, Soh HT. Rapid, sensitive, and quantitative detection of pathogenic DNA at the point of care through microfluidic electrochemical quantitative loop-mediated isothermal amplification. Angew Chem Int Ed Engl. 2012;51(20):4896–900.
26. Pearce DM, Shenton DP, Holden J, Gaydos CA. Evaluation of a novel electrochemical detection method for Chlamydia trachomatis: application for point-of-care diagnostics. IEEE Trans Biomed Eng. 2011;58(3):755–8.
27. Pearce DM, Styles DN, Hardick JP, Gaydos CA. A new rapid molecular point-of-care assay for Trichomonas vaginalis: preliminary performance data. Sex Transm Infect. 2013;89(6):495–7.
28. de Paz HD, Brotons P, Muñoz-Almagro C. Molecular isothermal techniques for combating infectious diseases: towards low-cost point-of-care diagnostics. Expert Rev Mol Diagn. 2014;14(7):827–43.
29. Centers for Disease Control and Prevention. Recommendations for the laboratory-based detection of Chlamydia trachomatis and Neisseria gonorrhoeae. MMWR Recomm Rep. 2014;63(RR-02):1–19.
30. Moazed TC, Kuo CC, Grayston JT, Campbell LA. Evidence of systemic dissemination of Chlamydia pneumoniae via macrophages in the mouse. J Infect Dis. 1998;177(5):1322–5. https://doi.org/10.1086/515280.
31. Cirino F, Webley WC, West C, Croteau NL, Andrzejewski C Jr, Stuart ES. Detection of Chlamydia in the peripheral blood cells of normal donors using in vitro culture, immunofluorescence microscopy and flow cytometry techniques. BMC Infect Dis. 2006;6:23. Published 2006 Feb 10
32. Kudratova ZE, Shamsiddinova MS Laboratory methods for diagnosing urogenital chlamydia. OAR [Internet] 2023.
33. Dowell SF, Peeling RW, Boman J, et al. Standardizing Chlamydia pneumoniae assays: recommendations from the Centers for Disease Control and Prevention (USA) and the Laboratory Center for Disease Control (Canada). Clin Infect Dis. 2001;33(4):492–503. https://doi.org/10.1086/322632.
34. López MÁC, Porteros HT, De La Iglesia SA, et al. Advantages of syndromic diagnostics: detection of the pathogens causing urethritis/cervicitis with the STI CNM real-time PCR kit from vitro S.A Pol. J Microbiol. 2024;73(4):529–34. https://doi.org/10.33073/pjm-2024-045.
35. da Silva FC, Kamuyu G, Michels B, et al. Candidate antibody reference reagents for Chlamydia trachomatis serology. Immunol Methods. 2024;534:113761. https://doi.org/10.1016/j.jim.2024.113761.
36. Ricard RM, Wobeser B. Molecular detection of Chlamydia abortus in endometrial biopsies of mares from western Canada. J Vet Diagn Invest. 2024;36(6):921–4. https://doi.org/10.1177/10406387241267864.
37. Baud D, Zufferey J, Hohlfeld P, Greub G. Performance of an automated multiplex immunofluorescence assay for detection of Chlamydia trachomatis immunoglobulin G. Diagn Microbiol Infect Dis. 2014;78(3):217–9. https://doi.org/10.1016/j.diagmicrobio.2013.11.022.
38. Baud D, Regan L, Greub G. Comparison of five commercial serological tests for the detection of anti-Chlamydia trachomatis antibodies. Comparative study. Eur J Clin Microbiol Infect Dis. 2010;29(6):669–75. https://doi.org/10.1007/s10096-010-0912-4.
39. Zinserling VA. School of infectious pathology of A.V. Zinserling: achievements and prospects. Arch Pathol. 2014;76(1):3–9. (in Russian)

40. Zinserling VA, Starshinova AA, Karev VE, et al. Granulomatous inflammation in mycoplasma and chlamydial infections. J. Infectol. 2015;7(4):5–9. https://doi.org/10.22625/2072-6732-2015-7-4-5-9. (in Russian)
41. Lienard J, Croxatto A, Aeby S, et al. Development of a new Chlamydiales-specifc real-time PCR and its application to respiratory clinical samples. J Clin Microbiol. 2011;49(7):2637–42.
42. Croxatto A., Rieille N., Kernif T. et. al. Presence of Chlamydiales DNA in ticks and fleas suggests that ticks are carriers of Chlamydiae. Ticks Tick Borne Dis 2014 5(4):359–365. doi: https://doi.org/10.1016/j.ttbdis.2013.11.009.
43. Arévalo F, Rayme S, Zurita F, et al. Immunohistochemical detection of Chlamydia trachomatis in sexually transmitted infectious proctitis. BMC Gastroenterol. 2022;22(1):171. https://doi.org/10.1186/s12876-022-02233-w.
44. He X, Madhav S, Hutchinson L, et al. Prevalence of Chlamydia infection detected by immunohistochemistry in patients with anorectal ulcer and granulation tissue. Hum Pathol. 2024;144:8–14. https://doi.org/10.1016/j.humpath.2023.12.009.

5 Clinical and Morphological Characteristics of Chlamydial Infections in Humans

Chlamydiosis is characterized by a wide variety of nosological (clinical) forms of diseases/conditions, amongst which the following main groups can be distinguished:

- Diseases of the genitourinary system and rectum (cervicitis, urethritis, salpingitis, prostatitis, epididymitis, proctosigmoiditis, lymphogranuloma venereum, etc.)
- Diseases associated with eye damage (trachoma, paratrachoma, etc.)
- Oral diseases (periodontitis, gingivitis, stomatitis) and others.

In this chapter, we consider the most studied variants of the disease, with respect to which we have our own experience.

5.1 Urogenital Chlamydia

Chlamydia has a tropism for columnar epithelium and is capable of affecting the mucous membrane of the urethra, cervical canal, fallopian tubes, endometrium, rectum, oropharynx and conjunctiva of the eyes, as well as epithelial cells of the lymphatic and blood vessels, leukocytes, monocytes, macrophages. In adult women, microorganisms are not capable of multiplying in the unchanged multilayered squamous epithelium of the vagina, since they exhibit high sensitivity to the acidic environment of its contents; therefore, the primary lesion is usually the mucous membrane of the cervix. In childhood and adolescence, *Chlamydia* can cause damage to the mucous membranes of the vulva and vagina, which is facilitated by the anatomical and physiological characteristics of the reproductive system of girls (imperfect physiological defence mechanisms, a small number of layers of the superficial epithelium, an alkaline reaction of vaginal discharge, an acid-base balance of cervicovaginal secretions close to alkaline).

Women with a history of chlamydial infection have a double risk of developing ovarian cancer. *Chlamydia* also increases the risk of developing cervical cancer, both in coinfection with the human papillomavirus and without it. *Chlamydia* suppresses the ability of the cell to correct defects and initiates premature cell exit from mitosis, inducing cervical metaplasia, which forms target cells for coinfection and persistence of the human papillomavirus [1–5].

Urogenital chlamydial infection is highly contagious: *C. trachomatis* is detected in 80% of women—sexual partners of men infected with *Chlamydia*. Very often (up to 80% of cases) *Chlamydia* is associated with pathogens of other STIs.

A distinction is made between acute and chronic chlamydiosis, in addition, there is also a recurrent form of this pathology.

The onset of acute (fresh), uncomplicated *Chlamydia* is noted immediately after the end of the incubation period, which can last for 1–2 days to a month. This form of the disease affects only

V. Zinserling et al., *Chlamydia Infections*, https://doi.org/10.1007/978-3-031-99642-9_5

the lower parts of the genitourinary system, and often proceeds with few symptoms. As a rule, the longer the incubation period, the weaker the symptoms. Therefore, at this stage, the disease is rarely diagnosed.

In the absence of timely treatment, the acute form becomes chronic and recurrent. It is characterized by damage to the upper genitourinary system, including the pelvic organs, as well as damage to other organs and systems. If the patient comes into contact with an infected partner after treatment, he will develop a repeated form of the disease, which is most dangerous due to its complications.

There is no generally accepted classification of urogenital chlamydial infection. The following forms of the disease are clinically distinguished:

- Chlamydial infections of the lower genitourinary tract: urethritis; cervicitis; cystitis; vulvovaginitis.
- Chlamydial infections of the pelvic organs and other genitourinary organs: paraurethritis; epididymitis; orchitis; prostatitis accompanying urethritis; vestibulitis; salpingo-oophoritis; endometritis.
- Chlamydial infection of the anorectal area.
- Chlamydial pharyngitis.
- Chlamydial sexually transmitted infections of other localizations (pelvic peritonitis, arthritis, pneumonia, perihepatitis).
- Chlamydial conjunctivitis.

Monoinfection with *C. trachomatis* is asymptomatic or asymptomatic.

The development of chronic chlamydiosis is determined to a greater extent by the adaptive properties of the pathogen and the formation of its persistent forms, which have very effective mechanisms for inactivating the protective factors of the host organism and using the regulatory pathways of the host cell to develop the infectious process. The pathogenetic significance of persistent forms of *Chlamydia* is determined, first of all, by the fact that they represent a form of long-term survival of the pathogen in the macroorganism with the preservation of pathogenic potential. At the same time, persistent forms of *Chlamydia* themselves are responsible for the development of severe immunopathological conditions due to the constant activation of immune system cells, maintenance of inflammation and the impact on many intracellular processes.

Chronic urogenital chlamydial infection causes a very wide range of complications associated with hematogenous dissemination of *C. trachomatis* from the primary site of infection to distant organs [6].

This leads to the development of serious diseases of both genital and extragenital localization, such as female and male infertility, pregnancy pathology, reactive arthritis, ophthalmochlamydia, perihepatitis, pelvic peritonitis [7–13].

For *C. trachomatis*, the generalization of the infectious process as a result of the spread of the pathogen by the hematogenous route was shown by A.L. Poznyak.

Recently, data have appeared that *C. trachomatis*, spreading haematogenously, can colonize the gastrointestinal tract organs in both animals and humans [14–16], which allows us to consider the gastrointestinal tract as a possible favourable niche for the long-term preservation of *Chlamydia*. However, at present, there is no information on the possible role of long-term colonization of the gastrointestinal tract organs by *Chlamydia* in the development of pathological changes in these organs and on the pathogenicity of *Chlamydia*. In addition, the features of chronic infection caused by *C. trachomatis* and associated with long-term persistence of the pathogen after an infection with extragenital localization of the pathogen have been practically not studied in humans. There is still little data on how widespread gastrointestinal tract colonization by *Chlamydia* is amongst people, whether long-term colonization is a carriage or an infectious process, and what consequences the presence of this pathogenic microorganism in the human intestinal microbiota can lead to [17–19].

All of the above determines the importance of the problem of controlling chronic chlamydial infections, for which antibacterial therapy must be adequate and based on accurate modern diagnostic methods.

5.1.1 Chlamydial Infections of the Lower Genitourinary Tract

In 70–95% of women, the disease is subjectively asymptomatic. In the acute course of the inflammatory process, the following subjective symptoms may be present: mucopurulent discharge from the urethra and/or genital tract, intermenstrual bloody discharge, pain during sexual intercourse (dyspareunia), discomfort or pain in the lower abdomen, itching, burning, pain during urination (dysuria).

In 50% of men, the disease is subjectively asymptomatic. In the acute course of the inflammatory process, the following subjective symptoms may be present: mucopurulent scant discharge from the urethra; itching, burning, pain during urination (dysuria); discomfort, itching, burning in the urethra; pain during sexual intercourse (dyspareunia); frequent urination and urgent urge to urinate (with proximal spread of the inflammatory process); pain in the perineum radiating to the rectum. *Chlamydia* may be detected during ejaculate examination (Fig. 5.1).

Subjective symptoms of chlamydial infection in childhood are similar to those in adults. A feature of the clinical course of the disease in girls is more pronounced subjective symptoms and damage to the mucous membranes of the vulva and vagina. In acute vaginitis in girls, the following subjective symptoms may be present: itching, burning, soreness in the vulva and vagina, mucopurulent discharge from the genital tract.

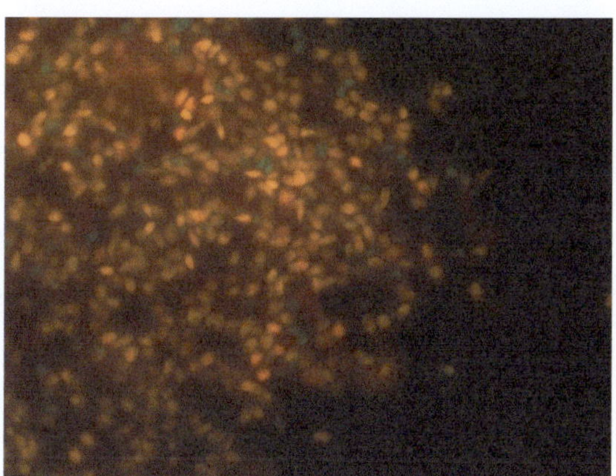

Fig. 5.1 *Chlamydia* in ejaculate. Direct IF

Objective symptoms in women with acute inflammatory process: hyperaemia and swelling of the mucous membrane of the external opening of the urethra, infiltration of the walls of the urethra, mucopurulent or mucous scanty discharge from the urethra, swelling and hyperaemia of the mucous membrane of the cervix, mucopurulent discharge from the cervical canal, erosion of the mucous membrane of the cervix; in acute vaginitis in girls: swelling and hyperaemia of the walls of the vagina, its vaults, mucopurulent discharge in the posterior vaginal vault.

Objective symptoms in men with an acute course of the inflammatory process: hyperaemia and swelling of the mucous membrane of the external opening of the urethra, infiltration of the walls of the urethra, mucopurulent or mucous scanty discharge from the urethra [20, 21].

5.1.2 Chlamydial Infections of the Pelvic Organs and Other Genitourinary Organs

Subjective symptoms in women:

- Vestibulitis: minor mucopurulent discharge from the genital tract, pain and swelling in the vulva.
- Catarrhal bartholinitis: minor mucopurulent discharge from the mouth of the Bartholin gland, pain and swelling in the area of the gland.
- Oophoritis: in the acute course of the inflammatory process—pain in the lower abdomen of a cramping nature, mucopurulent discharge from the genital tract; in the chronic course of the disease, subjective manifestations are less pronounced, a violation of the menstrual cycle is noted
- Endometritis: in the acute course of the inflammatory process—pain in the lower abdomen, usually of a pulling nature, mucopurulent discharge from the genital tract; in the chronic course of the disease, subjective

manifestations are less pronounced, post- and intermenstrual scanty bloody discharge is often noted.

Subjective symptoms in men during acute inflammatory process:

- Epididymoorchitis: mucopurulent discharge from the urethra, dysuria, dyspareunia, pain in the epididymis and inguinal region, often unilateral; pain in the perineum radiating to the rectum, lower abdomen, scrotum; pain can spread to the spermatic cord, inguinal canal, lumbar region, sacrum.
- Prostatitis associated with urethritis: pain in the perineum and lower abdomen radiating to the rectum, dysuria.

In both sexes, chlamydial lesions of the paraurethral glands are possible, with subjective symptoms: itching, burning, pain during urination (dysuria); mucopurulent discharge from the urethra; pain during sexual intercourse (dyspareunia); pain in the area of the external opening of the urethra. [22].

5.1.3 Chlamydial Infection of the Anorectal Area

In both sexes, the disease usually has a subjectively asymptomatic course. In the acute course of the inflammatory process, the following subjective symptoms may be present: with local lesion of the rectum— itching, burning in the anorectal area, minor discharge from the rectum of a yellowish or reddish colour; with localization of the process above the anus—painful tenesmus, pain during defecation, mucopurulent discharge from the rectum, often with an admixture of blood, secondary constipation.

Objective symptoms during the acute course of the inflammatory process: hyperaemia of the skin of the folds of the anus, mucopurulent discharge from the rectum [23–25].

Fig. 5.2 *Chlamydia* in a smear from the oral cavity. DIF

5.1.4 Chlamydial Pharyngitis

In both sexes, the disease usually has a subjectively asymptomatic course. In the acute course of the inflammatory process, the following subjective symptoms may be present: a feeling of dryness in the oropharynx, pain that intensifies when swallowing.

Objective symptoms in the acute course of the inflammatory process: hyperaemia and swelling of the mucous membrane of the oropharynx and tonsils [26, 27]. *Chlamydia* may be detected in smears from the oral cavity (Fig. 5.2).

5.1.5 Chlamydial Conjunctivitis

Subjective symptoms: slight pain in the affected eye, dryness and redness of the conjunctiva, photophobia, scanty mucopurulent discharge in the corners of the affected eye.

Objective symptoms during the acute course of the inflammatory process: hyperaemia and swelling of the conjunctiva of the affected eye, scanty mucopurulent discharge in the corners of the affected eye [28, 29].

5.1.6 Chlamydial Infections of the Pelvic Organs and Other Genitourinary Organs

Objective symptoms in women:

- Vestibulitis: minor mucopurulent discharge from the genital tract, hyperaemia of the external openings of the ducts of the vestibular glands, pain and swelling of the ducts upon palpation.
- Catarrhal bartholinitis: minor mucopurulent discharge from the mouth of the Bartholin gland, hyperaemia of the mouth of the gland, pain and swelling upon palpation.
- Salpingo-oophoritis: in the acute course of the inflammatory process—enlarged, painful to palpation fallopian tubes and ovaries, shortening of the vaginal vaults, mucopurulent discharge from the cervical canal; in the chronic course of the disease—minor pain, compaction of the fallopian tubes.
- Endometritis: in the acute course of the inflammatory process—a painful, enlarged uterus of a soft consistency, mucopurulent discharge from the cervical canal; in the chronic course of the disease—a dense consistency and limited mobility of the uterus.

Objective symptoms in men during acute inflammatory process:

Epididymoorchitis: mucopurulent discharge from the urethra, hyperaemia and swelling of the scrotum, upon palpation—enlarged, dense and painful testicle and its appendage

- Prostatitis accompanying urethritis: upon palpation—a painful, compacted prostate gland.

In persons of both sexes, chlamydial lesions of the paraurethral glands are possible, and the objective symptoms in the acute course of the inflammatory process are: mucopurulent discharge from the urethra, the presence of dense painful formations the size of a millet grain in the area of the excretory ducts of the paraurethral glands [30–33].

5.1.7 Chlamydial Sexually Transmitted Infections of Other Localizations

Disseminated chlamydial infection may develop pneumonia, perihepatitis and peritonitis (Fitz -Hugh-Curtis syndrome/FHCS). In some cases, the course of the disease may be complicated by reactive arthritis of chlamydial aetiology.

Chlamydial pelvic peritonitis has no specific symptoms and is characterized by severe abdominal pain, nausea, vomiting, weakness, bowel movement disorders, and a characteristic appearance—facies hypocratica, hectic body temperature, hypotension, oliguria, sharp abdominal pain upon superficial palpation, muscle tension in the lower abdominal wall and a positive symptom of peritoneal irritation.

Fitz -Hugh-Curtis syndrome (FHCS) is named after Thomas Fitz -Hugh Jr. [34] and Arthur Hale Curtis [35], who first reported the disease in 1934 and 1930, respectively. It was initially found to be caused by gonococci. Later, it became clear that *C. trachomatis* could also cause it [36, 37]. It is a rare disorder that occurs almost exclusively in women and is characterized by inflammation of the peritoneum lining the stomach and the tissue surrounding the liver (perihepatitis) [38]. The diaphragm may also be affected. Although FHCS is considered a disease entity, its boundaries are not entirely clear. Some authors consider FHCS to be a component or consequence of PID, whilst others consider it to be an acute perihepatitis only. There is also a third opinion, namely that the disease includes both acute and chronic perihepatitis. Although FCCS is primarily associated with PID, there are cases when it develops as an independent clinical picture [39]. Regardless of the discussions about the nature of this syndrome, its clinical characteristics are clearly defined. Acute perihepatitis is characterized by the sudden onset of severe pain in the right hypochondrium of the abdominal cavity, accompanied by a feeling of tension, increased heart rate and fever. Headaches, chills, night sweats, vomiting, nausea and malaise are most often noted. The pain may spread to other areas, including the right shoulder and the inner side of the right arm [38, 39]. FCCS often mimics acute cholecystitis [40, 41] or pancreatitis. It is possible that the infection spreads to the surrounding area, leading to the development of an adhesion process in the peritoneum located on the anterior wall of the liver. As a result, foci of encapsulated inflammation can form between the liver capsule and ligaments [42].

Over the years, various methods have been used to diagnose FCCS—cytology, serology, isolation of infectious agents, laparoscopy, visualization, paraclinical studies. Wolner-Hansen et al. [43] used laparoscopy and detected *C. trachomatis* in 31 of 52 women (59.6%) complaining of pain in the right upper quadrant of the abdomen. In patients with acute pain in the right hypochondrium and other symptoms characteristic of FCCS, Darougar S. et al. [44] isolated *Chlamydia* from various sites of the genitourinary system and found high titre of immunoglobulins IgG, IgM and IgA to *C. trachomatis*. Puolakkainen et al. [45] used a set of methods. High titres of chlamydial IgG was detected in 88–96% of patients by ELISA and in 50% by chlamydial membrane ELISA. Seroconversion was detected in 44% of patients. The authors recommend this diagnostic approach as convenient for identifying complaints associated with FCCS, which allows avoiding laparoscopy [45]. Puolakkainen et al. [46] detected *Chlamydia* in 40% and 78% of different parts of the genital tract, respectively, in patients with suspected acute perihepatitis. At the same time, this research group emphasizes the great importance of the diagnostic value of serological testing due to the significant difficulties in trying to isolate *Chlamydia* from the perihepatic space. In recent years, several publications have indicated the usefulness of computed tomography in the clinical diagnosis of FHCS [41, 47, 48]. Woo et al. [41] propose to use abdominal CT instead of abdominal sonography to facilitate diagnosis. According to Wang et al. [48], dynamic advanced multislice CT can accurately depict liver capsule lesions and possible pelvic inflammatory disease associated with SFCC, which indicate the source of infection and are of great practical significance for making early and accurate diagnoses and improving prognosis. The differential diagnosis should exclude a number of disease states that can mimic FCCS [48–56]: ectopic pregnancy; pyelonephritis; cholecystitis; viral hepatitis; renal colic; and pulmonary embolism [57–61].

5.1.8 Chlamydial Infection in Pregnant Women

Chlamydial infection can lead to miscarriage, development of fetoplacental insufficiency, intrauterine infection of the foetus, postpartum inflammatory diseases and neonatal infections.

In the first trimester of pregnancy, the most typical complications are threatened miscarriage, non-viable pregnancy and spontaneous abortion; in the second and third trimesters—threatened termination of pregnancy, tocolytic therapy for which usually gives an unstable effect. In the placentas of women with genital chlamydia, there is a violation of immune homeostasis with the formation of pathogenic immune complexes, including IgM, IgG, IgA and fixing the C3 fraction of complement as a pathogenicity marker. In case of infection of the amniotic membranes, polyhydramnios, specific placental damage (placentitis), placental insufficiency, faetal hypotrophy and hypoxia may develop. During an echographic examination of pregnant women with intrauterine infection, the following signs are revealed: polyhydramnios, oligohydramnios, hyperechoic suspension in the amniotic fluid, placental changes. When performing ultrasound placentography in women with infectious genital pathology, the following are detected: thickening of the placenta, heterogeneous echogenicity of the placental parenchyma, premature "aging" of the placenta, widening of the intervillous spaces, widening of the subchorionic space, thickening/doubling of the basal plate contour. For pregnant women with chlamydial infection and fetoplacental insufficiency, its primary manifestations are disturbances of intraplacental blood flow [62–67]. Placentitis and intrauterine infections, associated with urogenital chlamydia are described in Chap. 6.

5.2 Chlamydial Lesions of the Visual Organ (Boyko E.V., Poznyak A.L., Suetov A.A.)

Chlamydial infection, most commonly caused by *Chlamydia trachomatis* (C.trachomatis), can affect many structures and tissues of the visual organ and cause both acute and chronic pathological processes in them, leading to serious complications, such as, corneal scarring and blindness. The most important data on the epidemiology of trachoma were presented in Chap. 3.

The clinical manifestations of infections caused by *C. trachomatis* depend on the serovar and the characteristics of the immune response, whilst the literature identifies the main clinical forms of chlamydial damage to the visual organ: trachoma, paratrachoma in adults (chlamydial conjunctivitis, conjunctivitis with inclusions in adults), conjunctivitis with inclusions in newborns (paratrachoma in newborns), conjunctivitis in Reiter's disease, chlamydial uveitis, episcleritis [68].

Trachoma is a chronic keratoconjunctivitis caused by repeated episodes of infection with *C. trachomatis* serotypes A, B, Ba and C [69]. This ancient disease, described as early as 1500 BC in Ancient Egypt, comes from the Greek word for "rough," which is characteristic of the clinical picture of the active stage of the disease with pronounced changes in the subtarsal conjunctiva [70]. Today, trachoma is the leading infectious cause of blindness worldwide and remains prevalent in low-income countries, especially in sub-Saharan Africa [71]. According to the 2021 WHO report, about 125 million people live in trachoma-endemic areas and 1.9 million have severe visual impairment, including blindness [29, 72].

Pathophysiologically, trachoma involves two interrelated chronic processes: recurrent episodes of infectious inflammation with a frequently subclinical course of chlamydial inflammation: conjunctivitis and the cicatricial stage, which does not require the presence of an infectious agent, but, as a result of trichiasis and corneal opacity, usually leads to irreversible blindness. Primary infection causes bilateral mild mucopurulent conjunctivitis, which resolves spontaneously without consequences [29]. Repeated episodes of infection lead to the formation of a chronic immune response in the form of a cell-mediated delayed-type hypersensitivity reaction (type 4) [70]. This phase of the disease is characterized by the formation of subepithelial follicles and papillary hypertrophy in the subtarsal conjunctiva, mainly of the upper eyelid.

Quite often, fibrovascular infiltration of the upper parts of the cornea—pannus—is encountered. Conjunctival follicles in the upper limbal part, after their resolution, leave shallow depressions along the upper limbal edge of the cornea—Herbert's pits [70].

Repeated episodes of infection lead to conjunctival scarring, ranging from mild linear or stellate scars to thick, distorting fibrotic bands that appear as white lines (Arlt lines). Fibrous changes in the tarsal conjunctiva cause shortening and inversion of the upper eyelid (entropion), which causes a change in the direction of eyelash growth (trichiasis). Conjunctival scarring alters the volume and composition of the lacrimal fluid, which reduces the barrier properties of the mucosa: dry eye syndrome makes the corneal epithelium more susceptible to damage from inwardly curled eyelashes and additional infection by other pathogens, ultimately leading to corneal opacity [71].

In the simplified classification system of WHO, 2 forms of trachoma are distinguished: active and cicatricial [73]. Chronic follicular conjunctivitis is designated as the follicular type of active trachoma (FT). More pronounced inflammation with papillary hypertrophy is interpreted as an intense form of active trachoma, in which case there is involvement of small vessels with oedema, and in some severe cases, pronounced inflammatory thickening of the conjunctiva develops. Cicatricial trachoma includes the presence of visible scars on the tarsal conjunctiva, the development of entropion and trichiasis.

Pathophysiologically, a cascade of inflammatory reactions is triggered in tissues infected with *C. trachomatis*: vascular reactions with dilation of small vessels and capillaries, increased permeability of vascular walls, and exudation, consisting mainly of leukocytes, into the interstitial space are observed. Under the influence of proinflammatory cytokines produced by leukocytes, a mixed inflammatory cellular infiltrate is formed in the lamina propria of the conjunctiva, consisting of polymorphonuclear leukocytes, macrophages, plasma and dendritic cells [74, 75]. The accumulation of predominantly B cells, as well as CD8+ T cells and macrophages, forms lymphoid follicles, distorting the contour of the overlying conjunctival epithelium and clinically determined in active trachoma. Goblet cell loss and epithelial atrophy occur. Resolution of the infection is thought to depend on a cell-mediated immune response mediated through IFNγ produced by CD4+ T-helpers type 1 and decreasing with the elimination of the infectious agent [76, 77].

However, even after the infection has resolved, the inflammatory reaction continues—local tissues exhibit elevated levels of cytokines, cellular enzymes, growth factors and other proteins involved in regulating the state of the extracellular matrix. In the context of this chronic inflammatory environment, with the involvement and activation of leukocytes, the conjunctival tissue is repeatedly damaged and scar tissue is formed during the healing process. Thus, histological studies of the conjunctiva in chronic inflammation associated with trachoma reveal a significant content of natural killers, connective tissue growth factor and matrix metalloproteinases [78–80]. Fibrogenic growth factors have a profibrotic effect due to increased deposition of connective tissue elements by stromal fibroblasts. In this case, conjunctival fibroblasts cultured from individuals with trachomatous scarring have been shown to have an increased contractile phenotype, which probably causes increased eyelid contraction during the development of cicatricial trachoma [81]. In biopsies of cicatricial conjunctiva, destruction of the stromal architecture is observed, with its replacement by disorganized collagen. Along the basement membrane, loose collagen types 1 and 2 are replaced by collagen type 4, and vertically oriented collagen type 5 appears in the stromal structure of the lamina propria [82–84].

5.2.1 Paratrachoma (Chlamydial Conjunctivitis in Adults) and Chlamydial Conjunctivitis in Newborns (Inclusion Conjunctivitis)

The most common type of neonatal conjunctivitis worldwide is inclusion conjunctivitis. Inclusion conjunctivitis is caused by *C. trachomatis* serotypes D K, which form *chronic follicular conjunctivitis*. Although chlamydial infection typically affects the sexually active population, it can be transmitted to neonates from an infected mother during childbirth. Infants exposed to the organism from the mother's genital tract during childbirth develop chlamydial ophthalmia neonatorum. Approximately 30–50% of infants exposed at birth develop the disease. Neonatal chlamydial conjunctivitis occurs in 2–6% of all newborns.

Neonatal chlamydial conjunctivitis is an acute infection of the conjunctiva characterized by *swelling and erythema* of the eyelids, palpebral conjunctiva and *purulent* ocular discharge. It usually occurs 5–14 days after birth, although it may occur earlier. The infection is usually mild and self-limited. Rarely, severe disease may occur. Corneal scarring may be secondary to peripheral corneal pannus and conjunctival scarring [85, 86].

With chlamydial conjunctivitis the following changes are observed:

- Hyperplasia of the conjunctival epithelium, which leads to thickening of the mucous membrane.
- Infiltration of lymphocytes and plasma cells into the area of inflammation with the formation of follicles.

- Necrosis and desquamation of the superficial layers of the epithelium in some cases.

Uveitis is an inflammation of the vascular membrane of the eye, which can be caused by various infectious and non-infectious factors. One of the significant infectious agents causing uveitis is *Chlamydia*, especially *C. trachomatis*. Chlamydial uveitis can have both acute and chronic course; in addition, it can be both a primary and secondary disease arising against the background of systemic infections, whilst its features of pathogenesis and clinical course are due to the immune response of the body to the pathogen.

Acute anterior uveitis is the most common form of uveitis and is associated with HLA B27 in more than half of cases [87]. More than 55% of patients with acute anterior uveitis and positive B27 have concomitant systemic chronic bowel or joint diseases. The first episode of inflammation usually occurs in adolescence and subsequently occurs in the form of periodic relapses. Anterior uveitis often occurs with increased intraocular pressure and quickly leads to the development of multiple posterior synechiae with pupillary fusion. Hypopyon (purulent exudate) may appear in the anterior chamber and pronounced exudation in the posterior parts of the eyeball, which will correlate with the activity of inflammation.

The human leukocyte antigen (HLA) system, which is involved in the regulation of cellular immunity, has evolved in response to environmental factors/stresses. Thus, it has been shown that HLAB27 carriers are less effective in eliminating *Chlamydia* and some intestinal bacteria intracellularly, which creates a genetic predisposition to the development of the disease [88, 89]. Under the influence of HLA antigens, *Chlamydia* can probably lead to either a loss of tolerance to antigens present in plasma cells or a cross-reaction to bacterial antigens [90].

The combination of urogenital chlamydia with reactive arthritis and eye damage is usually classified as urethro-oculosynovial syndrome, formerly Reiter's syndrome [91]. The disease begins with urethritis, often with few symptoms. After 1–4 weeks, the eyes are involved in the pathological process in the form of mild conjunctivitis, which passes in 1–2 days, but in some cases with a severe course. Chlamydial conjunctivitis is prone to relapses and can be combined with anterior uveitis, less often with keratitis, neuritis and retinitis. After 1–1.5 months from the onset of urogenital chlamydia, joint syndrome in the form of arthritis of large and small joints of the lower extremities is added to the clinical picture [92]. It is possible to develop lesions of the skin and mucous membranes in the form of balanitis, keratoderma of the palms and feet, erythema with erosions on the mucous membranes of the oral cavity. The classic triad of the syndrome may be absent: in 40–60% of cases, there are no clinical signs of conjunctivitis [92].

Macroscopic changes are manifested by an increase in the thickness of the uveal membrane, signs of exudative inflammation, including oedema and hyperaemia. In severe processes, fibrous tissue may form.

Microscopic changes are manifested by an increase in the number of infiltrates in the area of the iris and ciliary body, an increase in the number of plasma cells and lymphocytes in the structures of the vascular membrane. Changes in the cells of the pigment epithelium are possible.

Chlamydial uveitis is a complex disease that requires a multidisciplinary approach. Understanding the pathomorphology of this condition is key to its effective diagnosis and treatment. Future research should be aimed at better understanding the pathogenesis and immune response to this infection, as well as developing new treatments and prevention methods.

5.2.2 Dry Eye Syndrome

Dry eye syndrome (DES) is one of the most common eye diseases, affecting 5–6% of the population [93]. The causes of the syndrome are decreased tear production, excessive evaporation, or abnormalities in the mucin or lipid components of the tear film. When the stability of the tear film is disrupted, the level of mucins decreases, the composition and concentration of microorganisms present in the conjunctival cavity changes, followed by activation of T cells and changes in the reactivity of the immune system. The combination of these and similar changes leads to the development of a subclinical chronic inflammatory condition of the ocular surface, often clinically similar to chronic conjunctivitis. At the same time, there are no significant diagnostic differences between DES and chronic conjunctivitis that can be identified without special examination methods. Furthermore, the associations found between some forms of conjunctivitis (particularly allergic) and dry eye syndrome suggest that chronic conjunctivitis may likely cause the development of dry eye syndrome [94]. However, in addition to allergy, chronic conjunctival inflammation may also be caused by persistent infection, which thus leads to the development of dry eye syndrome.

Thus, in a study of 114 patients aged 25–45 years, who were diagnosed with dry eye syndrome during a comprehensive examination, 63.2% of them had *C. trachomatis* pathogens detected in conjunctival scrapings using the DIF method (Fig. 5.3), whilst in the control group (98 patients without signs of dry eye syndrome), the detection rate was significantly lower—6.1% [95]. In addition to *C. trachomatis* pathogens, pathogens of other latent infections were also identified in the group—*M.hominis* and *U.urealiticum*.

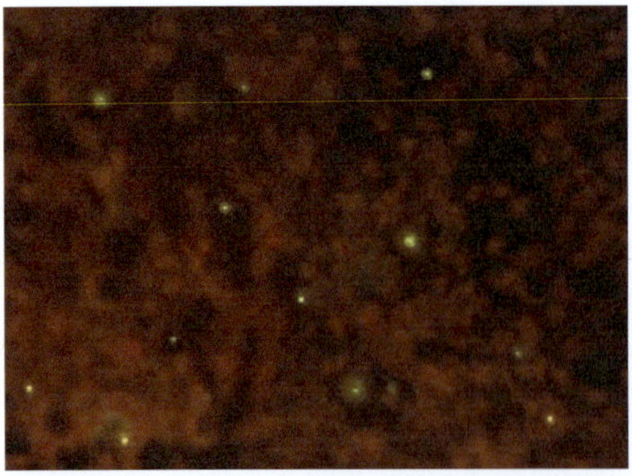

Fig. 5.3 *C. trachomatis* inclusions in conjunctival scraping of a patient with dry eye syndrome. DIF

In 90.2% of patients with dry eye syndrome, the duration of symptoms was at least 3 years, whilst the clinical manifestations of chronic conjunctival inflammation caused by *C. trachomatis, M. hominis and U. urealyticum* were completely masked by the symptoms of dry eye syndrome and differed from the manifestations of acute conjunctivitis (acute conjunctivitis was an exclusion criterion for inclusion in the study). It is important to note that not all patients who were infected suffered from dry eye syndrome (in particular, the infected control group did not have dry eye syndrome manifestations). The most probable causes may be (1) the early stage of the disease, (2) genetically determined features that determine the intensity of the inflammatory reaction of the host conjunctiva and (3) genetic variability of the pathogen, which is mainly characteristic of *C. trachomatis*.

Chronicity in the form of slowly progressive inflammation is a key role of *Chlamydia trachomatis* in the pathogenesis of dry eye syndrome, which develops after a latent period of 2–3 years against the background of morphological changes in the conjunctiva [96, 97]. Another study, which noted an improvement in the clinical course of dry eye syndrome in patients after treatment of chronic follicular conjunctivitis caused by *Chlamydia trachomatis*, also confirms this theory about the infectious cause of the development of dry eye syndrome [98].

This should be taken into account when identifying the causes of dry eye syndrome development amongst young individuals who do not have obvious risk factors for dry eye syndrome (age, history of refractive surgery, wearing contact lenses, systemic diseases or specific drug therapy, as well as obvious occupational risks) with dry eye syndrome symptoms masking chronic conjunctival infection.

5.2.3 Rhegmatogenous Retinal Detachment

Rhegmatogenous retinal detachment (RRD) is a vision-threatening disease characterized by separation of the inner neurosensory retina from the retinal pigment epithelium. The annual incidence of RRD is estimated at 6.9–18.2 cases per 100,000 people [99]. RRD is caused by a break in the area of atrophic changes in the retina and/or an area of pronounced traction of the vitreous body. Although the clinical picture of RRD is well known, the most fundamental causes of both retinal breaks and the changes in the retina and vitreous body that precede them remain poorly understood.

It has been hypothesized that chronic low-grade inflammation in the structures of the posterior segment of the eye, directly or indirectly caused by pathogens of latent infections, including *C. trachomatis*, may have pathogenetic significance in the development of vitreoretinal pathology [100].

In relation to RRD, the possibility of the influence of latent chlamydial infection on the pathogenesis of detachment was indirectly confirmed by the results of a clinical study involving 50 patients with RRD when analysing aspirates using PCR and DIF. In subretinal fluid (SRF), the pathogen *C. trachomatis* was detected in 50.8% and 71.4% of cases in eyes with RRD and only in 9.8% and 12.2% in the eyes of the control group. At the same time, in conjunctival scrapings, the pathogen in RRD was detected in 46.0% and 81.0% of cases, whilst in the control group, it was detected in 9.8 and 24.0% of cases [101]. In 61.9% of patients with RRD, pathogens were detected in the genitourinary system and in 63.5% in the blood. In this case, the patients did not have symptoms of acute conjunctivitis or acute inflammatory process in other ocular locations, and in a total of 90.5% of cases of RRD, at least one of the four samples (i.e. urethral swab, conjunctival scraping, genitourinary swab or blood) tested positive for *C. trachomatis* using the DIF method.

This is consistent with the fact that inflammation in general is of crucial importance in the pathogenesis of many vitreoretinal diseases, which causes retinal thinning, development of proliferative vitreoretinopathy with retinal tractions and subsequent retinal tears. There is sufficient evidence to prove the presence of high concentrations of proinflammatory cytokines such as (IL)-8, −10, −13, tumour necrosis factor-a (TNF-a) and interferon-g in the subretinal fluid of patients with RRD [102, 103]. It is possible that these inflammatory mediators accelerate the process of vitreous liquefaction and subsequent formation of holes in the retina.

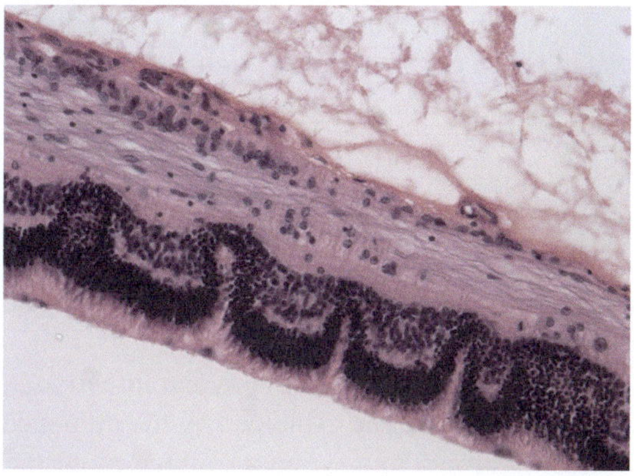

Fig. 5.4 Retinal detachment against the background of chorioretinitis caused by *C. trachomatis*, under experimental conditions. Folding at the level of the outer nuclear layer, plasma cells at the base of each fold. Neutrophils and lymphocytes in the neuroretina and preretinal vitreous body. Staining: haematoxylin and eosin, Magnification 200

An example of such a relationship may be retinal detachment against the background of infectious posterior or panuveitis (Fig. 5.4) [104]. At the same time, the role of latent infections, in which the infectious and inflammatory process occurs in a subclinical or asymptomatic form, remains insufficiently studied in the context of pathology of the vitreous body and the vitreoretinal interface. Primary infection with *C. trachomatis*, leading to self-limiting mucopurulent follicular conjunctivitis or developing into chronic inflammation of the conjunctiva, is capable of damaging not only epithelial, but also other tissues and structures of the body, including the posterior segment of the eye [102, 103]. There are studies proving that *C. trachomatis* can infect cells such as macrophages, neuroglial and synovial cells [103, 105, 106]. Repeated exposure to chlamydial antigens either as a result of re-infection or as a result of the occurrence of persistent or recurrent infections can serve as an antigenic stimulus for chronic inflammation.

The results obtained in the study also indicate that in RRD, chlamydial infection tends not only to cause local damage to the genitourinary tissues but also to cause bacteraemia and infect the eye. In addition, the results support the hypothesis that dissemination of the pathogen to the posterior segment structures of the eye or accessory organs may occur after primary infection of the conjunctiva [102].

The high frequency of chlamydial infection in eyes with RRD can be explained by the influence of latent chronic low-symptom infection on the development of vitreous body pathology and vitreoretinal interface. In this case, two options for the interaction of the infectious agent with the posterior part of the eyeball are possible: directly, in the form of damage by the pathogen to cells responsible for the synthesis and renewal of macromolecular structures of the vitreum, as well as those involved in the formation of the vitreoretinal contact—hyalocytes, Müller cells of the retina [107], or indirectly, through autoimmune mechanisms, maintaining an inflammatory reaction at a certain level with accompanying biochemical, metabolic shifts in the tissues. A similar possibility is demonstrated by our other work, where we studied clinical and histopathological changes, namely, in the retinal pigment epithelium, and proved the possibility of direct and indirect damage to the vitreous, retina, retinal pigment epithelium and choroid caused by *C. trachomatis*. When the chlamydial culture was injected subconjunctivally into rabbits, *C. trachomatis* antigens were detected in the vitreous, retina and choroid by direct ELISA (Figs. 5.5 and 5.6). When locally inoculated, chlamydial infection probably becomes disseminated, affecting the posterior segment of the eye regardless of the route of inoculation [102, 108].

Our other work proves the possibility of dissemination of *Chlamydia* from the primary source of infection in the visual organ to other organs: under experimental conditions, pathogens were detected in the brain, pancreas, prostate gland and urethra [109].

5.2.4 Retinal Pigment Epithelium Lesion

The retinal pigment epithelium, forming a monolayer between the choroid and the retina, performs many functions and is critically important in the pathogenesis of various diseases of the fundus. Previously, we conducted experimental studies on the infection of retinal pigment epithelium cultures with *C. trachomatis* (Fig. 5.7) [110]. As a result, we established for the first time that retinal pigment epithelium cells are sensitive to the pathogen, and the full life cycle of the pathogen is observed. Infection of cells with *C. trachomatis* triggered profibrogenic and proinflammatory

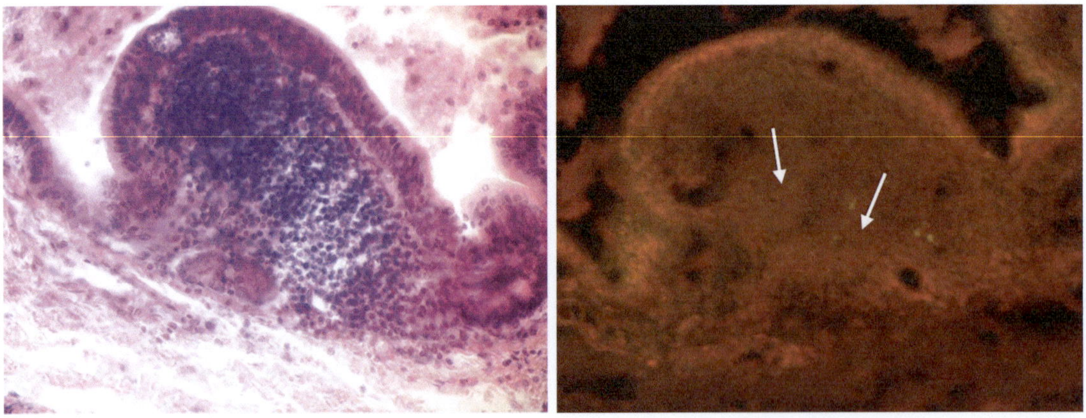

Fig. 5.5 Histological sections of the conjunctiva of a rabbit eye on the 189th day after subconjunctival administration of *C. trachomatis*: in addition to the inflammatory infiltrate, chlamydial antigens were detected with direct fluorescence. Staining: haematoxylin and eosin, direct fluorescence reaction. Magnification 200

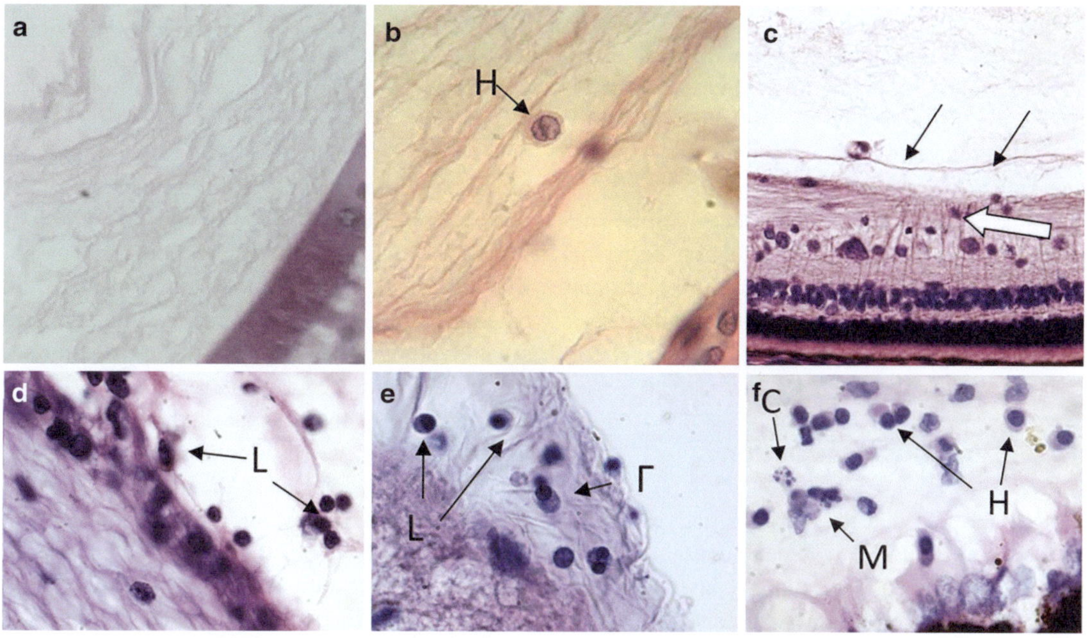

Fig. 5.6 Eye of an animal, challenged by *C. trachomatis L2* (128 d). (**a**) Disturbance of fibrillary structure of vitreous body x400. (**b**) In the background of disorganization of vitreous body fibres hyalocyte (H) with lobular nucleus without nucleolus, homogeneous light cytoplasm without inclusions and vacuolization. X 400. (**c**) Detachment of retinal matrix (black arrows) and lymphocytes in the inner layers of retina (white arrow). x 200. (**d**) Lymphocytic infiltration (L) of inner layers of retina and preretinal vitreum x1000. (**e**, **f**) Lymphocytes (L), monocytes (M), hyalocytes (H) and cells undergone cytolysis (C) at the bottom of vitreous body. X 1000. Stained by H.-E

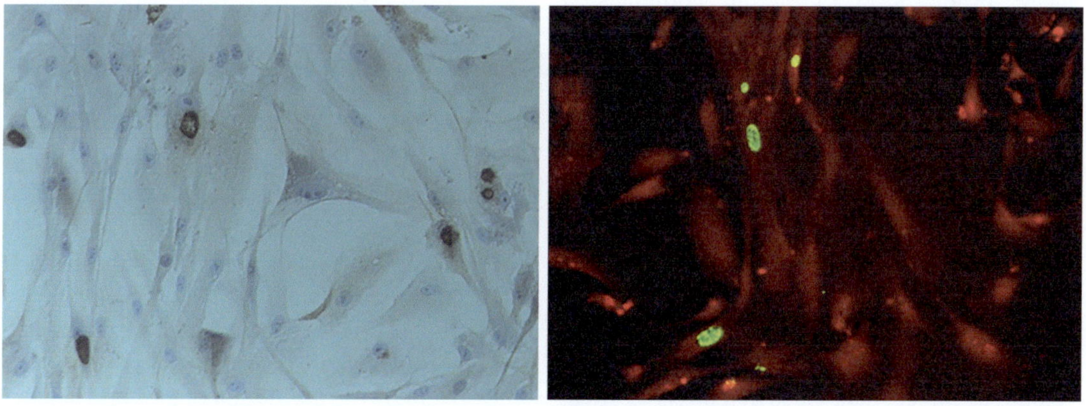

Fig. 5.7 Immunohistochemical staining and direct immunofluorescence reaction in retinal pigment epithelium culture and McCoy cell culture 48 hours after infection with *C. trachomatis*

changes in cells with the expression of signalling molecules, cytoskeletal components and extracellular matrix components, which was manifested in a selective increase in the expression of type IV collagen, type I collagen, IL-8, bFGF, and TGF-β.

Thus, experimental data for the first time substantiated the possibility of infection of retinal pigment epithelium cells with the possible participation of *C. trachomatis* in the pathogenesis of various vitreoretinal diseases.

5.2.5 Vitreous Destruction

Despite the fact that the vitreous body (V) consists of more than 99% water and contains a small number of cells, and its boundary layers perform a barrier function, it is nevertheless susceptible to various influences, which are clinically manifested in the form of dystrophic changes [111, 112]. It is known that the development of dystrophic processes caused by a violation of the structure and content of macromolecular components—collagen and hyaluronic acid—is influenced by a decrease in the synthesis of macromolecules against the background of a change in the level of steroid hormones, a decrease in the content of antioxidants and, as a consequence, an increased damaging effect of free radicals from the retina, as well as ionic shifts. The most discussed causes of such disorders are age-related changes, the presence of systemic diseases, previous severe inflammatory diseases of the retina and choroid, myopia [112]. At the same time, the role of latent infections, in which the infectious and inflammatory process has a subclinical or asymptomatic course, in the pathology of ST remains poorly studied.

Indirect clinical data on such a possible effect were obtained in relation to *C. trachomatis*. Thus, in a study including 312 volunteers aged 24 to 52 years, the frequency and nature of changes in the vitreous body were compared in patients with *C. trachomatis* infection diagnosed in the conjunctiva by the DIF method (165 people) and patients without infection (147 people) [113]. As a result, it was revealed that the infected people had a significantly higher frequency of dystrophic changes in the vitreous body ($p < 0.05$), especially at a younger age. In addition, in the group with *C. trachomatis*, only 19.39% of observations had a history of acute conjunctivitis of probable chlamydial aetiology; in 69.7% of observations, the lesion was of the nature of chronic conjunctivitis, often without any subjective manifestations. In other cases, despite the detection of the pathogen during examination, no signs of an inflammatory process in the conjunctiva were found.

Previously, experimental studies have shown that *Chlamydia*, when infecting the conjunctiva, is subsequently detected in the membranes of the eye, including penetrating the vitreous body, whilst clinically, from the posterior segment of the eye, manifestations of the infectious and inflammatory process were minimal, and the process itself often had a chronic course [108]. Considering that the result of chronic chlamydial infection is always a violation of metabolism and remodelling of the affected tissue [114], in the observed cases, a higher frequency of dystrophic changes in the vitreous body in infected eyes can be explained either by the presence of a latent infection in the structures of the posterior segment of the eye, or by the influence of autoimmune mechanisms as a consequence of chlamydial infection. In particular, changes can be caused by damage by the pathogen to cells responsible for the synthesis and renewal of macromolecular structures of the vitreum, as well as those involved in the formation of vitreoretinal contact—hyalocytes, Müller cells of the retina [107]. It should be noted that in the indicated cell types in experimental ophthalmochlamydiosis, intracellular forms of the pathogen were detected already on the 50th day after infection, whilst weak lymphocytic infiltration of the cortical layer of the vitreous body indicated the presence of an infectious-inflammatory process, but without clinical manifestations, and the outcome of the process was dystrophic changes, mainly destruction (Fig. 5.8) [108].

Unlike experimental models, in patients with *C. trachomatis* diagnosed in the conjunctiva, the infectious process could proceed over a longer

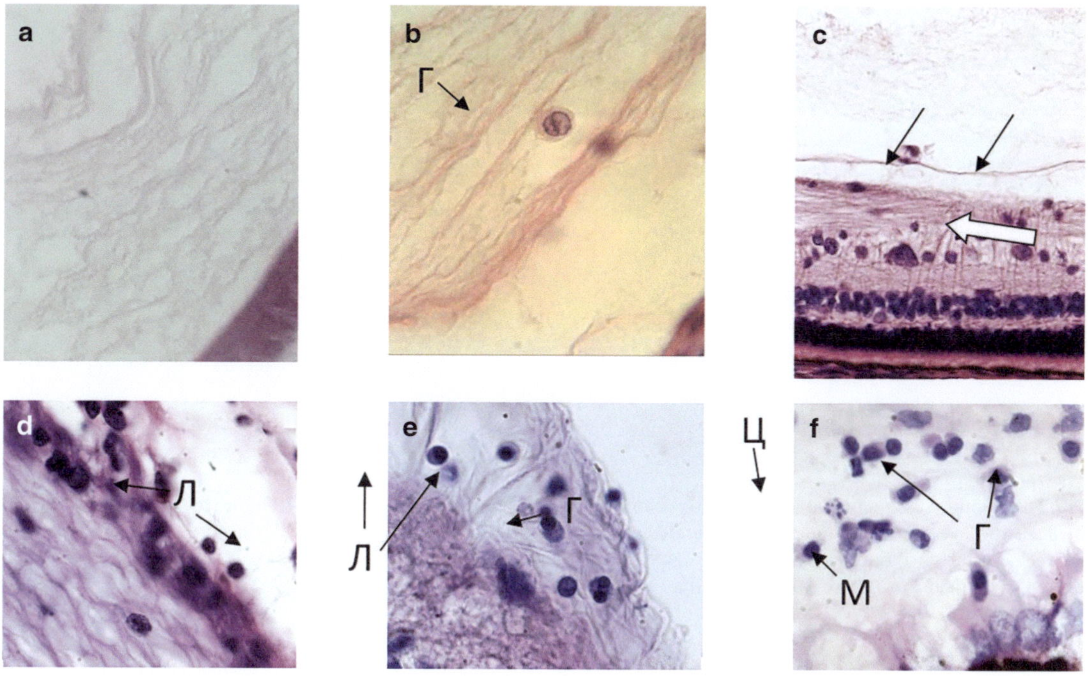

Fig. 5.8 Microscopic preparations of the eyeball of an animal infected with *C. trachomatis L2* (128 days after infection). (**a**) Disruption of the organization of the fibrillar structures of the vitreous body. Magnification 400. (**b**) Against the background of disorganization of the fibres of the vitreous body, a hyalocyte (D) with a lobed nucleus without nucleoli, homogeneous weakly stained cytoplasm without inclusions and vacuolization. Magnification 400. (**c**) Detachment of the retinal matrix (black arrows) and lymphocytes in the inner layers of the retina (white arrow). Magnification 200. (**d**) Lymphocytic infiltration (L) of the inner layers of the retina and preretinal vitreum. Magnification 1000. (**d**, **e**, **f**) E. Lymphocytes (L) and monocytes (M), as well as hyalocytes (H) and cells subjected to cytolysis (C) at the base of the vitreous body. Magnification 1000. Staining: haematoxylin and eosin

period—from several years to decades, whilst clinical manifestations were often limited to exacerbation of chronic conjunctivitis or acute conjunctivitis. In such conditions, the latent course of infection could be accompanied by the launch of the above-mentioned mechanisms of development of dystrophic changes in the vitreous body, including even without directly affecting the vitreous cells, but only maintaining an inflammatory reaction at a certain level with accompanying biochemical, metabolic shifts in the tissues.

5.2.6 Proliferative Vitreoretinopathy: The Importance of Latent Chlamydial Infection in the Course of the Disease

Experimental data indicate the possible influence of *C. trachomatis* not only on the development of dystrophic changes in the vitreous body and the pathogenesis of rhegmatogenous retinal detachment, but also on the development and course of its complication—proliferative vitreoretinopathy

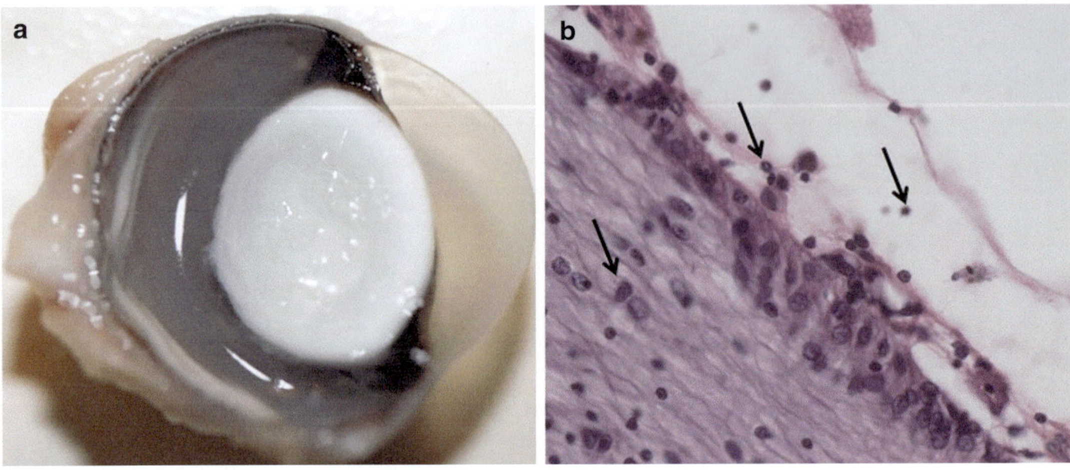

Fig. 5.9 Picture of chlamydial lesion of the posterior segment of the eye with minimal clinical manifestations at 8 weeks after the introduction of the infection: (**a**) Posterior segment of the eye without obvious inflammatory changes. Macropreparation. (**b**) Minor lymphocytic infiltration of the preretinal vitreum and retina (arrows). Staining: haematoxylin and eosin, magnification 600

(PVR), which is characterized by the formation and contraction of fibrous membranes in the vitreous body, retina and in the subretinal space [115].

Under experimental conditions, PVR was modelled in the eyes of rabbits that had been previously infected with *C. trachomatis* by intravitreal administration and in which the infection was either asymptomatic or had minimal clinical manifestations (Fig. 5.9), and during immunohistochemical examination, chlamydial inclusions were identified in both the inner and outer layers of the retina, as well as in cellular elements at the base of the vitreous body [116].

As a result, in infected eyes, PVR developed significantly more frequently and was more severe than in uninfected eyes, whilst in the vitreous body, chlamydial inclusions predominated in areas of proliferation with macrophages and lymphocytes as part of proliferates in the form of large intracellular formations (reticular bodies) located near the nucleus, small extracellular formations (elementary bodies), and also in the form of intracellular colonies.

It has been shown previously that the presence of extraocular foci of chronic infections causes a higher risk of PVR, whilst chronic inflammation, including that caused by infection, before the manifestation of PVR causes the "readiness" of intraocular structures for the proliferative process, which has been shown previously in experiments [117, 118]. In this case, the presence of a mild chronic infectious and inflammatory process in the posterior segment of the eye (i.e. subclinical uveitis) of chlamydial aetiology can also serve as an inducer of PVR. This is consistent with the results of the experiment, when in the control group (modelling of PVR without previously introduced infection), the wound process ended with scarring within the membranes without pronounced inclusion of the vitreous body in the proliferation processes. At the same time, in the experimental group, against the background of the presence of infection, the vitreous body was involved in the proliferative processes with the development of pronounced PVR. A similar course of the inflammatory process occurs in persistent chlamydial infections of various localizations, when infection-induced inflammation occurs predominantly in a proliferative form, causing tissue remodelling and fibrosis (e.g. in trachoma, joint diseases, urogenital pathology) [114].

In addition, the severe course of the inflammatory process with the previously performed introduction of chlamydial infection pathogens in the experiment allows us to talk about the possible aggravation of PVR in patients with persistent infections in the posterior segment of the eye (not only chlamydial, but also, possibly, other pathogens of viral and bacterial infections with properties similar to *Chlamydia* to cause subclinical inflammation, and the ability to persist). It can also be assumed that the presence of *C. trachomatis* infection stimulates PVR in traumatic and, probably, in rhegmatogenous retinal detachments. Antigenic stimulation in this case potentiates inflammation, and the pathogen, being absorbed by macrophages, is not eliminated [119]. On the other hand, in conditions of eye trauma, contamination with various pathogens with the development of an infectious and inflammatory process is possible. In the case of surgical interventions, contamination of the surgical wound is minimal, and hidden infectious agents (viral, bacterial) localized in the posterior segment of the eye come to the fore.

5.2.7 Data on the Impact of Chronic Chlamydial Infection on the Effectiveness of Antiglaucoma Surgery

Latent chronic infection of *C. trachomatis* in the conjunctiva, maintaining mild inflammation, can cause not only dry eye syndrome, but also affect the results of glaucoma surgery. Regardless of the type of intervention (penetrating or non-penetrating), a filtration cushion is formed during the operation, providing drainage of intraocular fluid and a corresponding decrease in intraocular pressure. One of the most common reasons for the insufficient effectiveness of antiglaucoma surgery is scarring in the intervention area: various approaches have been proposed for its treatment, including the use of antimetabolite applications. Scarring reflects excessive reparative regeneration and depends on the level of inflammatory and proliferative activity. Therefore, inflammatory changes in the conjunctiva (in particular, chronic conjunctivitis) are considered a risk factor for the failure of filtration surgery.

In a retrospective observational study of 50 eyes with primary open-angle glaucoma in 50 patients who underwent trabeculectomy without the use of cytostatics, the relationship between ineffective antiglaucoma surgery due to filtration bleb scarring and the detection of latent infection pathogens *C. trachomatis* and *B. fragilis*, as well as the level of cytokines IL-1β and IL-8 in tears was studied [120]. As a result, it was revealed that in the group of ineffective surgery (18 eyes), the frequency of detection of *C. trachomatis* and *B. fragilis* in conjunctival scrapings was 27.8% and 66.7%, significantly exceeding the frequency in the comparison group (0% and 9.4%). In addition, in scleroconjunctival biopsies from the scarring zone taken during reoperation, the pathogens *C. trachomatis* and *B. fragilis* were detected in 11.1% of cases, and the level of cytokines IL-1β and IL-8 in tears significantly exceeded (468.83 ± 80.43 and 107.89 ± 15.11 pg /ml, respectively) the indicators in the comparison group (22.34 ± 5.43 and 9.34 ± 2.83 pg /ml, respectively).

5.3 Chlamydial Lesions of the Nervous System (with the Participation of Vainshenker Yu. I., Mudritsky V.M.)

Recently, data have emerged on the possible involvement of various types of *Chlamydia* (*C. trachomatis, C. pneumoniae, C. psittaci*) in a whole spectrum of various diseases of the nervous system [121].

Functional insufficiency of the cranial and spinal nerves was noted: anisocoria, nystagmus, asymmetry of the nasolabial folds, neuropathy of the facial, glossopharyngeal and vagus nerves, neuralgia of the trigeminal nerve and the shoulder girdle, local hyperesthesia were detected. There are publications on chlamydial polyneuropathies and multiple mononeuropathies, Guillain -Barré type polyradiculoneuritis, meningoradiculitis.

Role of chlamydial infection in the development and course of brain lymphoma against the background of leukoencephalitis, multiple sclerosis, vasculitis, atherosclerosis of the cerebral arteries, etc. is discussed [122–126].

Cultural and PCR diagnostic methods for demyelinating diseases and CNS vasculitis associated with chronic persistent chlamydial infection, in half of the cases, are uninformative [127]. Researchers pay much attention to the characteristics of the course of latent chlamydial infection of the central nervous system [128].

It is rightly pointed out that damage to the nervous system is undoubtedly more common than it is diagnosed. However, information on the role of *Chlamydia* in neurological and psychiatric diseases remains fragmentary, unsystematized, controversial and sometimes exists in the form of isolated clinical observations, although the spectrum of neurological manifestations is quite wide. This can be explained by the absence of obvious clinical and neuroimaging manifestations of chlamydial infection of the central nervous system, as well as a lack of understanding of its pathogenetic significance in a variety of nosologies [129].

All representatives of the *Chlamydia* family pathogenic to humans, that is *C. trachomatis, C. pneumoniae* and *C. psittaci*, are capable of affecting cells of the nervous system. Their biological properties serve as a prerequisite for the variability of clinical manifestations of the infectious process and probable diagnostic difficulties. In this regard, it is necessary to note the diversity of interactions of the infectious agent with the host cell (reproduction, persistence with the development of aberrant reticular bodies and reactivation, in the Russian literature they also distinguish L-transformation) and inhibition or activation of apoptosis of the host cell depending on the conditions and form of existence of the pathogen.

The fundamental mechanism in the pathogenesis of chlamydial lesions of the nervous system is haematogenous dissemination of the pathogen from the primary foci of infection. *Chlamydia* can be found in monocytes, lymphocytes and macrophages, disrupt phagocytosis, spreading as part of these cells throughout the body, and have antigenic "mimicry." After infection, *Chlamydia* reproduce in the epithelial cells of the mucous membranes (primary focus), and their further spread occurs as per continuitatem, as well as haematogenous, lymphogenous [121, 130–132].

5.3.1 Chlamydial Lesions of the Peripheral Nervous System (PNS)

The spectrum of neurological manifestations associated with *Chlamydia* is quite wide, which also applies to damage to the peripheral nervous system. Damage to the PNS is associated with *Chlamydia psittaci* [133] and *Chlamydia pneumoniae* [134], as well as *Chlamydia trachomatis* [135, 136].

Studies specifically devoted to the study of chlamydial infection of the PNS are few in number and often have the character of describing individual clinical observations. In particular, there are indications of the detection of functional insufficiency of both cranial and spinal nerves: ptosis [137], anisocoria, nystagmus, asymmetry of the nasolabial folds, neuropathy of the facial, glossopharyngeal and vagus nerves, neuralgia of the trigeminal nerve and the shoulder girdle, local hyperesthesia [138–140] were detected. There are publications on chlamydial polyneuropathies and multiple mononeuropathies [140–142], polyradiculoneuritis of the Guillain -Barré type [143, 144], meningoradiculitis [145].

According to Mikhailenko et al. (1996) [135], amongst 242 patients with various mono- and polyneuropathies, an association with chlamydial infections was established with Guillain -Barré type polyradiculoneuritis ($n = 32$)—in 37.5% of cases, titre of specific antibodies 1:8–1:64; in polyneuropathy (alcoholic, diabetic, etc. ($n = 92$)—in 33.6%, 1:8–1:16; in cranial polyneuropathy ($n = 12$)—33.3%, 1:8–1:64; Tolosa-Hunt syndrome ($n = 8$)—37.5%, 1:16–1:64; facial nerve neuropathy ($n = 48$)—25%, 1:16–1:32; abducens nerve neuropathy (6)—33.3%, 1:32–1:64; trigeminal neuralgia ($n = 8$)—37.5%, 1:16–1:32; meningoradiculitis (36)—36.1%, 1:16–1:32. As a feature, these diseases were characterized by torpidity, protracted course and prolonged recovery. Additional antimicrobial therapy in these patients (doxycycline hydrochloride, tarivid (ofloxacin) before microbiological sanitization of blood and cerebrospinal fluid) increased the number of significant therapeutic results, and the regression of clinical and neurological symptoms partially correlated with the dynamics of immunoserological parameters.

Note that Mikhailenko et al. 1996 [135] diagnosed chlamydial infection based on the results of studying blood serum and cerebrospinal fluid only in cases of detection of: (a) five or more elementary chlamydial bodies (polyvalent luminescent chlamydial antibodies were used, revealing genus-specific antigen); (b) a titre of specific antibodies (to *Chlamydia* psittaci and trachomatis) of 1:8 or higher; (c) positive seroconversion after specific therapy. Interestingly, although in the control group ($n = 58$), the incidence of chlamydial infection was significantly less frequent, and the titres were lower, 15.5% with titres of 1:8 and < 1:8., the presence of chlamydial infection with damage to the nervous system cannot be excluded [Vainshenker Yu.I. (2020)]. Accordingly, the incidence of PNP associated with chlamydial The infection may be greater than the numbers presented.

According to Syniachenko 2022 [136], amongst patients with reactive chlamydial arthritis, peripheral neuropathy (PNP) occurred in 19% of cases, with mononeuropathy and polyneuropathy (1: 1) recorded with equal frequency with motor, sensory and mixed disorders in a ratio of 1: 3: 6. Autonomic disorders were detected in 53% of PNP cases (trophic, visceral and vascular in a ratio of 1: 3: 10). Carpal tunnel neuropathy—in 21% of PNP cases, Guillain -Barré syndrome—in 26% (or 5% of all RCA cases). Bilateral arm lesions were diagnosed in 69% of PNP cases, and leg lesions—in 88%. If the ratio of distal and distal-proximal neuropathy of the hands was 5:1, then of the legs—1:1. Positive sensory changes (paraesthesia, hyperesthesia, hyperalgesia) were 5 times more common than negative (hypoesthesia). Amongst movement disorders, convulsions were noted in 86% of cases of PSP, and restless legs syndrome—in every second such patient.

Although neuropathy is naturally considered a negative prognostic factor for the course of chlamydial reactive arthritis [Syngle et al. 2015], according to Syniachenko 2022, it was found that PNP correlates with clinical and laboratory signs of arthritis, and the high rate of progression of the latter is an unfavourable sign for the prognosis of the course of PNP. As was found, inflammatory immune proteins, vascular endothelial dysfunction and physicochemical surface-rheological properties of serum were involved in the pathogenesis of PNP, with seropositivity for Anti-CCP (Cyclic Citrullinated Peptide Antibodies) according to researchers, is a risk factor for the development of PNP.

It should be noted that in the last decade, coinfection of *C. pneumoniae* and *C. trachomatis* in the synovial fluid of patients with reactive arthritis has been confirmed [Di Pietro et al. 2019]. It is assumed that in the etiopathogenesis of this disease, *C. pneumoniae* can act synergistically with *C. trachomatis* through the development of chronic inflammation in the joint [146–148], and increasing the risk of developing the disease, as well as with other pathogens [146, 148]. By analogy, it seems to us that in the etiopathogenesis of at least severe forms of PNP, an association of different pathogens, including different types of *Chlamydia*, can play a role.

From the point of view of the route of infection of the PNS, the following clinical data are of interest. It was established (Mikhailenko et al. 1996) that the manifestations of clinical manifestations from the PNS were often preceded by episodes of “colds” and hypothermia, direct contact with sick domestic animals. In patients with damage to the PNS, damage to other organs or systems was usually noted: acute respiratory viral infection preceding the disease (in 68.6% of cases); acute conjunctivitis (in 6%); chronic blepharitis (in 14.4%); chronic tonsillitis (in 26.5%); chronic bronchitis (in 19.3%); urogenital diseases (in 73.5%); polyarthritis (in 22.9%), and there was also asthenic (astenovegetative) syndrome, which does not exclude pathology of the central nervous system [135].

Comparable data have been established O. Syniachenko [136], 2022 in the study of systemic pathology developing with reactive chlamydial arthritis (101 patients), along with damage to the PNS (19%). In 93–94% of patients, various urogenital diseases were encountered; ophthalmopathy (61%), skin syndrome, in particular psoriasis-like rash, erythema nodosum (21%), nephropathy (44%), heart damage (myocardial excitability and electrical conductivity disorders, chamber changes, valve fibrosis, diastolic dysfunction of the left ventricle—(58%), tendovaginitis (41%), enthesopathies (24%), sacroiliitis (59%), spondylopathy (32%).

Morphological changes, as well as the study of the route of infection, during the development of PNS lesions are based primarily on experimental data. It should be noted that the morphological manifestations of the infectious process in the CNS or PNS did not differ fundamentally depending on the route of infection (transnasal, including when modeling persistent infection, transconjunctival, intracerebral, intraperitoneal), and on the type of pathogen (*C. trachomatis, C. pneumoniae, C. psittaci*).

In the structures of the PNS (as well as the CNS), along with the detection of elementary bodies of *Chlamydia*, changes in cells and fibres of varying degrees of severity were detected,

Thus, according to Mikhailenko et al., 1996, in 50 Balb /C linear mice with intraperitoneal infection with C. psittaci and C. trachomatis with subsequent examination (light-optical and electron microscopy) of the roots of the equine tail and sciatic nerves at the height of clinical manifestations (3–6 days), the following changes were revealed [135].

Swelling of the endoneurium and perineurium was detected, in the vessels—stasis and moderate perivascular infiltration by lymphoid elements. In the endoneurium, perineurium, epineurium, as well as near the vessels, basophilic-metachromatic granularity was detected, similar granules were also found in the cells of the connective tissue around the vessels in the liver and spleen. Elementary bodies of *Chlamydia* were found in the axoplasm unmyelinated fibres and in myelinated fibres amongst curved myelin lamellae.

Polymorphic changes of varying severity were recorded in the lemmocytes of the myelin sheath. As an equivalent of tension and functional hyperactivity, large phagosomes with heterogeneous contents were found in the cytoplasm of lemmocytes, determining their uneven electron density. With more pronounced pathology, destruction of changes in the organelles of the cytoplasm and the cell nucleus was recorded. The nucleus disintegrated into fragments, amongst which mitochondria altered in the form of vacuoles were found. Irregularly shaped lipids, large phagosomes with heterochromic (granular) contents, altered fragments of the endoplasmic reticulum, and various vesicles (in the form of multivesicular bodies, in the form of chains along the cell membrane) were found in the cytoplasm of lemmocytes. Clusters of ribosomes sometimes formed irregularly shaped electron-dense figures with an indefinite and uneven localization in the cytoplasm, which gave the latter a heterogeneous appearance.

The structure of the synapses was disrupted: the characteristic thickenings at the point of contact between the pre- and postsynaptic membranes were absent, and the shape and electron density of the contents of the synaptic vesicles changed.

The axoplasm of the fibres, especially the non-myelinated ones, was often oedematous and contained myelin-like and layered structures (modified remnants of mitochondria and endoplasmic reticulum). Some mitochondria showed only moderate deformation, whilst others were transformed into electron-transparent vacuoles, retaining only the double mitochondrial membrane.

Various variants of myelin fibre debonding were found: divergence of curved but maintaining the same electron density lamellae; thinning and interruption of lamellae in areas of curvature; adhesion of lamellae across the entire cross-section or in the outer part of the myelin sheath, and irregularly shaped granular formations protruded toward the axial cylinder. In adjacent areas, a picture of vesicular degeneration was often determined, and elementary chlamydial bodies were sometimes found in the zone of granular degeneration. In fibres with pronounced myelin changes, the axial cylinders did not remain intact either, some of which had a "empty" appearance, whilst in others, altered mitochondria and endoplasmic reticulum were detected.

Although, taking into account clinical data, the PNS lesion is more often a part of a generalized infection, which, however, does not exclude the potential possibility of isolated PNS lesion. In particular, in an experimental study of the participation of *Chlamydia* in late-onset Alzheimer's disease [149, 150], it was finally proven that CNS infection (*C. pneumonia, C. muridarum*) can occur through the olfactory and trigeminal nerve. This work confirmed the possibility of developing "isolated" cranial neuropathy, at least before the development of systemic pathology.

It is suggested that the olfactory and trigeminal nerve glial cells are directly infected [151]. Olfactory nerve glia, olfactory ensheathing cells (OECS), are known to be the main phagocytes of the olfactory nerve [152, 153]. Olfactory nerve sheath cells can ingest bacteria and mount a potent innate immune response to pathogens [154–157]. Trigeminal nerve glia are trigeminal Schwann cells (TgSCs), which can also ingest bacteria [157]. However, Schwann cells have been shown to have a significantly lower immune response to pathogens than olfactory nerve sheath cells [154]. Those olfactoryglia demonstrated less infection and a stronger immune response than trigeminal glia.

Olfactory nerve glial cells (OECs) are thought to be the key phagocytes in this nerve and play a key role in defence against microorganisms [153, 155, 157]. The ability to infect and survive within OECS, rather than being phagocytosed and degraded by the cells, is thought to be a feature of microorganisms that can invade the primary olfactory nervous system [158, 159]. Trigeminal Schwann cells (TgSCs) can also phagocytose microorganisms [157]; however, Schwann cells have also been shown to express lower levels of mRNA for factors.

5.3.2 *Chlamydia*: A Key Microorganism of Hidden Encephalitis in Patients in Prolonged Disorders of Consciousness (PDoC)

In a special work provided by YI Vainshenker were examined 68 patients in PDoC (28 [23, 37] yo, men −48, women—20) aetiology of brain injury was: traumatic −50 patients, non-traumatic (hypoxia, stroke, etc.)—18 patients. Levels of consciousness within the framework of PDoC: in vegetative state (VS)—43, in minimally conscious state (MCS)—25 patients duration of pDoc >2 months (maximum 10 years) before brain damage, all patients were healthy all patients had no typical signs of encephalitis.

During microbiological studied (by culture and PCR): *Chlamydia* spp. *(C. trachomatis, C. pneumoniae, C. psittaci*) were found in various biomaterials in 56% (38/68) of patients (for comparison: *Mycoplasma* spp.: 38%, *Ureaplasma* spp.: 28%). Repeated studies (laboratory, morphological) were required for the diagnostic detection of *Chlamydia* spp. in 1/4 of cases. Detectability of *Chlamydia* spp. in various biomaterials (the ratio) liquor: blood: mucous membranes—1.2: 1.2: 1. The presence of *Chlamydia* spp. correlated with inflammatory demyelination ($P < 0.01$) (with "diagnostically hidden forms" in the liquor $P < 0.001$). Paradoxically, the presence of Chlamydia spp. corresponded to a relatively favourable prognosis ($P < 0.01$) both for improving consciousness and survival of patients (taking into account etiotropic therapy).

Dependence of the results on the treatment option: with standard therapy (ST) and additional treatment, including *Chlamydia* infection (hidden pathogens therapy, HPT) are presented in Figs. 5.10, 5.11, 5.12 and 5.13.

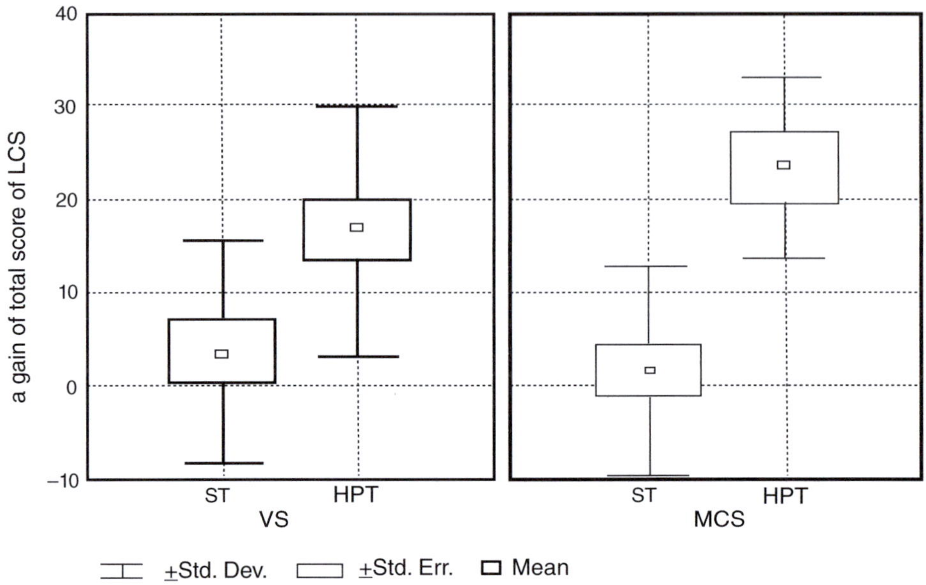

Fig. 5.10 Change of consciousness in patients in a vegetative state (VS) and minimally conscious state (MCS) 3 months after the start of therapy (improvement with HPT), Levenstein communication scale

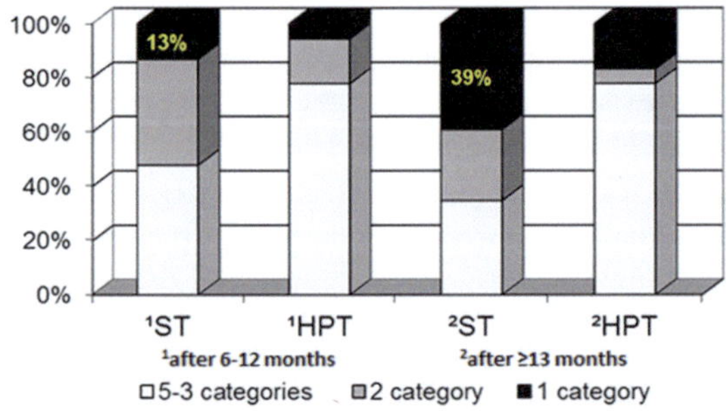

Fig. 5.11 Long-term outcomes (mortality increase with ST), Glasgow Outcome scale

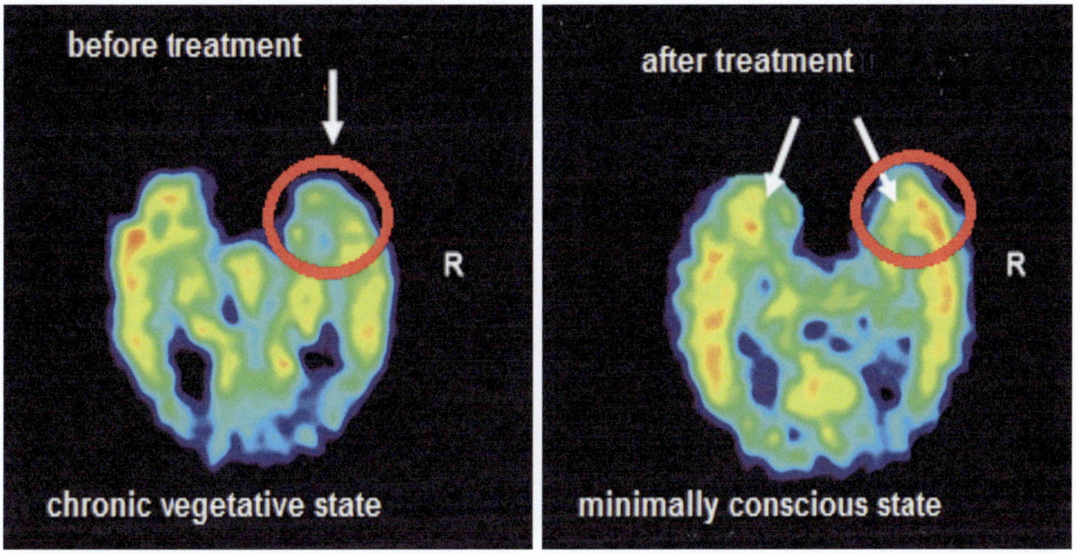

Fig. 5.12 Improving brain metabolism (PET 18 FDG) 3 months after the start of *Chlamydia* infection treatment (HPT)

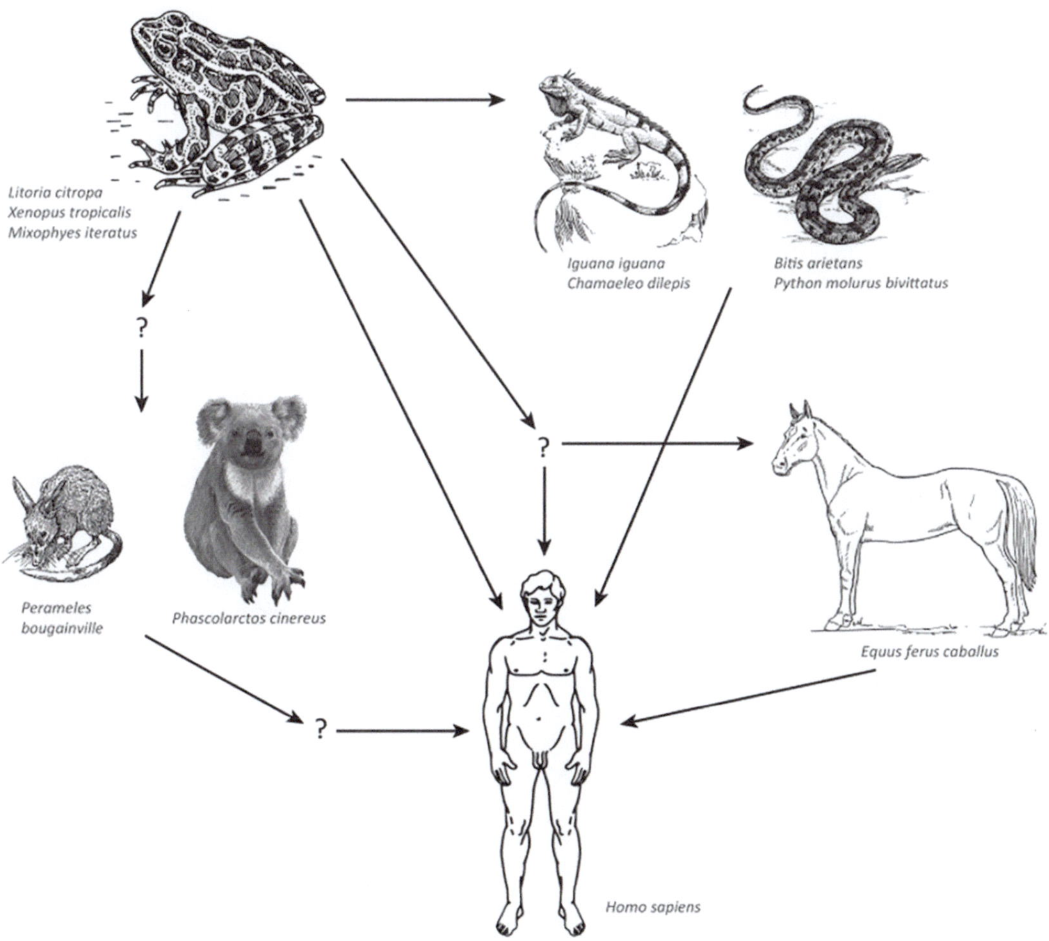

Fig. 5.13 Distribution of *C. pneumoniae* in animal and human populations. (From Ref. [169])

5.4 Pneumochlamydiosis

5.4.1 *Chlamydia*-Related Diseases *Pneumoniae*

C. pneumoniae is a pathogen that causes diseases in humans and animals. It has a global distribution in the animal kingdom. This pathogen infects both domestic and wild animals (Fig. 5.14). Chlamydia in a koala (*Phascolarctos cinereus)* was first described in 1974 and was later found to be caused by two different strains of *C. psittaci*, with the type 1 strain being reclassified as *C. pneumoniae* in 1994. Evidence of *C. pneumoniae* infection in animals other than the koala has emerged with the discovery of *C. pneumoniae* in horses, frogs and reptiles [160–163]. As with human disease, *C. pneumoniae infections* in animals present with vascular and respiratory pathologies, but conjunctival, genitourinary and systemic manifestations of the disease are not uncommon.

C. pneumoniae was initially discovered in humans in association with acute respiratory infections and community-acquired (atypical) pneumonia.

Atypical pneumonia, which may result from chlamydial infection, has been reported in adults and infants since the 1930s. Early work attempted to characterize these infections as chlamydial due to poor diagnostic tools, but they were eventually recognized and named *Chlamydia psittaci* TWAR [164, 165].

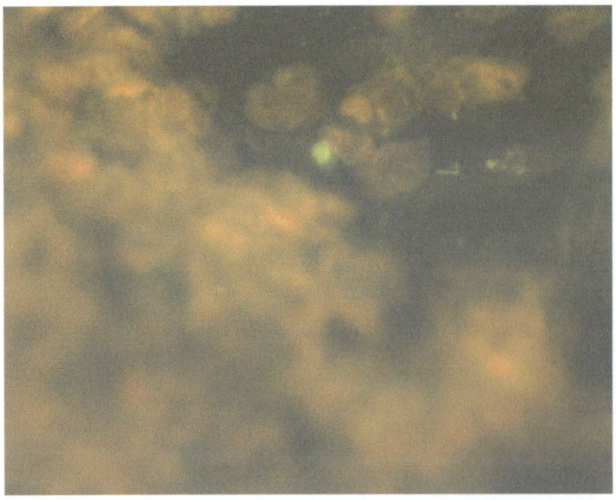

Fig. 5.14 Chl. Trachomatis antigen in a smear from joint fluid DIF

An epidemic of mild pneumonia affecting young adults was discovered during routine radiological screening in Finland in 1978 [166]. This was apparently the first epidemic associated with *C. pneumoniae*, setting the stage for what would become the starting point of numerous studies linking infection with this pathogen to a range of illnesses and, ultimately, to a similar number of hosts.

Pathogenic to humans strain (formerly TWAR) upon further study was named *C. pneumoniae* (see Chap.1) [167, 168].

Molecular typing studies indicate that animal strains are the ancestors of human strains and that *C. pneumoniae* jumped from animals to humans in at least one relatively recent zoonotic event. Whole-genome analyses appear to support this concept—the human strains are highly conserved, whereas the only animal strain that has been fully sequenced has a larger genome with several notable differences. Compared to *Chlamydia trachomatis*, *C. pneumoniae* exhibits significant differences in their cellular biology, development and genome structure [146, 170].

In the late 1980s and 1990s, *C. pneumoniae* was frequently found in association with a number of respiratory infections [171–173].

Although some diagnostic techniques were clearly more reliable than others [174], these studies nonetheless demonstrated that *C. pneumoniae* is a widespread pathogen in humans. Adding to this puzzle is the more recent realization that worldwide, the incidence of *C. pneumoniae respiratory infections* appears to have declined dramatically [175]. Epidemics of *C. pneumoniae pneumonia* still occur, and are most often reported in military settings [176–178].

One explanation is that the mild course of respiratory disease caused by *C. pneumoniae* leads to its underdiagnosis by physicians in terms of verification of the etiologic agent, but this does not explain the apparent decrease in the detection of this pathogen in daily practice [179]. On the other hand, it may mean that people have developed a certain level of immunity to *C. pneumoniae*.

The relationship between *C. pneumoniae* and atherosclerosis is perhaps less clear. Although a causal relationship is yet to be determined, there is no doubt that *C. pneumoniae DNA* can be reliably detected in coronary (and other) plaques [180–182], and animal models do suggest a causal or exacerbating relationship [183] (See Chap. 8).

Standardization of experimental methods and a larger patient sample will undoubtedly contribute to understanding the true prevalence of *C. pneumoniae* in humans and its association with respiratory disease, as well as the multitude of chronic diseases to which this bacterial pathogen is associated.

It is currently believed that *C. pneumoniae* infection (pneumochlamydiosis) occurs in latent (asymptomatic) and manifest forms. The incubation period is presumably up to a month.

There is currently no generally accepted clinical classification either in Russia or in other countries. This is due to the lack of knowledge as well as the state and the level of understanding of the disease at the moment. The working classification we propose takes into account the views of various authors (Table 5.1).

The latent form of the infectious process can be primary, developing after infection, and secondary, after the disease. With prolonged persistence of *Chlamydia*, relapses of the disease and the development of chronic forms of the disease are possible. The culture of *Chlamydia* can be isolated from nasopharyngeal swabs even 12 months after the disappearance of clinical manifestations, whilst serological reactions can remain negative.

Manifest Chlamydia pneumoniae can be acute or chronic. Clinical manifestations ***of the acute form*** vary from mild acute respiratory disease (*nasopharyngeal form:* rhinitis, pharyngitis, otitis media, sinusitis, adenoiditis) to massive damage to the lung tissue with the development of respiratory failure (*pneumonic form).*

The onset of the disease in the overwhelming majority of cases is acute, manifested by a syndrome of general infectious intoxication (chills, fever, headache, myalgia, arthralgia without organic damage and dysfunction; dizziness, nausea, vomiting, loss of appetite are possible).

Most patients show signs of pharyngitis, bronchitis or pneumonia (catarrhal syndrome) from

Table 5.1 Clinical classification of pneumochlamydia

Form of the disease	Severity of the current	Phase of the infectious process (according to serological criteria)	Functional disorders
Asymptomatic (latent): Manifest acute pulmonary: Nasopharyngeal, Pneumonic. Manifest chronic extrapulmonary: Damage to the respiratory system (sinusitis, recurrent obstructive bronchitis, bronchial asthma, pneumosclerosis, chronic obstructive disease, lung cancer, sarcoidosis) Cardiovascular (endocarditis, damage to the vascular endothelium with subsequent atherosclerotic changes, contributing to the development of coronary disease, coronary heart disease, myocardial infarction, aortic aneurysm) Nervous system (serous meningitis, meningoencephalitis, myelitis, cerebrovascular disease, multiple sclerosis, Guillain–Barré syndrome, Alzheimer's disease, schizophrenia, etc.) Connective tissue (reactive vasculitis, arthritis, erythema nodosum)	Light, Average, Heavy Without complications, With complications	Primary infection (acute course) Reinfection Chronic course (exacerbation, remission, persistence) Carriage	Respiratory failure Heart failure Heart rhythm disturbance

Ref. [184]

the first few days. Rhinitis, sinusitis and otitis are possible.

Chlamydial bronchitis is characterized by a low-productive cough that persists during the convalescence period for several weeks. In pneumonia, the cough is unproductive or produces a scanty amount of mucous sputum, dyspnoea, chest pain, focal shortening of percussion sound, harsh or weakened breathing, dry or moist wheezing are possible.

There may be an increase in the submandibular, cervical and sometimes axillary lymph nodes (polylymphadenopathy). Tachycardia is characteristic, and in severe cases, muffled heart sounds. There is a tendency towards hypotension.

The exact frequency of detection of *C. pneumoniae* in community-acquired pneumonia (CAP) is unknown, but it is believed to be at least 10% [185–192] (See also Chap. 3).

The main diagnostic criteria for manifest forms of pneumochlamydia are as follows:

- Indication of contact with a patient with acute respiratory disease/pneumonia, outbreak in a group.
- Protracted, usually not severe course of the disease.
- Febrile fever at the onset of the disease, subsequently with a tendency to long-term continuous or periodic subfebrile temperature.
- Catarrhal syndrome at the onset of the disease in the form of pharyngitis.
- Damage to the respiratory tract with an emphasis on pneumonia and/or bronchitis in the early stages of the disease, the absence of clear physical and radiological signs of pulmonary tissue infiltration.
- Presence of non-respiratory syndromes.
- Long recovery, asthenovegetative syndrome during the convalescence period.
- Absence of neutrophilic leukocytosis, tendency to leukopenia, with possible normal ESR in the development of pneumonia.
- Negative result in microscopy of a sputum smear stained by Gram and in standard bacteriological examination of sputum.
- Radiological data in the form of peribronchial and perivascular infiltration.
- Lack of effect from beta-lactam therapy.

The prognosis is usually favourable, with a mortality rate of less than 1%.

Mixed infection, for example a combination with pneumococcus or the presence of severe concomitant diseases, increases the risk of death. Relapses and chronicity of the process are possible.

Differential diagnostics is carried out with acute respiratory diseases of viral and bacterial aetiology. The disease is often interpreted as an undifferentiated ARI, occurs with subfebrile body temperature, less pronounced intoxication and catarrhal syndrome with a protracted course. The clinic of the pneumonic form of pneumochlamydia also has a lot in common with pneumonia of other aetiologies (ornithosis, mycoplasma, pneumococcal, etc.). Pneumochlamydiosis differs from the pneumonic form of ornithosis by the presence of damage to the upper respiratory tract, relatively less pronounced intoxication. It differs from community-acquired pneumonia of other aetiologies by an unproductive cough, scanty auscultatory data; it can be characterized by the presence of extrapulmonary manifestations—skin, joint, neurological. Pneumonia is often mild, but is characterized by a slow and long recovery.

In a blood test, the number of leukocytes is usually normal; there may be a moderate shift in the leukocyte formula to the left due to band elements, and a normal or moderately increased ESR. Urinalysis may reveal febrile albuminuria and cylindruria. Chest radiography reveals interstitial pneumonia in most patients [193].

Complicated course is mainly found in the chronic form of pneumochlamydiosis. Severe course with fatal outcome is more often observed in elderly people and in people with chronic diseases of the cardiovascular system and respiratory tract.

Diagnosis of pneumochlamydia is based on identifying the characteristics of clinical and instrumental data and is confirmed by specific laboratory diagnostics (see Chap. 4).

Chronic pneumochlamydiosis. Chronic chlamydial infection increases the risk of developing pathology of the respiratory, cardiovascular, nervous systems, and connective tissue. Currently, numerous researchers are examining its role in a wide range of chronic diseases (see Chap. 8).

C. pneumoniae research has been active since its description as an acute respiratory pathogen in humans in the late 1980s, and although its discovery in chronic diseases such as atherosclerosis, asthma, and Alzheimer's disease has important implications for the diagnosis and treatment of these diseases, a firm causal relationship with any of these pathologies has not yet been established. Importantly, *C. pneumoniae is ubiquitous* in human tissues, and once infected, *C. pneumoniae* readily spreads from the respiratory system through the bloodstream. The detection of *C. pneumoniae* in the brain, heart, vasculature, and joints appears to confirm this. *C. pneumoniae infection* is predominantly asymptomatic, and a single individual may be infected multiple times during their lifetime. Often, *C. pneumoniae* is not tested for at the onset of disease, and indeed its association with chronic disease is established after the disease has progressed significantly. If *C. pneumoniae* infection were definitely associated with underlying chronic diseases, we might expect a much higher incidence of multiple morbidities in a larger percentage of the population—this has not been demonstrated so far.

5.4.2 Ornithosis

The first information about ornithosis dates back to 1875, when Jurgensen pointed out a possible connection between atypical pneumonia in people and infection from sick parrots. In 1895, Morange proposed the term psittacos. The epidemic of 1929–1930 affected many countries, more than 800 people fell ill and was associated with the import of sick parrots from Brazil. In 1930–1932, the viral nature of the disease was suggested. In 1942, Meyer KF p proposed to use the term ornithosis for diseases not associated with parrots.

Ornithosis, also known as psittacosis (parrot fever), is a zoonotic disease caused by *Chlamydia psittaci*, a bacterium that commonly infects birds [194–197].

The disease is transmitted from birds to humans and causes a variety of clinical manifestations, from mild non-specific illness (with chills and headache), atypical pneumonia to severe systemic fulminant disease with multiple organ failure (pneumonia, hepatosplenomegaly, serous meningitis) and, in rare cases, death [198–200].

Subclinical infection (about 70%) is also common, and it is likely that many human cases remain undiagnosed and therefore unreported [201].

Transmission *of C. psittaci* is an emerging public health risk, particularly for healthcare workers and their close contact [202, 203]. (See Chap. 3).

The incubation period for ornithosis is from 5 to 14 days.

Pneumonic (typical) forms. The onset of the disease is manifested by febrile fever of a remittent or permanent nature and general intoxication syndrome, joint pain, nausea and vomiting, and abdominal pain.

In mild cases, the symptoms of intoxication are moderate, the fever lasts no more than a week; in severe cases, it resolves after 3–4 weeks.

Unlike acute respiratory infections, lesions of the upper respiratory tract in ornithosis are weakly expressed, although discomfort in the throat and hyperaemia of the pharynx are often noted and may be the only manifestation of ornithosis, which some authors interpret as a flu-like variant of the disease.

From the 2nd–3rd day of the disease, a low-productive cough joins in. On the 5th–7th day of the disease, with the onset of the peak period, signs of pneumonia are revealed (productive cough with mucous sputum, possibly the appearance of blood streaks in the sputum, haemoptysis, and with bacterial association—mucous -purulent sputum), whilst dyspnoea is not expressed, a change in the percussion sound over the lungs is rarely detected. Dry wheezing can be detected during auscultation. Physical signs are often less pronounced than radiological ones, and do not correspond to the severity of the patient's condition. A tendency to relative bradycardia, a decrease in blood pressure, and muffled heart sounds is noted. Liver enlargement is often detected, less often splenomegaly. Lymphadenopathy is possible.

The clinical picture of ornithosis is dominated by mild and moderate pneumonic forms of the disease.

Severe pneumonia is diagnosed when one or more of the following symptoms or signs are present: altered consciousness; respiratory rate ≥ 30 breaths/min; PaO2 < 60 mmHg; PaO2/FiO2 < 300 mmHg, requiring mechanical ventilation; arterial systolic blood pressure < 90 mmHg; septic shock; chest radiograph showing bilateral or multiple lobar involvement, or involvement increasing by ≥50% within 48 h of admission; urine output <20 mL/h or < 80 mL/4 hours, or in combination with acute renal failure requiring dialysis.

Atypical forms. In meningopneumonia meningeal symptoms (severe headache, vomiting, stiff neck, Kernig's, Brudzinski's, etc. symptoms) join the symptoms of intoxication and lung damage at the end of the 1st—beginning of the 2nd week of the disease. The disease occurs in moderate and severe forms. Fever persists for 3–4 weeks. Sanitation of the cerebrospinal fluid occurs after 5–6 weeks and later.

With ornithosis meningitis, as with meningopneumonia, meningeal symptoms appear, but there is no damage to the lungs.

Ornithosis without lung damage develops with alimentary infection. The onset is acute, with febrile fever of a constant and remitting type and signs of general infectious intoxication. By the end of the first week, an enlargement of the liver and spleen is determined. A dull rash (Horder's spots) may appear, similar to roseola in typhoid fever.

During the early convalescence period, in the absence of adequate etiotropic therapy, patients may experience *a relapse of the disease* with a new wave of fever, between two fever waves there is a period of apyrexia of at least 2 days, fever of at least 38 °C, lasting at least 2 days and exacerbation of existing or the appearance of new inflammatory foci in the lungs. *Exacerbation* of the disease is possible even against the background of an active process, more often on the 2–3rd week of the disease, body temperature rises, intoxication symptoms increase, new organ lesions may appear.

Asymptomatic (inparticular) form usually discovered during investigations of epidemic outbreaks.

Chronic form can develop after both pneumonic and atypical forms of acute ornithosis. It is described as pneumonia with broncho-obstruction phenomena, as well as without lung damage and other focal lesions with a disease duration of 6 months to several years, with periodic exacerbations or a continuous course, accompanied by subfebrile temperature, intoxication and hepatosplenic syndrome.

The main criteria that are taken into account when assessing the severity of ornithosis are: duration and nature of fever; degree of intoxication; prevalence and nature of the process in the lungs; damage to other organs and systems along with the lungs; degree and nature of disorders in them; presence and nature of complications; concomitant diseases [204].

Complications and critical conditions. Myocarditis with the development of acute heart failure, thrombophlebitis with subsequent pulmonary embolism, and pulmonary infarction can lead to death.

It is possible to develop haemorrhagic syndrome (hemorrhagic exanthema, haemorrhages into visible mucous membranes, nosebleeds), up to a full-blown picture of DIC syndrome, which is often combined with septic shock.

Other complications include: adult respiratory distress syndrome, septic shock, idiopathic cardiomyopathy, endocarditis, myocarditis, pericarditis, pancreatitis, thyroiditis, iridocyclitis, keratitis, anaemia, autoimmune hepatitis, spondylodiscitis. Neurological disorders include encephalitis, cranial nerve damage (including sensorineural hearing loss) and cerebellum, and myelitis. Reactive arthritis, renal damage (acute glomerulonephritis, tubulointerstitial nephritis, renal tubular necrosis, acute kidney injury), erythema multiforme, and erythema nodosum have been reported [205–208].

Ornithosis can cause severe complications during pregnancy and often leads to the development of DIC syndrome, liver dysfunction, placentitis and spontaneous abortion.

Differential diagnostics. Polymorphism of clinical manifestations and the absence of pathognomonic symptoms significantly complicates the clinical diagnostics of ornithosis, especially its sporadic cases; therefore, the collection of an epidemiological anamnesis (it is necessary to take into account possible contacts, including professional ones, with birds and animals) and laboratory diagnostics are of great importance in establishing a diagnosis [209, 210].

The main diagnostic criteria for manifest forms of ornithosis are as follows:

- Epidemiological history data (contact with birds and animals).
- Febrile fever of a constant or remittent type.
- Combination of pneumonia with splenomegaly.
- Lung damage without signs of acute inflammation of the upper respiratory tract.
- Relative bradycardia, hypotension.
- Moderate leukopenia or normocytosis.
- Increase in ESR to 40–60 mm/h.
- Lack of effect from beta-lactam therapy.

Differential diagnostics of ornithosis is carried out with acute respiratory infections, respiratory mycoplasmosis, pneumochlamydios, legionellosis, community-acquired pneumonia, typhoid-paratyphoid diseases, pulmonary tuberculosis, leptospirosis, malaria, etc.

The pneumonic form of ornithosis is characterized by the absence of pronounced signs of damage to the upper respiratory tract. This is a significant difference from acute respiratory infections of viral aetiology (influenza, parainfluenza, adenovirus and respiratory syncytial infections). The addition of pneumonia symptoms is not accompanied by increased intoxication; there is a discrepancy between the relatively minor changes in the lungs and the pronounced manifestations of intoxication. Liver enlargement is characteristic in most patients. The pneumonic form of ornithosis lasts longer than pneumonia of other aetiologies; relapses and late myocarditis (in the 3rd–5th week) may be observed.

Meningopneumonia and ornithosis meningitis should be differentiated from meningitis of other aetiologies (tuberculosis, enterovirus, mumps, lymphocytic choriomeningitis, etc.). Compared with other serous meningitis, ornithosis meningitis is characterized by a longer febrile period, slow disappearance of meningeal symptoms and relatively slow sanitation of cerebrospinal fluid.

The typhoid-like form requires differential diagnosis with typhoid-paratyphoid diseases, brucellosis, tularaemia, bacterial endocarditis and sepsis.

Recent publications have also reported co-infection with *SARS-CoV-2*.

Laboratory and Instrumental Diagnostics. In the blood test, the total number of leukocytes is normal or slightly increased (leukocytosis at the height of the disease is evidence of a secondary infection); lymphocytosis, monocytosis (absolute and relative), significant (40–60 mm/h) increase in ESR, eosinophilia—during the recovery period.

Urine analysis shows no characteristic changes; signs of toxic kidney damage may appear (single erythrocytes, cylinders, traces of protein).

When examining sputum, an increased number of leukocytes (including monocytes), eosinophils and alveolar macrophages, alveolar epithelium and sometimes erythrocytes are detected.

In patients with severe disease, the levels of neutrophils, D- dimer, lactate dehydrogenase, interleukin (IL)-2, IL-6 and IL-10 are significantly higher, whilst the number of lymphocytes, CD3+ T cells and CD4+ T cells, the ratio of CD4+ /CD8+ T cells and the level of albumin are significantly lower than in patients with mild disease, inflammatory markers such as procalcitonin (PCT), C-reactive protein (CRP), kidney and liver function tests [211].

Radiographic data in the lungs during the development of pneumonia are characterized by interstitial changes (increased pulmonary pattern, peribronchial or perivascular infiltration, which is manifested by a reticular pattern, band-like darkening along the vessels and bronchi with the most frequent localization of the process in the root areas and in the lower lobes of the lungs). Against this background, infiltrates of various sizes and shapes, single or multiple, may appear. Involvement of peribronchial lymph nodes, lymph nodes of the roots of the lungs and exudative pleurisy are possible. Radiographic changes resolve within an average of up to 6 weeks, but sometimes up to 20 weeks.

Chest computed tomography scans of patients with severe disease can demonstrate extensive areas of lung tissue consolidation; ground-glass opacities may be present with an increased risk of multilobular involvement and pleural effusion [212, 213].

If *meningitis* develops, pleocytosis in the cerebrospinal fluid is moderate, usually does not exceed 300–500 cells in 1 μl: in the first few days, neutrophils predominate in it, then lymphocytes (up to 80–90%), the sugar and chloride content is normal, the protein level is slightly increased. Changes in the cerebrospinal fluid can persist for 3–4 weeks.

The diagnosis of ornithosis in humans is considered established upon laboratory confirmation using serological and molecular genetic methods.

Historically, confirmation of diagnosis was based on clinical manifestations and a positive serologic test on paired sera. However, serologic tests show cross-reactivity with other chlamydial species. Therefore, it is now advisable to consider serologic testing only as an adjunctive test to other, more reliable tests, such as nucleic acid amplification tests (PCR, real-time PCR). In addition to high sensitivity and specificity for *C psittaci*, nucleic-acid-based tests allow genotyping of strains.

Metagenomic next-generation sequencing (mNGS) enables rapid and accurate detection of potential pathogens. It is increasingly used to diagnose infectious diseases, especially when traditional diagnostic methods have limitations. Studies have shown that mNGS is the most promising method for comprehensive diagnosis of infections, especially severe pneumonia [214–216].

Cultivation of *C. psittaci* from respiratory secretions is possible, but difficult, and is generally carried out only in specialized laboratories due to the high infectivity of this pathogen (in the Russian Federation it belongs to the II pathogenicity group).

The material for testing for ornithosis is blood serum, sputum, bronchoalveolar lavage, cerebrospinal fluid; cadaveric material—blood, exudate, biopsies of organs and tissues (lungs, heart, etc.).

Currently, the prognosis of the disease is good. Before the advent of antimicrobials, 15–20% of people with ornithosis died, but with the advent of antibiotics, mortality has become extremely rare (case fatality rate is less than 1%). There are published reports of adverse pregnancy outcomes associated with ornithosis infection during pregnancy, but the diagnosis in these cases was made mainly on the basis of serologic testing.

When conducting etiotropic therapy, most patients respond with positive dynamics within 48–72 hours. Relapses and chronicization of the process are possible. Chronic forms can end with the body being freed from *Chlamydia* after several years, ending with complete recovery or with the formation of residual effects in the form of nonspecific pneumonia, obstructive bronchitis and pneumosclerosis.

In severe forms of ornithosis, recovery is slow, long-term (1.5–2.5 months) asthenic syndrome (tendency to hypotension, fatigue, vegetative-vascular changes—hyperhidrosis of the palms, tremor of the fingers), impaired respiratory function, residual changes in the lungs according to X-ray data are preserved. After ornithosis pneumonia, the pulmonary pattern may remain enhanced for several years.

The terms of patient discharge are determined by clinical recovery, not earlier than the 10th day of normal body temperature, normalization of X-ray and laboratory data, including cerebrospinal fluid sanation in meningitis. Approximate terms of temporary disability are 15–30 days.

C. psittaci detected as a monoinfection or in combination with *C. trachomatis*. This indicates a possible role of *C. psittaci* in the etiopathogenesis of trachoma [217].

The importance of *C. psittaci* and other chlamydiae in the development of cancer has been debated. The organism has been identified in MALT lymphomas of the ocular adnexa [218, 219]. It has been reported that patients with MALT lymphomas have *C. psittaci* in both tumour tissue [220] and peripheral blood mononuclear cells [218]. *C. psittaci* appears to be present as a viable bacterium in lymphomatous tumours [221], preferentially occurring in organs exposed to external antigen, where monocytes/macrophages may act as major reservoirs for the pathogen. It has been suggested that persistent *C. psittaci* infections may play a key role in the development of MALT lymphomas, supported by the fact that suppression of *C. psittaci* with doxycycline is accompanied by detectable regression of the lymphoma. MALT lymphomas are most frequently found in Germany (47%), the East Coast of the United States (35%) and the Netherlands (29%). Clearly, further studies are needed to demonstrate a causal relationship between the presence of *C. psittaci* in affected tissues and the development of MALT lymphomas [222].

Promising areas of research on ornithosis are as follows:

- Epidemiological studies: to identify epidemiological differences between *C. psittaci* and *C. trachomatis* to determine whether detection *of C. psittaci should be included* in routine clinical practice.
- Highly sensitive detection methods: to develop and optimize detection methods with higher sensitivity for rapid, accurate and convenient diagnosis of *C. psittaci infection.*
- Studies in cell or animal models: evaluate the need to use primates and non-human primates as experimental models and explore more cost-effective and ethical alternative animal models to study the mechanism of infection and therapeutic effects *of C. psittaci.*

Birds are the natural host of *C. psittaci*, but no studies have been conducted using avian cells. Although the prospects, utility and value of using avian cells are unclear, the feasibility of using avian cells or birds in *C. psittaci research has not been determined.*

- Identification and functional study of virulence factors: Further studies should focus on the virulence factors *of C. psittaci*, including specific proteins, lipopolysaccharides, secretion systems, etc., and how they affect the invasive capabilities of the bacterium and its survival in host cells. This will help to identify the specific mechanisms of disease pathogenesis [222–224].

Mortality during previous epidemic outbreaks reached 20–40%. The lungs are enlarged in volume and weight with atelectasis or pycnotic areas and numerous, poorly defined foci of consolidation, mostly lobular in nature, often merging with each other, sometimes capturing an entire lobe. Sometimes lobar pneumonia with dense fibrinous exudate occurs, without signs of its resorption. Histologically, there is severe plethora, sometimes thrombosis of the capillaries of the alveolar septa, which are thickened. The contents of the alveoli may be serous-haemorrhagic or with the participation of fibrin and leukocytes. A significant number of macrophages are large in size, with division figures, partly hyperchromic nuclei, vacuolated cytoplasm. In the cytoplasm are phagocytized erythrocytes, nuclear detritus, elementary bodies. The accompanying bacterial infection leads to purulent changes. In experimental psittacosis of monkeys, McGavran established that the process in the lungs begins with the respiratory bronchioles and reaches its maximum extent on the 14–16th day after infection, the resorption of exudate ends on the 5th week. Inclusions were determined in the cytoplasm of the alveolar epithelium and mononuclear cells [224].

In the myocardium, there are dystrophic changes, small haemorrhages, oedema of the interstitial tissue with accumulation of large mononuclear cells [225, 226].

5.5 Arthropathy Associated with Chlamydial Infection

The problem of joint damage associated with the inflammatory process in the genitourinary tract is one of the important sections of modern medicine. Most researchers attach key importance *to C. trachomatis* in the development of this pathology [227, 228].

It is an obligate intracellular microbe with adaptation to existence inside and outside the cell. Urogenital chlamydial infection (UCI) is one of the most common sexually transmitted infections and affects mainly young people. Despite its long history and numerous publications, the incidence of arthropathies against the background of UCI both in Russia and abroad has not been reliably established [229–231].

Studies in the United States of patients who underwent UCI showed that 3.0–8.1% of patients developed arthritis [232, 233]. At the same time, the role of *C. pneumoniae* in these lesions requires evaluation.

Many aspects of this complex pathology remain unclear and insufficiently studied [230, 231, 233]. CI may not only be a trigger for the development of reactive arthritis, but also be the cause of "septic" inflammation of the joints. According to various authors, the pathogen forms a primary inflammatory focus in the genitourinary tract and with the development of the inflammatory process, failure of nonspecific resistance factors, haematogenous dissemination of *Chlamydia* occurs with damage to various organs and tissues [234, 235].

After the pathogen penetrates the joint cavity, synovial membrane or periarticular tissues, chlamydial synovitis and arthritis develop. *Chlamydia* can infect chondrocytes and cause their death, which over time can lead to cartilage destruction and joint dysfunction. Detection of DNA and RNA, as well as metabolically active *Chlamydia species* spp. in the joints has created a terminological and nosological problem. At the same time, there are significant disagreements on the issue of the diagnostic significance of individual clinical manifestations [230, 231, 233]. Many experts are convinced that the presence of manifestations of arthritis is necessary for the diagnosis of arthropathy. There are differences of opinion on the issue of what type of joint damage is related to the diagnosis of "reactive arthritis" (ReA). Most authors advocate the presence of oligoarthritis (inflammation of 2–3 joints) or monoarthritis, but others believe that any variant is possible, including polyarthritis (inflammation of 4 or more joints) [233].

Given the diversity of symptoms, in which articular syndrome predominates, patients, as a rule, seek help from different specialists and undergo treatment with different diagnoses. This prevents adequate therapy, especially in the early stages of the pathological process, as well as the implementation of measures to prevent the development of systemic manifestations of urogenital chlamydia. The position that joint damage against the background of urogenital infections is an integral part of the group of spondyloarthropathies (SpA) remains valid and, therefore, should correspond to the known features of this group of diseases both in clinical and immunogenetic (association with HLA-B27) manifestations. However, HLA-B27 is detected only in 60–80% of patients [91, 236].

The issue of etiotropic therapy of UHI as a cause of arthropathy is also currently debatable worldwide. Optimal therapy periods for various forms and types of arthropathy have not yet been determined. Sometimes only chronicization of the process is achieved against the background of relief of the main clinical symptoms without final sanitation of the affected tissues from *Chlamydia* [233]. The lack of clinical guidelines and, therefore, physician awareness, also perpetuates this problem.

Thus, the study of various variants of the course of inflammatory joint diseases, against the background of UHI and the evolution of the disease, the determination of prognostic significant factors is of great practical importance for the development of a system of the most rational therapeutic measures for each individual patient.

We have analysed the results of our own studies on inflammatory joint diseases against the background of CI. Personal experience was accumulated through direct consultation and management of a large sample of patients with this pathology over 25 years in various medical organizations in St. Petersburg [12]. When diagnosing arthropathy, we took into account the presence of a connection between the development of joint syndrome and urogenital symptoms: 80% of patients had previous urogenital pathology at the time of inclusion in the study, and 20% indicated the presence of genitourinary diseases in their anamnesis.

The association between infections and joint inflammation has existed since ancient times, and in the time of Hippocrates (c. 460 BC), the presence of joint inflammation in young men after their first sexual experience was already described. This implied the presence of septic or reactive arthritis, possibly secondary to a gonococcal infection, either of intestinal or urogenital origin. Apparently the first known description of urethro-oculosynovial syndrome was given in 1496 by one of Columbus's physicians [237]. Descriptions of similar patients were found in the literature later on: Pieter van Forest (1507), Pierre Martin de la Martiniere (1664), T. Sydenham (1686), W. Musgrave (1715), M. Stoll (1776), F. Swediaur's (1798), B. Brody (1818), E. Vidal (1893), N. Fiessinger, H. Leroy (1916), I. Paronen (1948), V. Wright, W. B. Reed (1964) [238]. In Russia, the first descriptions were presented in 1900 by V. Stanislavsky. After the isolation of the causative agent of gonorrhoea by A. Neisser in 1879, a group of people with arthritis was identified within the framework of disseminated gonococcal infection.

Reiter's syndrome/disease "also became widespread and was used to describe arthritis in combination with conjunctivitis, urethritis and possible lesions of the skin and mucous membranes that developed after a previous intestinal or genitourinary infection. In recent years, this term has fallen out of use for obvious reasons [238–240].

The term "reactive arthritis" was proposed in 1969 by Finnish authors. P. Ahvonen et al. described ReA induced by *Yersinia* infection, characterized clinical symptoms, including extra-articular ones, and verified the pathogen using serological methods. The type of etiologic association determined the approach to terminology used to describe joint lesions [229]. The introduction of the term "reactive arthritis" to denote joint inflammation observed after infection with *Y.enterocolitica* or *C.trachomatis* and some other pathogens, in which the pathogen can be isolated from the synovial fluid extremely rarely, and the association with HLA-B27 became historical milestones for the classification and attribution of the former Reiter's syndrome to spondyloarthritis.

According to the Russian Ministry of Health, in 2019, the primary incidence of reactive arthritis (ReA) amongst the adult population ranged from 10.1 to 57.2 cases per 100 thousand population, with significant differences across federal districts [230, 241]. Data from foreign studies are also contradictory. In Norway, the incidence of urogenic ReA is 4–5 per 100 thousand, which is similar to the situation in Finland and the USA [233, 242].

In Sweden, the annual incidence of reactive arthritis is 28 cases per 100,000 people. In Germany, 30% of patients with asymptomatic arthritis ReA was diagnosed with chlamydial infection, and *C. trachomatis* was detected in 42% of cases of undifferentiated spondyloarthritis [243].

In the Middle East and Africa region, a lack of epidemiological data has prevented researchers from estimating prevalence [233].

The main reason for the differences in epidemiological data in statistical reports of individual regions of the Russian Federation and other countries, according to most authors, is the lack of a unified classification and generally accepted diagnostic criteria for the disease [230, 233]. Arthropathy occurs more often in individuals aged 18 to 40 years, with a peak at the age of 20 to 29 years. However, children are also considered a target, but their prevalence is low. The risk of developing arthropathy against the background of genitourinary infections is higher in men than in women, with a ratio of 9:1 [235]. The research groups that determined the main stages of implementing approaches to the terminology and classification of ReA were predominantly European.

The relationship between infection and arthritis was critically reviewed at a symposium organized by WHO and the Arthritis and Rheumatism Research Council in London in 1974. The consensus document classified the relationship between infection and joint disease into four main categories [244].

Group 1 (infectious arthritis or septic arthritis) was defined by the presence of infection in the body and identification of the infectious agent or microbial product in the joint. Group 2 (postinfectious arthritis) was characterized by the presence of infection and identification of bacterial antigens in the joint (e.g. arthritis secondary to meningococcemia). Group 3, ReA, was defined as an inflammatory process of the joint in which there is a known history of infection in the genitourinary tract or in the intestine, but the causative agent or its products are not detected in the joints. Group 4 was characterized by a joint syndrome (inflammatory process) in the absence of a history of infectious disease and in which neither the infectious agent nor its products or antigens are detected or identified in the joint (e.g. rheumatoid arthritis) [244].

The literature also contains the terms "urogenic reactive arthritis," "sexually acquired arthritis"—SARA (sexually acquired reactive arthritis), "chlamydial arthritis," "*Chlamydia*-induced arthropathy" [229, 245].

But only molecular biological studies opened up a new pathogenetic understanding of ReA, through the intra-articular detection of waste products of various microorganisms. Therefore, it was proposed to abandon the distinction between post-infectious arthritis and ReA and to prefer the term "ReA" for both [237]. This gave rise to a terminological and nosological problem.

On the one hand, there are generally accepted diagnostic criteria for classical HLA-B27-associated ReA, classified as SpA. At the same time, a significant number of patients with this pathology are not carriers of HLA-B27. The ambiguity of the name reflects the continuing imprecision and low level of objectivity of clinical and epidemiological studies of this phenomenon. On the other hand, an increasing number of pathogens are considered triggers of arthritis and are also considered under the term "ReA" (Table 5.2). Since the beginning of the SARS-CoV-2 pandemic, cases of acute arthritis have been described that have also been classified as ReA due to comparable clinical features [229].

The course of CI, both in general and in cases of joint damage, is largely determined by the ability of the pathogen to form aberrant (persistent) forms. The presence of these forms is associated with a number of problems in the examination and treatment of patients [246, 247].

"Persistence" is a term intended primarily to denote altered metabolic and other characteristics underlying the altered developmental cycle, and at the same time reflecting the tendency of microorganisms to long-term infection of tissues at the sites of their spread [57, 248, 249]. *Chlamydia* in the persistent state are characterized by high resistance to antibacterial therapy. In principle, *Chlamydia* can be determined in the joint fluid (Fig. 5.14).

Dissemination of *C. trachomatis* from the primary site of infection is due to their penetration into polymorphonuclear leukocytes, monocytes and dendritic cells. Circulating cells carry the pathogen and initiate both inflammation and an immune response to infection, which is accompanied by the expression of co-stimulatory molecules and the secretion of proinflammatory cytokines. Chlamydiosis is characterized by the ability to long-term persistence—maintaining viability without the production of infectious bodies, both in monocytes and in human dendritic cells, which is accompanied by an increase in the expression of the Ct604 gene, encoding the heat shock protein HSP 60, which is involved in maintaining the state of persistence [250].

The complex network of cytokines that mediate the pathological process will vary depending on the stage of the disease. In the acute phase, bacterial clearance may be facilitated by the production of IL-12, IL-23, and IL-6, as well as IFN γ and IL-17. Regulatory T cells may produce IL-10, which may lead to bacterial persistence in the mucosa. If the disease becomes chronic, IL-6, IL-17, IFN γ and TNF α may lead to chronic inflammation in the joint. This inflammation may be enhanced by the persistence of bacterial antigens in the joint [57, 251].

Table 5.2 Infectious agents that are rare triggers for reactive arthritis

Entry gate of infection	Microbial agent	Microbial products in the joint	Presence of HLA-B27
Urogenital tract	*G. vaginalis*	No data	Yes
	HIV	Positive culture, a single case	Yes, amongst Caucasians
	M. genitalium/ hominis/orale	DNA, coinfections	Yes, an isolated case
	N.gonorrhoeae[a]	DNA	No
	U. urealyticum	DNA, coinfections	No
Gastrointestinal tract	*Blastocystosis*[a]	No data	Yes, an isolated case
	C. difficile	No data	No
	C.cayetanensis[a]	No data	No
	E. coli	No data	Yes, there are several cases
	H. alvei	No data	No
	H. pylori	No data	No
	Microsporidia	Antigens, DNA, positive culture	Yes, an isolated case
	Strongyloides stercoralis[a]	Larva and antigen in synovial membrane, single case	Yes, an isolated case
	T. whippelii[b]	DNA, rRNA, positive culture	No
	Cryptosporidium	No data	No
	E.histolytica[a]	Positive culture, a single case	No
	E.hartmanni[a]	No data	Yes, an isolated case
	G. lamblia[a]	No data	Yes, there are several cases
Respiratory tract	*β-hemolytic Group A streptococcus*	No data	Yes, there are several cases
	M. tuberculosis[a]	Synovial T cells reactive to mycobacterial heat shock protein 65 kDa	Yes, there are several cases
	M.pneumoniae	No data	Yes, there are several cases
	N. meningitidis	Immune complexes	Yes, an isolated case
Leather, soft tissues	*B. henselae*	No data	No
	B. burgdorferi[b]	DNA	No
	P. acnes	Positive culture	Yes, an isolated case
	P.aeruginosa	DNA	No
	R. conorii[a]	Immune complexes	No
	S.aureus	No data	Yes, there are several cases
	S.epidermidis	No data	There is a single case
	S.haemolyticus	No data	Yes, an isolated case

[a]Effective antimicrobial therapy for ReA has been documented in case reports
[b]Effective antimicrobial therapy for ReA has been confirmed by double-blind controlled studies

A special place in the etiopathogenesis of arthritis, according to a number of researchers (Yeoh N., Burton JP, Suppiah P., Reid G., Stebbings S.), is occupied by the intestinal microflora. This direction remains developing and may become the key to new therapeutic interventions in the future. There is a complex relationship between the immune system and the intestinal microbiome [252]. Intestinal dysbiosis promotes an increase in the translocation of the intestinal wall for microorganisms that make up the intestinal microbiocenosis and their molecular components, stimulates the mechanism of translocation of intestinal microbiota components and immune cells into the joints, leading to the development and intensification of the inflammatory process in reactive and infectious arthritis [252].

In terms of pathogenesis, clinical picture and course, arthropathy against the background of UHI is similar to both sexually transmitted infections and diffuse connective tissue diseases [253]. The disease is characterized by a variety of clinical manifestations and variability of the course. The most common clinical picture of ReA is usually the acute form. Some patients recover spontaneously within the first 6 months, whilst others (10–30% of patients) usually develop chronic ReA. Depending on the form (acute or chronic), ReA is characterized by joint and extra-articular symptoms. Chronic ReA, along with peripheral arthritis, is characterized by sacroiliitis and damage to the visual organs [233].

Joint syndrome is the leading one in this pathology, as it determines the severity of the inflammatory process, its course and prognosis. The variety of clinical manifestations of arthropathy fits into 4 clinical variants: arthralgia; mono- and oligoarthritis; spondyloarthritis; polyarthritis. According to the duration of joint syndrome, the following are distinguished: acute course (joint syndrome up to 2 months); subacute (joint pain up to a year); chronic (duration of the disease more than 12 months).

The clinical form of arthropathy, occurring in the form of arthralgia, is characterized by the appearance of pain in the joints that is not intense, but painful, persistent or recurring, sometimes migrating, limiting the range of motion and tolerance to stress mainly in the lower limbs. At the same time, no visual changes in the joints are observed. There is no swelling, hyperaemia and hyperthermia, that is, there are no signs of arthritis and synovitis. This clinical picture is explained by the pathology of the tendons (enthesitis and enthesopathies), and not by damage to the tissues of the joint itself, its synovial membrane. The most common manifestations of enthesiopathies are pain in the heel (talalgia) and in the Achilles tendon, caused by calcaneal bursitis and Achilles bursitis. Dactylitis of one or more toes often develops with the formation of a sausage-shaped deformation, which is the result of inflammatory changes in the periarticular structures. In some cases, amyotrophy develops quite quickly.

Arthropathy, occurring as mono- (10%) or oligoarthritis (70%), is the most common. The typical picture of the disease is when the joints are affected, but the spine and sacroiliac joints are not involved in the process. As a rule, the joint syndrome is of a ladder- like nature with all the signs of arthritis and synovitis. The pain is intense both in the projection of the affected joint and around it, and may be accompanied by fever, mainly in the evening. More typical is the development of periarticular oedema, to a greater extent along the ligamentous apparatus and at the sites of tendon attachment.

An ambiguously interpreted form of arthropathy is polyarthritis (10–14%). Joint syndrome can begin with any joint of the upper and lower extremities. It is important to take into account the asymmetry of the process in the clinical and, especially, radiological sense. The same ladder-like type of lesion is characteristic, only in this case not one, but more than four joints or a group of joints are affected.

The most affected joints are the knee (52.12–64.7%), ankle joint (50–57%), metatarsophalangeal joint (41–48%) and wrist joint (44–48%) [12, 233].

Damage to the sciatic joints and/or spine is preferably confirmed by MRI examination)—a group of diseases when the patient's peripheral joints and spine are affected. Pain in the lower back and rigidity of the corresponding muscles are typical for the onset of the disease; signs of sacroiliitis are observed in 10–14% of patients.

Studies by various authors have shown that synovial tissue samples from patients with confirmed ReA were positive for ocular (trachoma) but not genital serovars, the latter of which were thought to cause ReA after urogenital infections [11, 254]. This observation led to the suggestion that ocular strains are arthritogenic and probably more prone to dissemination than genital strains; this may also explain the fact that many patients develop ocular disease.

Lesions of the visual organ occur in 20–25% of patients with chlamydial arthropathy. The occurrence of ophthalmopathy is one of the early signs of the disease. They often occur in the form of conjunctivitis (up to 90% of cases) and are manifested by eye pain, photophobia, blepharospasm, dry eye syndrome, and develop following inflammation of the urogenital system and can disappear after 2–3 days (but still more often after 2–3 weeks). In other cases, iritis, iridocyclitis and keratitis are diagnosed, much less often choroiditis, hypopyon, hyphema, corneal ulceration, cataract, glaucoma and even diffuse eye damage leading to vision loss. It should be noted that amongst patients with anterior uveitis, chlamydial infection is diagnosed in every fifth case. Rarely, corneal ulceration and keratitis may be observed; optic neuritis and posterior uveitis have been described.

Of the skin manifestations, the most frequently observed are blennorrhagic keratoderma, circinate balanitis, aphthous ulcers (up to 60%) and erythema nodosum (rare). Keratoderma occurs in 20% of patients with ReA. Circinate balanitis occurs in 10–40% of ReA cases.

Pericarditis is more common in the chronic stage of ReA, whilst heart block and valvular disease may occur in acute ReA.

Opinions on the combination of the triad ("urethro—oculo -synovial syndrome") or tetrad (+ lesions of the skin and mucous membranes) differ these days. In cases of incomplete form, verification of the diagnosis is significantly more complicated. In domestic and American classifications of rheumatic diseases, it is designated as arthritis combined with spondylitis (spondyloarthritis); a number of authors classify the disease as spondyloarthritis, others consider it one of the forms of reactive arthritis.

Evaluation of the activity of inflammatory phenomena in joint damage against the background of CI is a complex problem. Common laboratory parameters (ESR, C-reactive protein, sialic acids) are not informative enough and often (54.5%) do not correspond to the severity of clinical manifestations of the disease. The results of the study of synovial fluid are nonspecific and are characteristic of inflammatory arthritis with an increased number of leukocytes (usually from 2000 to 4000 leukocytes per ml) with a predominance of neutrophils.

Laboratory diagnostics of CI includes a number of methodological approaches. Polymerase chain reaction is most often used, the immunofluorescence method has not lost its importance and only in some laboratories, the culture method of diagnostics is used. Serological blood testing for the determination of immunoglobulins IgG, IgM, IgA to *C. trachomatis* is also available.

Serologic testing for *C. trachomatis* is of limited value due to serologic cross-reactivity between *C. trachomatis* and *C. pneumoniae*, inability to differentiate past from current infection, and the absence of antibodies or the presence of low titres in lower urinary tract infections. Patients are serologic positive and negative based on antibody production. The absence of antibodies in a patient's serum is a prognostically unfavourable marker for the course of the disease [252].

The diversity of methodological possibilities, on the one hand, contributes to improving the quality of diagnostics and, on the other hand, leads to different interpretations of patient examination results by specialists. None of the listed methodological approaches ensure 100% reliability of the results obtained in this category of patients. To unify the interpretation of examination results, it is proposed to use diagnostic algorithms, but they can hardly be considered flawless. Therefore, today, it is advisable to consider the complex use of two methods based on different principles as the "gold standard." The choice of diagnostic method for CI should be significantly influenced by the clinical form of the disease: the nature of the inflammation (acute, chronic) and topical diagnosis (in men—urethritis, epididymitis, orchiepididymitis, prostatitis, paraurethritis and proctitis; in women —cervicitis, urethritis, bartholinitis, cystitis, salpingitis, salpingo-oophoritis, endometritis, pelvic peritonitis; as well as conjunctivitis, nasopharyngitis, respiratory allergosis), the prevalence of the inflammatory process—generalized (common) forms of *Chlamydia* (urethra-oculosynovial syndrome), the purpose of the examination (laboratory confirmation of the diagnosis or mass screening of risk groups). There is a high dependence of the research results on the following factors: compliance with the requirements for the technique of collecting clinical material from primary and secondary foci of chlamydial infection by the doctor lesions; correct storage and delivery of material to the laboratory; timely conduct of the study; logistical support for the laboratory study; the level of qualification of the medical personnel conducting the study, etc.

The possibility of the presence of coinfection with *C. pneumoniae* and *C. trachomatis* has been established in the synovial fluid of patients with rheumatoid arthritis, suggesting their synergism in the development of inflammation in the joint [147, 255].

Reports of mixed infections *with Chlamydia, T. vaginalis, M. hominis, U. urealyticum, B. fragilis* in patients, as well as our own studies (A.L. Poznyak) indicate the need to study the impact of co-infections on clinical and laboratory diagnostics and treatment of arthritis [256]. Arthritogenic potential data pathogens are not fully studied [11].

A positive result for chlamydial nucleic acids by polymerase chain reaction (PCR) in a joint is probably of diagnostic importance, but current methods used to detect *Chlamydia* in the genitourinary tract are not validated for diagnostic purposes in synovial specimens.

The percentage of complications leading to disability in joint damage is the highest amongst all extragenital pathologies of CI [257]. There is insufficient data on the long-term results of monitoring patients, the dynamics and outcome of the joint syndrome. In approximately 15–20% of cases, the disease becomes chronic, requiring constant treatment. There is a risk that arthropathy can lead to chronic destructive arthritis [258]. However, the hypothesis that early effective etiotropic treatment of CI prevents the development of joint damage requires further study [229].

A 2019 Canadian Rheumatology Review found that nonsteroidal anti-inflammatory drugs were used as first-line treatment for reactive arthritis in all cases, and intra-articular steroid injections and disease-modifying antirheumatic drugs were common. Two-thirds of practitioners reported occasional or frequent use of monoclonal antibodies in chronic forms. The use of TNF inhibitor biologics represents the most significant change in the therapeutic management of reactive arthritis in recent years [229]. A randomized trial comparing two antibiotic combinations (doxycycline + rifampicin and azithromycin + rifampicin) with placebo for 6 months in 42 patients with chronic ReA infected with *Chlamydia* (PCR positive) showed a higher percentage of patients with its effectiveness. The response to the antibiotic combination was higher than to placebo (63% vs. 20%) [229].

C. trachomatis are capable *of* persisting for many years in the monocytes of the synovial tissue of the joint, which necessitates a differentiated approach to the treatment of such lesions. It is obvious that the synovial tissue in this case is not sterile, with persistent *C. trachomatis*, in which the development cycle stops at a late stage of elementary body formation, the number of which decreases and aberrant forms of reticular bodies are formed. *Chlamydia* in the state of persistence are characterized by high resistance to antibacterial therapy, and amongst the biovariants of *C. trachomatis*, persistence in synovial tissue is characteristic of serovars that cause eye diseases, which is assumed to be due to more effective dissemination of these serovars from the primary infection site.

The use of animal models that allow control of the time between infection and the onset of joint syndrome may allow progress in understanding the mechanisms of the disease on the one hand and in evaluating new treatments on the other

[259]. New pathophysiological data will shed light on the interactions amongst microbiological agents, HLA-B27, mucosal and intestinal microbiota, cell subsets and cytokine production.

An important area of promising clinical and applied research is the development of scientifically based diagnostic criteria covering the entire spectrum of pathogens known today, which is important for understanding the pathophysiology of these lesions, analysing the characteristics of the clinical course depending on the trigger factors for the formation of structural changes in the joints and spine.

The development of new practical and sensitive methods for detecting *Chlamydia* in blood samples will allow simpler, faster and more specific diagnostics in patients from whom joint samples cannot be obtained.

Future studies of the pathogen–host interaction in relation to the intestinal microbiome promise to make an important contribution to elucidating the pathogenesis of the disease. To date, the role of microbial factors, primarily the intestinal microbiome, in the development of reactive and infectious arthritis has been proven.

Advances in recent decades, particularly in the identification of infectious agents and their antigens using molecular biology, genetic and immunological tests, make it necessary to clarify the relationship between infection and arthritis.

The expansion of the use of the term "ReA" in the literature contradicts the generally accepted classification of spondyloarthritis: even if from a historical point of view, the original distinction between reactive and post-infectious arthritis is no longer justified.

Comprehensive clinical and laboratory studies, including synovial fluid, blood cell testing for chlamydemia and careful patient monitoring, are necessary to differentiate chlamydial joint lesions from diseases that may have similar clinical features. Further and, importantly, additional studies are needed to determine the wide variety of arthritis pathogens.

New classification and diagnostic criteria, as well as updated treatment recommendations, are needed to improve our understanding of this pathology.

5.6 Periodontitis (Together with A.F. Eliseeva)

Amongst periodontal diseases, the first place belongs to chronic generalized periodontitis (CGP). The leading role in the formation of the inflammatory process in the oral cavity belongs to resistant obligate anaerobic and microaerophilic microflora. The influence of cardiovascular diseases on dental diseases has been discussed in the works of scientists in many countries. It has often been noted that patients with cardiovascular pathology experience changes in the haemodynamics of both the periodontium and the body as a whole. At the same time, the presence of foci of chronic infection in the oral cavity (in particular, periodontal pockets, abundant supra- and subgingival dental deposits) can affect the systemic health of the human body. Numerous studies have proven an increased risk of developing cardiovascular diseases with poor oral hygiene and the presence of inflammatory periodontal diseases, which is explained by the effect of the chronic inflammatory process on the rheological properties of the blood. An important feature of the functioning of the organs and tissues of the oral cavity is the fact that everything that happens in the mouth is carried out in the constant presence of various associations of microorganisms, which are either the cause or participant in pathological processes in the body.

Over the past decades of research, there have been reports of an association between inflammation in periodontal tissues and cardiovascular pathology. In the last decade, there have been a large number of studies on the relationship between the degree of damage to the periodontal complex and a number of somatic diseases, primarily cardiovascular diseases.

When examining periodontal biopsy material in patients with ischaemic heart disease and atherosclerosis, we determine the following changes: pronounced inflammatory infiltrate, cellular elements are located both within the epithelial layer and in the proper plate of the gingival mucosa in the form of diffuse infiltration, single elements are located intraepithelially, pronounced acanthosis. There is a significant infiltration by leukocytes: polymorphic cells with a predominance of neutrophils.

Morphological changes in the coronary vessels are similar, but microscopically less informative, due to the peculiarity of the structure, and are manifested, as a rule: vasculitis, oedema, infiltration of mast cells and monocytes. In the control group in periodontal biopsies, the cells of the inflammatory infiltrate are located exclusively in the proper plate of the gingival mucosa with a tendency to perivascular localization, acanthosis is weakly expressed. The inflammatory infiltrate, in most cases moderate: it is composed of exclusively mononuclear with the dominance of lymphocytes and macrophages. During the morphological study in both groups, a wide microbial spectrum was detected. The data are confirmed by PCR diagnostics. In the microbial associations of periodontal pockets, representatives classified by WHO as specific pathogens of periodontal infection dominate: Porphyromonas gingivalis, treponema denticole, tannerella forcythensis. Along with periodontopathogens, we have identified *Chlamydia trachomatis* in a large percentage of studies, which was an unexpected finding for us. Thus, in the group with combined pathology, the presence of *Chlamydia trachomatis* was detected in 88% of cases, without cardio-vascular diseases pathology, it was detected in 76% of observations. In patients who had suffered a myocardial infarction, a high prevalence of chlamydial infection was most often noted. The authors also identified a familial nature of cardiovascular pathology, in particular, coronary heart disease, which may probably be associated with early infection of children in families where parents suffer from various forms of chlamydial infection. Diagnosis of *Chlamydia trachomatis* was confirmed by a morphological method when staining the biopsy with PAS and Romanovsky, real-time PCR and immunofluorescence testing.

Example

Patient M., 46 years old. Considers himself ill since 2006, when weakness and squeezing chest pains first appeared. During the year, he noted minor pressing pains in the heart area, but did not consult a doctor. Pathogenetic therapy was not carried out. He has noted periodontal diseases for 15 years and a familial nature of the diseases. He has not been seen by a dentist: periodontist. At the time of examination, the patient complained of bleeding, sore gums, loose teeth and bad breath.

Main diagnosis: Ischaemic heart disease: angina pectoris III–IV FC. intramural anterior widespread MI from 2009. Paroxysmal form of atrial fibrillation. Hypertension stage III. Chronic generalized periodontitis of severe severity.

Research results and analysis data: The patient does not smoke. Height 178 cm, weight 75 kg. Normosthenic constitution. Heart sounds on auscultation are muffled, rhythmic. No murmurs. Heart rate is 74 per minute. The borders of the heart on percussion are expanded to the left by 1.5 cm. Peripheral oedema is not pronounced. Working pressure 130/100 mm Hg. An increase in blood pressure is observed up to 150/115 mm Hg.

Clinical examination revealed: mucous membrane of interdental papillae and gingival margin is oedematous, hyperaemic, bleeds on probing. Gum colour is pink. Mucous membrane is dry, tongue is coated with plaque, hyperplasia of filiform and fungiform papillae. Exposure of tooth necks, non-carious lesions of hard tissues, accompanied by hyperesthesia. Periodontal pockets up to 6.5 mm are probed, discharge from the periodontal pocket is serous—purulent. There is a periodontal abscess, multiple soft and hard supra and subgingival dental deposits. There is grade III tooth mobility. Gum recession according to Miller P. D. (1985) III. On the orthopantomogram, uneven bone resorption is more than 1/3. Severe periodontitis is diagnosed. PCR data (Table 5.3).

Table 5.3 PCR data

Aggregatibacteria actinomycetemcomitans	+
Porphyromonas gingivalis	+
Tannerella forcythensis	–
Treponema denticola	–
Prevotella intermedia	+
Chlamydia trachomatis	+ +

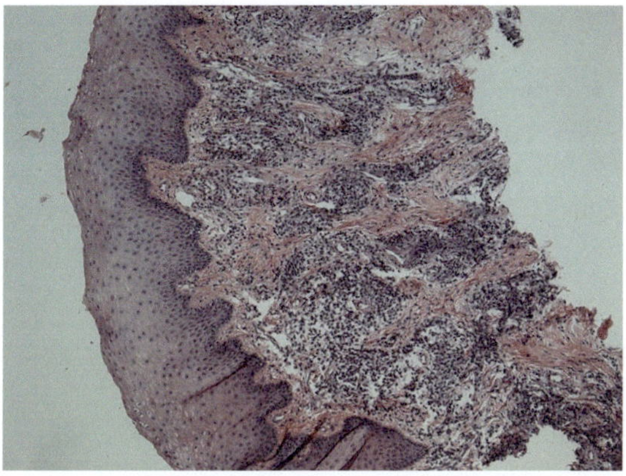

Fig. 5.15 Periodontal biopsy of patient M., 46 years old. Pronounced mononuclear infiltration. Haematoxylin and eosin staining, magnification 100

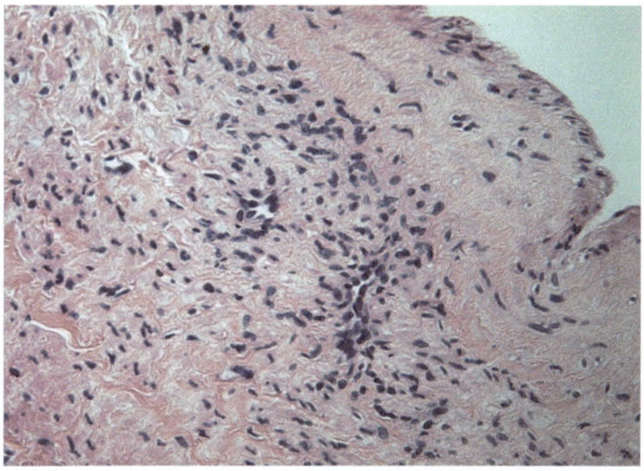

Fig. 5.17 Biopsy of coronary vessels in the same patient. Mononuclear infiltration of the coronary artery wall. Haematoxylin and eosin staining, magnification 340

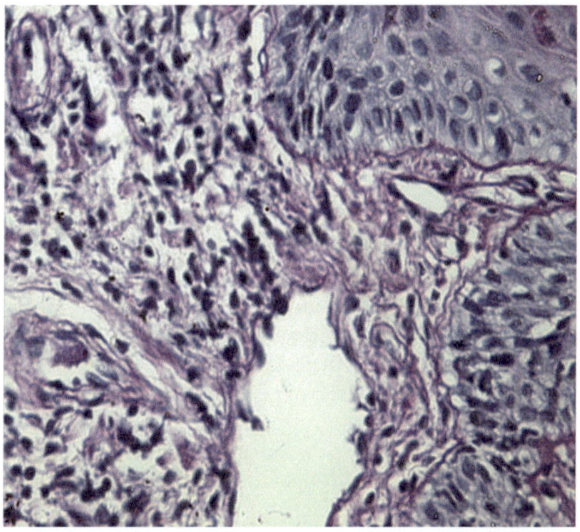

Fig. 5.16 Periodontal biopsy of patient M., 46 years old. Mononuclear infiltration with intracytoplasmic PAS-positive inclusions PAS staining, magnification 640

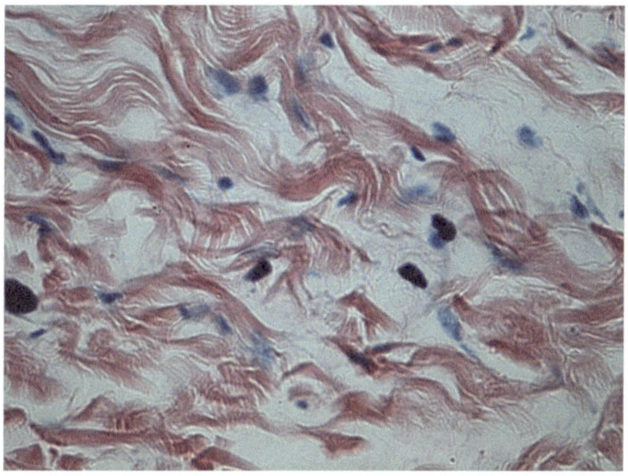

Fig. 5.18 Biopsy of coronary vessels of patient M., 46 years old. An increased number of mast cells are visible. Romanovsky staining, magnification 340

Histological examination of periodontal biopsy significant inflammatory infiltration with predominantly mononuclear infiltration was revealed (Fig. 5.15). Extra- and intracellular PAS-positive inclusions were determined (Fig. 5.16). On the coronary, in the artery biopsy of the same patient, mononuclear inflammatory infiltration was also found (Fig. 5.17) with the detection of mast cells in the vessel wall (Fig. 5.18).

Conclusion, *Chlamydia trachomatis* is capable of exerting a pathological effect on the vessel walls directly and indirectly, but its role in the aetiology of cardiovascular diseases requires additional, more in-depth studies. Since the microbial factor is dominant in the aetiology of periodontitis, we have suggested a mixed nature of the infection. In the vessels, especially in both the periodontium and coronary arteries, an inflammatory reaction of varying severity is expressed, which occurs in 94% of cases against the background of an immunopathological reaction.

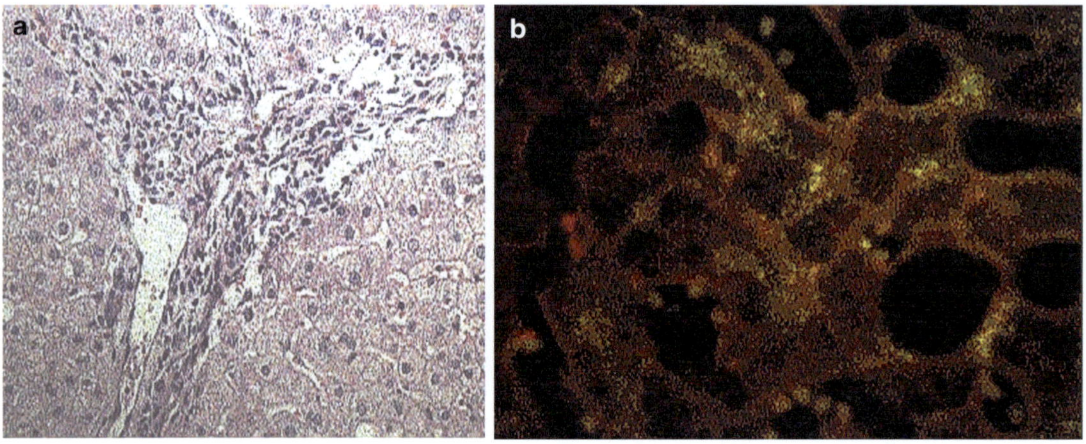

Fig. 5.19 Observation with long-term hepatitis of probable chlamydial aetiology. (**a**) Haematoxylin-eosin staining. Magnification 200. (**b**) Direct immunofluorescence. Magnification 1000

5.7 Other Organ Lesions

There are isolated publications that demonstrate the possibility of detecting *Chlamydia* in serous membranes (peritonitis) [260].

In some cases, we have determined the chlamydial aetiology of lymphadenitis and hepatitis in the long-term course of inflammatory processes of previously unknown aetiology (Fig. 5.19).

References

1. Trabert B, Waterboer T, Idahl A, et al. Antibodies against Chlamydia trachomatis and ovarian cancer risk in two independent populations. J Natl Cancer Inst. 2019;111(2):129–36. https://doi.org/10.1093/jnci/djy084.
2. Franchini APA, Iskander B, Anwer F. The role of Chlamydia trachomatis in the pathogenesis of cervical cancer. Cureus. 2022;14(1):e21331. https://doi.org/10.7759/cureus.21331.
3. Honkila M, Wikstrom E, Renko M, et al. Probability of vertical transmission of Chlamydia trachomatis estimated from national registry data. Sex Trans Infect. 2017;93(6):416–20. https://doi.org/10.1136/sextrans-2016-052884.
4. White JA, Dukers-Muijrers NH, Hoebe CJ, et al. European guideline on the management of Chlamydia trachomatis. Int J STD AIDS. 2025;2025:9564624251323678. https://doi.org/10.1177/09564624251323678.
5. Nwokolo NC, Dragovic B, Patel S, et al. 2015 UK national guideline for the management of infection with Chlamydia trachomatis. Int J STD AIDS. 2016;27(4):251–67. https://doi.org/10.1177/0956462415615443.
6. Zhou Z, Tian Q, Wang L, et al. Chlamydia spreads to the large intestine lumen via multiple pathways. Infect Immun. 2021;89(10):e0025421. https://doi.org/10.1128/IAI.00254-21.
7. El-Din AN, Sorour H, Fattouh M, El-Hamd MA. Evaluation of the role of Chlamydia trachomatis in primary male infertility. Int J Clin Pract. 2021;75(10):e14702. https://doi.org/10.1111/ijcp.14702.
8. Rodrigues R, Sousa C, Barros A, Vale N. Chlamydia trachomatis: from urogenital infections to the pathway of infertility. Genes (Basel). 2025;16(2):205. https://doi.org/10.3390/genes16020205.
9. Moazenchi M, Totonchi M, Yazdi RS, et al. The impact of Chlamydia trachomatis infection on sperm parameters and male fertility: a comprehensive study. Int J STD AIDS. 2018;29(5):466–73. https://doi.org/10.1177/0956462417735245.
10. Sarkar K, Saini V. Current topics in Chlamydia trachomatis infections. In: Understanding sexually transmitted diseases—prevention, symptoms, and treatment options. https://doi.org/10.5772/intechopen.1007204.
11. Carlin E, Marzo-Ortega H, Flew S. British Association of Sexual Health and HIV national guideline on the management of sexually acquired reactive arthritis 2021. Int J STD AIDS. 2021;32(11):986–97. https://doi.org/10.1177/09564624211020266. Epub 2021 May 20
12. Lobzin YV, Sidorchuk SN, Poznyak AL. Clinical and laboratory diagnostics of chlamydia-induced arthropathies. Epidemiol Infect Dis. 2010;6:48–51.

13. Nishida H, Takahashi Y, Takehara K, et al. Chlamydia peritonitis mimicking juvenile carcinomatous peritonitis diagnosed by exploratory laparoscopy: a case report. Pathogens. 2023;12(1):94. https://doi.org/10.3390/pathogens12010094.
14. Wang L, Zhu C, Zhang T, et al. Nonpathogenic colonization with Chlamydia in the gastrointestinal tract as Oral vaccination for inducing transmucosal protection. Infect Immun. 2018;86(2):e00630-17. https://doi.org/10.1128/IAI.00630-17.
15. Howe SE, Shillova N, Konjufca V. Dissemination of Chlamydia from the reproductive tract to the gastro-intestinal tract occurs in stages and relies on Chlamydia transport by host cells. PLoS Pathog. 2019;15(12):e1008207. https://doi.org/10.1371/journal.ppat.1008207.
16. Bondareva NE, Koroleva EA, Zigangirova NA. The role of chlamydia colonization of the gastrointestinal tract in the development and maintenance of chronic chlamydial infections. Mol Genet Microbiol Virol. 2018;36(4):177–81. https://doi.org/10.17116/molgen201836041177 2020.
17. Zhong G. Chlamydia spreading from the genital to gastrointestinal tracts —a two-hit hypothesis. Trends Microbiol. 2018;26(7):611–23. https://doi.org/10.1016/j.tim.2017.12.002. Epub 2017 Dec 27
18. Rank RG, Yeruva L. Hidden in plain sight: chlamydial gastrointestinal infection and its relevance to persistence in human genital infection. Infect Immun. 2014;82(4):1362–71. https://doi.org/10.1128/IAI.01244-13. Epub 2014 Jan 13
19. Tian Q, Zhou Z, Wang L, et al. Gastrointestinal coinfection promotes chlamydial pathogenicity in the Genital Trac t. Infect Immun. 2020;88(4):e00905–19. https://doi.org/10.1128/IAI.00905-19. Print 2020 Mar 23
20. Lee Y-S, Lee K-S. Chlamydia and male lower urinary tract diseases. Korean J Urol. 2013;54(2):73–7. https://doi.org/10.4111/kju.2013.54.2.73.
21. Miller KE. Diagnosis and treatment of Chlamydia trachomatis infection. Am Fam Physic. 2006;73(8):1411–6.
22. Bryan ER, Kollipara A, Trim LK, et al. Hematogenous dissemination of Chlamydia muridarum from the urethra in macrophages causes testicular infection and sperm DNA damage. Biol Reprod. 2019;101(4):748–59. https://doi.org/10.1093/biolre/ioz146.
23. de Vries HJC, Nori AV, Larsen HK, et al. 2021 European guideline on the management of proctitis, proctocolitis and enteritis caused by sexually transmissible pathogens. J Eur Acad Dermatol Venereol. 2021;35(7):1434–43. https://doi.org/10.1111/jdv.17269.
24. Llata E, Braxton J, Asbel L, et al. Rectal Chlamydia trachomatis and Neisseria gonorrhoeae infections among women reporting anal intercourse. Obstet Gynecol. 2018;132(3):692–7. https://doi.org/10.1097/AOG.0000000000002804.
25. Chandra NL, Broad C, Folkard K, et al. Detection of Chlamydia trachomatis in rectal specimens in women and its association with anal intercourse: a systematic review and meta-analysis. Sex Transm Infect. 2018;94(5):320–6. https://doi.org/10.1136/sextrans-2017-053161.
26. Karlsson A, Österlund A, Forssén A. Pharyngeal Chlamydia trachomatis is not uncommon any more. Scand J Infect Dis. 2011;43(5):344–8. https://doi.org/10.3109/00365548.2011.553243.
27. Chan PA, Robinette A, Montgomery M, et al. Extragenital infections caused by Chlamydia trachomatis and Neisseria gonorrhoeae: a review of the literature. Infect Dis Obstet Gynecol. 2016;2016:5758387. https://doi.org/10.1155/2016/5758387.
28. Petrovay F, Németh I, Balázs A, Balla E, et al. Chlamydial conjunctivitis: prevalence and serovar distribution of Chlamydia trachomatis in adults. J Med Microbiol. 2015;64(9):967–70. https://doi.org/10.1099/jmm.0.000115.
29. Satpathy G, Behera HS, Ahmed NH. Chlamydial eye infections: current perspectives. Review. Indian J Ophthalmol. 2017;65(2):97–102. https://doi.org/10.4103/ijo.IJO_870_16.
30. den Heijer CDJ, Hoebe CJPA. Driessen JHM Chlamydia trachomatis and the risk of pelvic inflammatory disease, ectopic pregnancy, and female infertility: a retrospective cohort. Clin Infect Dis. 2019;69(9):1517–25. https://doi.org/10.1093/cid/ciz429.
31. Yang X, Siddique A, Khan AA, et al. Chlamydia trachomatis infection: their potential implication in the etiology of cervical cancer. J Cancer. 2021;12(16):4891–900. https://doi.org/10.7150/jca.58582.
32. Hill AV, Perez-Patron M, Tekwe CD, et al. Chlamydia trachomatis is associated with medically indicated preterm birth and preeclampsia in young pregnant women. Sex Transm Dis. 2020;47(4):246–52. https://doi.org/10.1097/OLQ.0000000000001134.
33. Paavonen J, Fortner RT, Lehtinen M, Idahl A. Chlamydia trachomatis, Pelvic inflammatory disease, and epithelial ovarian cancer. J Infect Dis. 2021;224(12 Suppl 2):S121–7. https://doi.org/10.1093/infdis/jiab017.
34. Fitz HT. Acute gonococcal peritonitis of the right upper quadrant in women. JAWA. 1934;102:2094–5.
35. Curtis AHA. Cause of adhesion in the right upper quadrant. JAWA. 1930;94:1221–2.
36. Huang HH, Tsai CM, Tyan YS. Unusual cause should be kept in mind of abdominal pain in female patient. Fitz-Hugh-Curtis Syndrome Gastroenterol. 2011;140:e7–8.
37. Antonie F, Billion C, Vic C. Chlamydia trachomatis Fitz-Hugh-Curtis syndrome in a female adolescent. Arch Pediatr. 2013;20:289–91.

38. Anonymous. Fitz Hugh Curtis syndrome. Danbury: National Organization for Rare Disorders (NORD); 2017.
39. Popov G, Martinov S, Dimitrov K. Sexually transmitted chlamydial infections. Sofia: Medicine and Physical Culture Publisher; 1989. p. 166.
40. Piscaglia F, Vidili G, Ugolini G, et al. Fitz Hugh Curtis syndrome mimicking acute cholecystitis: value of new ultrasound findings in the differential diagnosis. Ultraschall Med. 2005;26:227–30.
41. Woo S, Kim JI, Cheung DY, et al. Clinical outcome of Fitz Hugh Curtis syndrome mimicking acute biliary disease. World J Gastroenterol. 2008;14:6975–80.
42. Peter NG, Clark LR, Jaeger R. Fitz Hugh Curtis syndrome: a diagnosis to consider in women with right upper quadrant pain. Cleveland Clin J Med. 2005;71:233–9.
43. Wolner-Hansen P. Proceedings of Scandinavian Symposium on C. trachomatis in genital and related infections. 1982;32:77–82.
44. Darougar S, Forsey T, Wood JJ, et al. Chlamydia and the Curtis-Fitz Hugh syndrome. Br J Ven Dis. 1981;57:391–4.
45. Puolakkainen M, Saikku P, Leinonen M, et al. Comparative sensitivity of different sertological tests for detecting chlamydial antibodies in perihepatitis. J Clin Pathol (London). 1985;1985(38):929–32.
46. Paavonen J, Saikku P, Von Knorring JK, et al. Association of infection with C. trachomatis with Fitz Hugh Curtis syndrome. J Inf Dis. 1981;114:176.
47. Le Moigne F, Lamboley JL, Vitry T. Usefulness of contrst -enhanced CT scan for diagnosis of Fitz-Hugh–Curtis syndrome. Gastroenterol Clin Biol. 2009;33:1176–8.
48. Wang PY, Zhang L, Wang X, et al. Fitz-Hugh-Curtis syndrome: clinical diagnostic value of dynamic enhanced MSCT. J Phys Ther Sci. 2015;27:1641–4.
49. de Boer JP, Verpalen IM, Gabriëls RY, et al. Fitz-Hugh-Curtis syndrome resulting in nutmeg liver on computed tomography. Radiol Case Rep. 2019;14(8):930–3. https://doi.org/10.1016/j.radcr.2019.04.008.
50. Lee SH, Yang JI, Choi JS. A case of Fitz-Hugh-Curtis syndrome in a male patient. Kosin Med J. 2018;33(2):223. https://doi.org/10.7180/kmj.2018.33.2.223.
51. Gomes RRA. Rare case of Chlamydia trachomatis associated Fitz-Hugh-Curtis syndrome masquerading acute cholecystitis. J Gynecol Res Rev Rep. 2020;2(4):1–3. https://doi.org/10.47363/JGRRR/2020(2)122.
52. Cugliari M, Pandit T, Pandit R. Small bowel obstruction and appendicitis in patient with Fitz-Hughes-Curtis syndrome. J Med Cases. 2022;13(7):335–40. https://doi.org/10.14740/jmc3947.
53. Santoscoy F, Paes FM. Goyenechea MR computed tomography findings in Fitz-Hugh-Curtis syndrome. J Case Rep Images Obstet Gynaecol. 2018;4:100039Z08JS2018. https://doi.org/10.5348/100039Z08JS2018CL.
54. Marbet UA, Stalder GA, Vogtlin J, et al. Diffuse peritonitis and chronic ascites due to infection with Chlamydia trachomatis in patients without liver disease: new presentation of the Fitz-Hugh-Curtis syndrome. Br Med J (Clin Res Ed). 1986;293(6538):5–6. https://doi.org/10.1136/bmj.293.6538.5.
55. Laura A, Alejandro J, Arroyo T. Diagnosis and treatment of Fitz-Hugh-Curtis syndrome: review of current literature. Int J Med Sci Clin Res Stud. 2023;03(05) https://doi.org/10.47191/ijmscrs/v3-i5-16.
56. Ekabe CJ, Kehbila J, Njim T, et al. Chlamydia trachomatis-induced Fitz-Hugh-Curtis syndrome: a case report. Case Rep BMC Res Notes. 2017;10(1):10. https://doi.org/10.1186/s13104-016-2357-z.
57. Carter JD, Hudson AP. The evolving story of Chlamydia-induced reactive arthritis. Curr Opin Rheumatol. 2010;22:424–30.
58. Bojovic J, Strelic N, Pavlica L. Reiter's syndrome—disease of young men—analysis of 312 patients. Med Pregl. 2014;67:222–30.
59. Taylor-Robinson D, Keat A. Observations on Chlamydia trachomatis and other microbes in reactive arthritis. Int J STD AIDS. 2015;26:139–44.
60. Kaga M, Ito S, Ueda T. Two cases of Perihepatitis with the liver capsule irritation sign: a new physical examination technique. Cureus. 2023;15(1):e34327. https://doi.org/10.7759/cureus.34327.
61. Kumar P, Khanna G, Batra S. Chlamydia trachomatis elementary bodies in synovial fluid of patients with reactive arthritis and undifferentiated spondyloarthropathy in India. Int J Rheum Dis. 2016;19(5):506–11. https://doi.org/10.1111/1756-185X.12364.
62. Tjahyadi D, Ropii B, Tjandraprawira KD, et al. Female urogenital chlamydia: epidemiology, chlamydia on pregnancy, current diagnosis, and treatment. Review. Ann Med Surg. 2022;75:103448. https://doi.org/10.1016/j.amsu.2022.103448.
63. Chen CO, Balaram K, Hackney DN. Chlamydia trachomatis and adverse pregnancy outcomes: meta-analysis of patients with and without infection. Meta-analysis. Matern Child Health J. 2018;22(6):812–21. https://doi.org/10.1007/s10995-018-2451-z.
64. Simons JL, McKenzie JS, Wright NC, et al. Chlamydia prevalence by age and correlates of infection among pregnant women. Sex Transm Dis. 2021;48(1):37–41. https://doi.org/10.1097/OLQ.0000000000001261.
65. Adachi K, Nielsen-Saines K, Klausner JD. Chlamydia trachomatis infection in pregnancy: the global challenge of preventing adverse pregnancy and infant outcomes in sub-Saharan Africa and Asia. Biomed Res Int. 2016;2016:9315757. https://doi.org/10.1155/2016/9315757.
66. Salari N, Olfat N, Ghasemi H, et al. The global prevalence of Chlamydia trachomatis genital infection in pregnant women: a meta -analysis. Arch Gynecol

Obstet. 2025;311:529–42. https://doi.org/10.1007/s00404-024-07928-x.
67. Glazkova LK, Bashmakova NV, Motornyuk YI, Remizova II. Features of the course of chlamydial infection in pregnant women, improvement of diagnostics and treatment. STD. 2002;2:15–20.
68. Boyko EV, Poznyak AL, Ageev VS, Sidorchuk SN, Khlopunova OV. Ophthalmochlamydia in young people: etiology, pathogenesis, clinical forms, diagnostics (literature review). Bull Ophthalmol. 2008;124(1):50–3.
69. Ramadhani AM, Derrick T, Holland MJ, Burton MJ. Blinding trachoma: systematic review of rates and risk factors for progressive disease. PLoS Negl Trop Dis. 2016;10(8):e0004859. https://doi.org/10.1371/journal.pntd.0004859.
70. Mabey DC, Solomon AW, Foster A. Trachoma. Lancet. 2003;362(9379):223–9. https://doi.org/10.1016/S0140-6736(03)13914-1.
71. Solomon AW, Burton MJ, Gower EW, Harding-Esch EM, Oldenburg CE, Taylor HR, Traoré L. Trachoma. Nat Rev Dis Primers. 2022;8(1):32. https://doi.org/10.1038/s41572-022-00359-5.
72. Asgedom YS, Melaku T, Gebrekidan AY, Meskele M, Asnake G, Alemu A, Efa AG, Haile KE, Kassie GA. Prevalence of active trachoma among 1–9 years of age children in Ethiopia: a systematic review and meta-analysis. BMJ Open. 2024;14(7):e079623. https://doi.org/10.1136/bmjopen-2023-079623.
73. Thylefors B, Dawson CR, Jones BR, West SK, Taylor HR. A simple system for the assessment of trachoma and its complications. Bull World Health Organ. 1987;65(4):477–83.
74. El-Asrar AM, Van den Oord JJ, Geboes K, Missotten L, Emarah MH, Desmet V. Immunopathology of trachomatous conjunctivitis. Br J Ophthalmol. 1989;73(4):276–82. https://doi.org/10.1136/bjo.73.4.276.
75. Hu VH, Massae P, Weiss HA, Cree IA, Courtright P, Mabey DC, Bailey RL, Burton MJ. In vivo confocal microscopy of trachoma in relation to normal tarsal conjunctiva. Ophthalmology. 2011;118(4):747–54. https://doi.org/10.1016/j.ophtha.2010.08.029.
76. Burton MJ, Bailey RL, Jeffries D, Mabey DC, Holland MJ. Cytokine and fibrogenic gene expression in the conjunctivas of subjects from a Gambian community where trachoma is endemic. Infect Immun. 2004;72(12):7352–6. https://doi.org/10.1128/IAI.72.12.7352-7356.2004.
77. Ramadhani AM, Derrick T, Macleod D, Massae P, Mtuy T, Jeffries D, Roberts CH, Bailey RL, Mabey DCW, Holland MJ, Burton MJ. Immunofibrogenic gene expression patterns in Tanzanian children with ocular Chlamydia trachomatis infection, active trachoma and scarring: baseline results of a 4-year longitudinal study. Front Cell Infect Microbiol. 2017;7:406. https://doi.org/10.3389/fcimb.2017.00406.
78. Hu VH, Luthert PJ, Derrick T, Pullin J, Weiss HA, Massae P, Mtuy T, Makupa W, Essex D, Mabey DC, Bailey RL, Holland MJ, Burton MJ. Immunohistochemical analysis of scarring trachoma indicates infiltration by natural killer and undefined CD45 negative cells. PLoS Negl Trop Dis. 2016;10(5):e0004734. https://doi.org/10.1371/journal.pntd.0004734.
79. Derrick T, Luthert PJ, Jama H, Hu VH, Massae P, Essex D, Holland MJ, Burton MJ. Increased epithelial expression of CTGF and S100A7 with elevated subepithelial expression of IL-1 β in trachomatous Trichiasis. PLoS Negl Trop Dis. 2016;10(6):e0004752. https://doi.org/10.1371/journal.pntd.0004752.
80. Hu VH, Weiss HA, Ramadhani AM, Tolbert SB, Massae P, Mabey DC, Holland MJ, Bailey RL, Burton MJ. Innate immune responses and modified extracellular matrix regulation characterize bacterial infection and cellular/connective tissue changes in scarring trachoma. Infect Immun. 2012;80(1):121–30. https://doi.org/10.1128/IAI.05965-11.
81. Kechagia JZ, Ezra DG, Burton MJ, Bailly M. Fibroblasts profiling in scarring trachoma identifies IL-6 as a functional component of a fibroblast-macrophage pro-fibrotic and pro-inflammatory feedback loop. Sci Rep. 2016;6:28261. https://doi.org/10.1038/srep28261.
82. Al-Rajhi AA, Hidayat A, Nasr A, Al-Faran M. The histopathology and the mechanism of entropion in patients with trachoma. Ophthalmology. 1993;100(9):1293–6. https://doi.org/10.1016/s0161-6420(93)31485-5.
83. Abu El-Asrar AM, Geboes K, Al-Kharashi SA, Tabbara KF, Missotten L. Collagen content and types in trachomatous conjunctivitis. Eye. 1998;12(4):735–9. https://doi.org/10.1038/eye.1998.179.
84. Stephens RS. The cellular paradigm of chlamydial pathogenesis. Trends Microbiol. 2003;11(1):44–51. https://doi.org/10.1016/s0966-842x(02)00011-2.
85. Chang K, Cheng VY, Kwong NS. Neonatal haemorrhagic conjunctivitis: a specific sign of chlamydial infection. Hong Kong Med J. 2006;12(1):27–32.
86. Grygiel-Górniak B, Folga BA. Chlamydia trachomatis-an emerging old entity? Microorganisms. 2023;11(5):1283. https://doi.org/10.3390/microorganisms11051283.
87. Inman RD, Whittum-Hudson JA, Schumacher HR, Hudson AP. Chlamydia and associated arthritis. Curr Opin Rheumatol. 2000;12(4):254–62. doi: 10.1097/00002281-200007000-00004
88. Haller-Schober EM, El-Shabrawi Y. Chlamydial conjunctivitis (in adults), uveitis, and reactive arthritis, including SARA. Sexually acquired reactive arthritis. Best Pract Res Clin Obstet Gynaecol. 2002;16(6):815–28. https://doi.org/10.1053/beog.2002.0320.
89. Bănicioiu-Covei S, Vreju AF, Ciurea PL. Correlations between infection patterns and

eye damage in reactive arthritis. Rom J Morphol Embryol. 2019;60(2):601–4.
90. Wakefield D, Penny R. Cell-mediated immune response to chlamydia in anterior uveitis: role of HLA B27. Clin Exp Immunol. 1983;51(2):191–6.
91. Vlasenko A, Kireeva E. Urethrooculosynovial syndrome (Reiter's disease). Doctor. 2017;10:19–22.
92. Amor B. Reiter's syndrome. Diagnosis and clinical features. Rheum Dis Clin North Am. 1998;24(4):677–95. https://doi.org/10.1016/s0889-857x(05)70037-5.
93. Craig JP, Nichols KK, Akpek EK, Caffery B, Dua HS, Joo CK, Liu Z, Nelson JD, Nichols JJ, Tsubota K, Stapleton F. TFOS DEWS II definition and classification report. Ocul Surf. 2017;15(3):276–83. https://doi.org/10.1016/j.jtos.2017.05.008.
94. Hom MM, Nguyen AL, Bielory L. Allergic conjunctivitis and dry eye syndrome. Ann Allergy Asthma Immunol. 2012;108(3):163–6. https://doi.org/10.1016/j.anai.2012.01.006.
95. Boiko EV, Pozniak AL, Maltsev DS, Suetov AA, Nuralova IV. High frequency of latent conjunctival C. trachomatis, M. hominis, and U. Urealyticum infections in young adults with dry eye disease. J Ophthalmol. 2014;2014:154627. https://doi.org/10.1155/2014/154627.
96. Boyko EV, Chernysh VF, Poznyak AL, Ageyev VS. On the role of chlamydial infection in the development of dry eye syndrome. Bull Ophthalmol. 2008;124(4):16–9.
97. Abdelfattah MM, Khattab RA, Mahran MH, Elborgy ES. Evaluation of patients with dry eye disease for conjunctival Chlamydia trachomatis and Ureaplasma urealyticum. Int J Ophthalmol. 2016;9(10):1457–65. https://doi.org/10.18240/ijo.2016.10.15.
98. Krásny J, Hrubá D, Netuková M, Kodat V, Tomásová BJ. Chlamydia pneumoniae v etiologii keratoconjunctivitis sicca u dospělých patient (pilot) studie [Chlamydia pneumoniae in the etiology of the keratoconjunctivitis sicca in adult patients (a pilot study)]. Cesk Words Oftalmol. 2009;65(3):102–6.
99. Kuhn F, Aylward B. Rhegmatogenous retinal detachment: a reappraisal of its pathophysiology and treatment. Ophthalmic Res. 2013;51(1):15–31. https://doi.org/10.1159/000355077.
100. Yoshimura T, Sonoda KH, Sugahara M, Mochizuki Y, Enaida H, Oshima Y, et al. Comprehensive analysis of inflammatory immune mediators in vitreoretinal diseases. PLoS One. 2009;4(12):e8158. https://doi.org/10.1371/journal.pone.0008158.
101. Boyko EV, Poznyak AL, Ageyev VS. Relationship between rhegmatogenous retinal detachment and chlamydial infection: diagnostics and detection rate of the pathogen. Bull Ophthalmol. 2008;124(5):52–5.
102. Boiko EV, Pozniak AL, Maltsev DS, Suetov AA, Nuralova IV. Chronic ocular Chlamydia trachomatis infection in rabbits: clinical and histopathological findings in the posterior segment. Invest Ophthalmol Vis Sci. 2014;55(2):1176–83. https://doi.org/10.1167/iovs.13-13416.
103. Hanada H, Ikeda- Dantsuji Y, Naito M, Nagayama A. Infection of human fibroblast-like synovial cells with Chlamydia trachomatis results in persistent infection and interleukin-6 production. Microb Pathog. 2003;34(2):57–63. https://doi.org/10.1016/s0882-4010(02)00189-4.
104. Boiko EV, Pozniak AL, Maltsev DS, Suetov AA, Nuralova IV. High frequency of latent Chlamydia trachomatis infection in patients with rhegmatogenous retinal detachment. Int J Ophthalmol. 2016;9(6):863–8. https://doi.org/10.18240/ijo.2016.06.13.
105. Jendro MC, Fingerle F, Deutsch T, Liese A, Köhler L, Kuipers JG, Raum E, Martin M, Zeidler H. Chlamydia trachomatis-infected macrophages induce apoptosis of activated T cells by secretion of tumor necrosis factor-alpha in vitro. Med Microbiol Immunol. 2004;193(1):45–52. https://doi.org/10.1007/s00430-003-0182-1.
106. Levitt D, Danen R, Levitt P. Selective infection of astrocytes by Chlamydia trachomatis in primary mixed neuron-glial cell cultures. Infect Immun. 1986;54(3):913–6. https://doi.org/10.1128/iai.54.3.913-916.1986.
107. Suetov AA, Boyko EV. Hyalocytes of the vitreous body and their importance in ocular pathology. Bull Ophthalmol. 2018;134(6):94–101. https://doi.org/10.17116/oftalma201813406194.
108. Boyko EV, Chepur SV, Poznyak AL, Nuralova IV, Suetov AA, Maltsev DS, Ageev BS, Shestaev AY. Features of damage to the structures of the posterior segment of the eye in experimental chlamydial infection. Bull Ophthalmol. 2010;126(1):27–32.
109. Boyko EV, Poznyak AL, Nuralova IV, Maltsev DS, Suetov AA, Ageev VS, Yakushev DY. On the development of multiorgan chlamydial lesions in primary local infection of the eye in an experiment. Arch Pathol. 2011;73(6):15–8.
110. Boiko E, Maltsev D, Savicheva A, Shalepo K, Khusnutdinova T, Pozniak A, et al. Infection of human retinal pigment epithelium with Chlamydia trachomatis. PLoS One. 2015;10(11):e0141754. https://doi.org/10.1371/journal.pone.0141754.
111. Foos RY, Wheeler NC. Vitreoretinal juncture. Synchysis senilis and posterior vitreous detachment. Ophthalmology. 1982;89(12):1502–12. https://doi.org/10.1016/s0161-6420(82)34610-2.
112. Sebag J. Structure, function, and age-related changes of the human vitreous. Bull Soc Belge Ophthalmol. 1987;223(Pt 1):37–57. https://doi.org/10.1007/978-1-4757-1901-7_3.
113. Boyko EV, Poznyak AL, Suetov AA, Maltsev DS. Dystrophic changes in the vitreous body in ophthalmochlamydia. Bull Ophthalmol. 2012;128(6):45–9.
114. Lobzin YV, Lyashenko YI, Poznyak AL. Chlamydial infections. Tome: St. Petersburg "Publishing house"; 2003.

115. Charteris DG. Proliferative vitreoretinopathy: revised concepts of pathogenesis and adjunctive treatment. Eye. 2020;34(2):241–5. https://doi.org/10.1038/s41433-019-0699-1.
116. Boyko EV, Poznyak AL, Suetov AA, Maltsev DS, Nuralova IV. The role of intraocular Chlamydia infection trachomatis in the development of proliferative vitreoretinopathy (experimental study). Bull Ophthalmol. 2015;131(1):50–7. https://doi.org/10.17116/oftalma2015131150-56.
117. Boyko EV, Shishkin MM, Ryabous EA, Lepneva SV. Morphological changes in eye structures during modeling of proliferative vitreoretinopathy. Bull Ophthalmol. 2010;126(4):25–30.
118. Pastor JC, de la Rúa ER, Martín F. Proliferative vitreoretinopathy: risk factors and pathobiology. Prog Retin Eye Res. 2002;21(1):127–44. https://doi.org/10.1016/s1350-9462(01)00023-4.
119. Chlamydia SRS. Intracellular biology, pathogenesis, and immunity. Washington, DC: ASM Press; 1999. p. 321p.
120. Boiko EV, Pozniak AL, Iakushev DI, Maltsev DS, Suetov AA, Nuralova IV. Latent infections as a risk factor for Posttrabeculectomy bleb failure. J Glaucoma. 2016;25(3):306–11. https://doi.org/10.1097/IJG.0000000000000212.
121. Zinserling VA. Infectious lesions of the Central nervous system. Springer. https://doi.org/10.1007/978-3-030-96260-9.
122. Stratton CW, Wheldon DB. Multiple sclerosis: an infectious syndrome involving Chlamydophila pneumonia. Trends Microbiol. 2006;14(11):474–9.
123. Fainardi E, et al. Under the microscope: focus on Chlamydia pneumoniae infection and multiple sclerosis. Curr Neurovasc Res. 2008;5(1):60–70.
124. Wagner AD, Gerard HC, Fresemann T. Detection of Chlamydia pneumoniae in giant cell vasculitis and correlation with the topographic arrangement of tissue-infiltrating dentritic cells. Arthrit Rheum. 2000;43(7):1543–51.
125. Wohlschlaeger J, Wimmer ML, Nagler DK, et al. Identification of Chlamydia pneumoniae in intracranial and extracranial arteries in patients with stroke and in controls: combined immunohistochemical and polymerase chain reaction analyses. Hum Pathol. 2005;36(4):395–402.
126. Stratton CW, Sriram S. Association of Chlamydia pneumonia with central nervous system disease. Microbes Infect. 2003;5(13):1249–53.
127. Robertson DK, et al. Inclusion biogenesis and reactivation of persistent Chlamydia trachomatis requires host cell sphingolipid biosynthesis. PLoS Pathol. 2009;5(11):e1000664. https://doi.org/10.1371/journal.ppat.1000664.
128. Fukano H. Comparison of five PCR assays for detecting Chlamydia pneumoniae DNA. Microbiol Immunol. 2004;48(1):441–8.
129. Zinserling VA, Vainshenker YI. Chapter 11: Hidden encephalitis in prolonged disorders of consciences. In: Zinserling VA, editor. Infectious lesions of the central nervous system. Springer; 2022. p. 271–9. doi: 10.1007/978-3-030-96260-9.
130. Zigangirova NA, Petyaev IM, Pashko YP, et al. Generalization of infection in patients with urogenital chlamydia. Clin Microbiol Antimicrob Chem. 2007;9(4):351–60.
131. Contini C., Seraceni S., Cultrera R. et al. Chlamydophila pneumoniae infection and its role in neurological disorders. Interdiscip Perspect Infect Dis. 2010.
132. Boyko EV, Poznyak AL, Nuralova IV, et al. On the development of multiorgan chlamydial lesions in primary local infection of the eye in an experiment. Arch Pathol. 2011;6:15–8.
133. Punter MNM, Varma AR. Myeloradiculitis with meningoencephalopathy and optic neuritis in a case of previous Chlamydia psittaci infection. BMJ Case Rep. 2010;2010:bcr1220092521. https://doi.org/10.1136/bcr.12.2009.2521.
134. Coste S, De Greslan T, Renard JL, et al. Acute polyradiculoneuropathy after Chlamydia pneumoniae infection. [article in French]. Rev Neurol (Paris). 2002;158(3):361–3.
135. Mikhaylenko AA, Onishchenko LS, Nuralova IV, Borzenko OV. Pathology of the peripheral nervous system of chlamydial nature. Neurol Bull. 1996;28(1—2):5–8.
136. Syniachenko O, Selezneva SV, Zapada AV. Peripheral neuropathy in chlamydia reactive arthritis. Actual Infectol. 2016;4(3.12):27–32. https://doi.org/10.22141/2312-413x.3.12.2016.81708.
137. Baguley S, Greenhouse P. Non-genital manifestations of Chlamydia tracomatis. C Clin Med. 2003;3:206–8. https://doi.org/10.7861/clinmedicine.3-3-206.
138. Boganes M, Strnad A. Neurological manifestations of ornithosis. J Neuropathol Psychiatr. 1960;60(10):1297–9.
139. Furst W, Kovac W, Moritsch H. Enten als Virusreservoir für Ornithoseerkrankungen des Menschen. Wien. klin Wo- chenschr. 1957;69(13):223–8.
140. Schmechel H. Ophtalmoplegia totalis im Verlauf einer Ornithose. Dtsch. Gesundh.-Wes. 1965;20(39):1804–6.
141. Pap L, Munich D. Über einen von Polyneuritis und Nervenlahmungen infolge humaner Ornitosis. Dtsch Zschr inn Med. 1963;18(23):1079–83.
142. Popec K. Die nevrologische Bedeutung der Ornitose. Zschr. arztl. Fortbild. 1963;57(119):1051–7.

143. Haidl S, Ivarsson S, Bjerre I, Persson K. Guillain-Barré syndrome after Chlamydia pneumoniae infection. N Engl J Med. 1992;326(8):576–7.
144. Uzun N. Chlamydia infection's role in neurological diseases. In: Sarier M, editor. Chlamydia—secret enemy from past to present [Internet], Infectious diseases. IntechOpen; 2023. https://doi.org/10.5772/intechopen.106108.
145. Michel D, Antoine JC, Pozzetto B, et al. Lumbosacral meningoradiculitis associated with Chlamydia pneumoniae infection. J Neurol Neurosurg Psychiatry. 1992;55:511.
146. Di Pietro M, Filardo S, Romano S, Sessa R. Chlamydia trachomatis and Chlamydia pneumoniae interaction with the host: latest advances and future prospective. Microorganisms. 2019;7(5):140. https://doi.org/10.3390/microorganisms7050140.
147. Telyatnikova N, Gaston JSH. Prior exposure to infection with Chlamydia pneumoniae can influence the T-cell-mediated response to Chlamydia trachomatis. FEMS Immunol Med Microbiol. 2006;47(2):190–8. https://doi.org/10.1111/j.1574-695X.2006.00080.x.
148. Strelić N, Bojović J, Pavlica L, et al. Detection of bacteria and analyses of Chlamydia trachomatis viability in patients with postvenereal reactive arthritis. Intern Med J. 2014;44(12a):1247–51. https://doi.org/10.1111/imj.12580.
149. Nazareth L, Walkden H, Chacko A, et al. Chlamydia muridarum can invade the central nervous system via the olfactory and trigeminal nerves and Infect peripheral nerve glial cells. Front Cell Infect Microbiol. 2021;10:607779. https://doi.org/10.3389/fcimb.2020.607779.
150. Chacko A, Delbaz A, Walkden H, et al. Chlamydia pneumoniae can infect the central nervous system via the olfactory and trigeminal nerves and contributes to Alzheimer's disease risk. Sci Rep. 2022;12(1):2759. https://doi.org/10.1038/s41598-022-06749-9.
151. Dando SJ, Mackay-Sim A, Norton R, et al. Pathogens penetrating the central nervous system: infection pathways and the cellular and molecular mechanisms of invasion. Clin Microbiol Rev. 2014;27(4):691–726. https://doi.org/10.1128/CMR.00118-13.
152. Su Z, Chen J, Qiu Y, et al. Olfactory ensheathing cells: the primary innate immunocytes in the olfactory pathway to engulf apoptotic olfactory nerve debris. Glia. 2013;61(4):490–503. https://doi.org/10.1002/glia.22450.
153. Nazareth L, Lineburg KE, Chuah M, et al. Olfactory ensheathing cells are the main phagocytic cells that remove axon debris during early development of the olfactory system. J Comp Neurol. 2015;523(3):479–94. https://doi.org/10.1002/cne.23694.
154. Vincent AJ, Choi-Lundberg DL, Harris JA, West AK, Chuah MI. Bacteria and PAMPs activate nuclear factor κB and Gro production in a subset of olfactory ensheathing cells and astrocytes but not in Schwann cells. Glia. 2007;55(9):905–16. https://doi.org/10.1002/glia.20512.
155. Harris JA, West AK, Chuah MI. Olfactory ensheathing cells: nitric oxide production and innate immunity. Glia. 2009;57(16):1848–57. https://doi.org/10.1002/glia.2089.
156. Herbert RP, Harris J, Chong KP, et al. Cytokines and olfactory bulb microglia in response to bacterial challenge in the compromised primary olfactory pathway. J Neuroinflam. 2012;9:109. https://doi.org/10.1186/1742-2094-9-109.
157. Panni P, Ferguson IA, Beacham I, et al. Phagocytosis of bacteria by olfactory ensheathing cells and Schwann cells. Neurosci Lett. 2013;539:65–70. https://doi.org/10.1016/j.neulet.2013.01.052.
158. Macedo-Ramos H, Ruiz-Mendoza S, Mariante RM, et al. Streptococcus pneumoniae resists intracellular killing by olfactory ensheathing cells but not by microglia. Sci Rep. 2016;6:36813. https://doi.org/10.1038/srep36813.
159. Walkden H, Delbaz A, Nazareth L, et al. Burkholderia pseudomallei invades the olfactory nerve and bulb after epithelial injury in mice and causes the formation of multinucleated giant glial cells in vitro. PLoS Negl Trop Dis. 2020;14(1):e0008017. https://doi.org/10.1371/journal.pntd.0008017.
160. Cockram FA, Jackson ARB. Isolation of a Chlamydia from cases of keratoconjunctivitis in koalas. Aust Vet J. 1974;50:82–3.
161. Girjes AA, et al. Two distinct forms of Chlamydia psittaci associated with disease and infertility in Phascolarctos cinereus (Koala). Infect Immun. 1988;56:1897–900.
162. Girjes AA, et al. Remarkable sequence relatedness in the DNA encoding the major outer membrane protein of Chlamydia psittaci (koala type-I) and Chlamydia pneumonia. Gene. 1994;138:139–42.
163. Bodetti TJ, et al. Molecular evidence to support the expansion of the hostrange of Chlamydophila pneumoniae to include reptiles as well as humans, horses, koalas and amphibians. Syst Appl Microbiol. 2002;25:146–52.
164. Smadel JE. Atypical pneumonia and psittacosis. J Clin Invest. 1943;22:57–65.
165. Puolakkainen M, et al. Chlamydial pneumonitis and its serodiagnosis in infants. J Infect Dis. 1984;149:598–604.
166. Saikku P, et al. An epidemic of mild pneumonia due to an unusual strain of Chlamydia psittaci. J Infect Dis. 1985;151:832–9.
167. Grayston JT, et al. Chlamydia pneumoniae SP-Nov for Chlamydia SP strain TWAR. Int J Syst Bacteriol. 1989;39:88–90.
168. Allegra L, Blasi F. Chlamydia pneumoniae. Springer; 1999. p. 205p.
169. Roulis E, Polkinghorne A, Timms P. Chlamydia pneumoniae: modern insights into an ancient pathogen. Trends Microbiol. 2013;21(3):120–8. https://doi.org/10.1016/j.tim.2012.10.009. Epub 2012 Dec 5

170. Roulis E, Bachmann NL, Myers GSA, et al. Comparative genomic analysis of human Chlamydia pneumoniae isolates from respiratory, brain and cardiac tissues. Genomics. 2015;106(6):373–83.
171. Hahn DL, et al. Chlamydia pneumoniae as a respiratory pathogen. Front Biosci. 2002;7:E66–76.
172. Grayston JT, et al. A new respiratory tract pathogen: Chlamydia pneumoniae strain TWAR. J Infect Dis. 1990;161:618–25.
173. Falck GÑ, et al. Prevalence of Chlamydia pneumoniae in healthy children and in children with respiratory tract infections. Pediatr Infect Dis J. 1997;16:549–54.
174. Benitez AJ, et al. Comparison of real-time PCR and a microimmunofluorescence serological assay for detection of Chlamydophila pneumoniae infection in an outbreak investigation. J Clin Microbiol. 2012;50:151–3.
175. Kumar S, Hammerschlag MR. Acute respiratory infection due to Chlamydia pneumoniae: current status of diagnostic methods. Clin Infect Dis. 2007;44:568–76.
176. Oktem IMA, et al. PCR and serology were effective for identifying Chlamydophila pneumoniae in a lower respiratory infection outbreak among military recruits. Jpn J Infect Dis. 2007;60:97–101.
177. Sevketbeyoglu H, et al. Outbreak of Chlamydia pneumoniae infection in a military unit: the distribution of lobar and segmental infiltration. Nobel Med. 2012;8:26–31.
178. Coon RG, et al. Chlamydophila pneumoniae infection among basic underwater demolition/SEAL (BUD/S) candidates, Coronado, California. Mil Med. 2011;176:320–3.
179. Senn L, et al. Does respiratory infection due to Chlamydia pneumoniae still exist? Clin Infect Dis. 2011;53:847–8.
180. Edvinsson M, et al. Presence of Chlamydophila pneumoniae DNA but not mRNA in stenotic aortic heart valves. Int J Cardiol. 2010;143:57–62.
181. Dabiri H, et al. Detection of Chlamydia pneumoniae in atherosclerotic plaques of patients in Tehran. Iran Jpn J Infect Dis. 2009;62:195–7.
182. Borel N, et al. Evidence for persistent Chlamydia pneumoniae infection of human coronary atheromas. Atherosclerosis. 2008;199:154–61.
183. Watson C, Alp NJ. Role of Chlamydia pneumoniae in atherosclerosis. Clin Sci. 2008;114:509–31.
184. Savenkova MS, Savenkov MP. Topical issues concerning treatment of intracellular bacterial pathogens in children. Russian J Woman Child Health. 2020;3(4):326–35.
185. Pacheco A, González- SJ, Arocena C, et al. Community acquired pneumonia caused by Chlamydia pneumoniae strain TWAR in chronic cardiopulmonary disease in the elderly. Respiration. 1991;58(5–6):316–20. https://doi.org/10.1159/000195952.
186. Cosentini R, Blasi F, Raccanelli R, et al. Severe community-acquired pneumonia: a possible role for Chlamydia pneumonia. Respiration. 1996;63(2):61–5. https://doi.org/10.1159/000196519.
187. File TM, Plouffe JF, Breiman RF, Skelton SK. Clinical characteristics of chlamydia pneumoniae infection as the sole cause of community-acquired pneumonia get access arrow. Clin Infect Dis. 1999;29(2):426–8. https://doi.org/10.1086/520227.
188. Marrie TJ, Peeling RW, Reid T, De Carolis E. Chlamydia species as a cause of community-acquired pneumonia in Canada. Eur Respir J. 2003;21(5):779–84. https://doi.org/10.1183/09031936.03.00095403.
189. Sohn JW, Park SC, Choi Y-H, et al. Atypical pathogens as etiologic agents in hospitalized patient with community-acquired pneumonia in Korea: a prospective multi-center study. J Korean Med Sci. 2006;21(4):602–7. https://doi.org/10.3346/jkms.2006.21.4.602.
190. Al- Aydie SN, Obeidat NM, Al-Younes HM. Role of Chlamydia pneumoniae in community-acquired pneumonia in hospitalized Jordanian adults. J Infect Dev Cries. 2016;10(3):227–36. https://doi.org/10.3855/jidc.6590.
191. Vieyra JM, Ranero ADC, Reyes DP, et al. Chlamydophila pneumoniae-associated community-acquired pneumonia in pediatric patients of a tertiary care hospital in Mexico: molecular diagnostic and clinical insights. Sci Rep. 2023;13(1):21477. https://doi.org/10.1038/s41598-023-48701-5.
192. Levin NF, Skipsky IM, Radchenko VG, et al. Clinical and morphological features of pneumonia caused by Chlamydia: case analysis. Pulmonology. 2009;2:124–6.
193. Liu B, Lyu Z, Zhang X. Chlamydia Pneumonia. In: Li H, Liu J, Li L, editors. Radiology of infectious and inflammatory diseases, vol. 3. Singapore: Springer; 2023. https://doi.org/10.1007/978-981-99-4614-3_10.
194. Wang J, Wang B, Xiao J, et al. Chlamydia psittaci: a zoonotic pathogen causing avian chlamydiosis and psittacosis. Virulence. 2024;15(1):2428411. https://doi.org/10.1080/21505594.2024.2428411.
195. Sachse K, Laroucau K, Vanrompay D. Avian Chlamydiosis. Curr Clin Micro Rpt. 2015;2:10–21. https://doi.org/10.1007/s40588-014-0010-y.
196. Krawiec M, Piasecki T, Wieliczko A. Prevalence of Chlamydia psittaci and other Chlamydia species in wild birds in Poland. Vector Borne Zoonotic Dis. 2015;15(11):652–5. https://doi.org/10.1089/vbz.2015.1814. Epub 2015 Oct 26
197. Caspe SG, Hill H. Chlamydiosis in animals. Animals (Basel). 2024;14(21):3130. https://doi.org/10.3390/ani14213130.

198. Hogerwerf L, De Gier B, Baan B, Van der Hoek W. Chlamydia psittaci (psittacosis) as a cause of community-acquired pneumonia: a systematic review and meta-analysis. Epidemiol Infect. 2017;145(15):3096–105. https://doi.org/10.1017/S0950268817002060. Epub 2017 Sep 26
199. Abd El-Ghany WA. Avian chlamydiosis: a worldwide emerging and public health threat. Adv Anim Vet Sci. 2020;8(s2):82–97. https://doi.org/10.17582/journal.aavs/2020/8.s2.82.97.
200. Huang H, Liu Y, Liu Y, et al. Analysis and perception of chlamydia psittaci pneumonia: novel insights into the rare disease in infectiology. Infect Drug Resist. 2024;17:5261–75. https://doi.org/10.2147/IDR.S486895. eCollection 2024
201. Dembek ZF, Mothershead JL, Owens AN, et al. Psittacosis: an underappreciated and often undiagnosed disease. Pathogens. 2023;12(9):1165. https://doi.org/10.3390/pathogens12091165.
202. Zhang Z, Zhou H, Cao H, et al. Human-to-human transmission of Chlamydia psittaci in China, 2020: an epidemiological and aetiological investigation. Lancet Microbe. 2022;3:e 512–e520.
203. Liu S, Cui Z, Carr MJ, et al. Chlamydia psittaci should be a notifiable infectious disease everywhere Lancet Microbe 2022.; published online Nov 10. https://doi.org/10.1016/S2666-5247(22)00306-8 .
204. Jia Q, Sun J, Wang D, et al. Clinical features and prognostic predictors of C. psittaci pneumonia: a systematic review and individual patient meta-analysis. BMC Pulm Med. 2025;25(1):55. https://doi.org/10.1186/s12890-025-03511-5.
205. Zhao D, Zhang L, Sun Q, Cheng J. A case report of Chlamydia psittaci infectious endocarditis complicated with pneumonia. Case Rep Infect Dis. 2025;2025:7536462. https://doi.org/10.1155/crdi/7536462.
206. Zhou Y, Zou Y, Zhou L, et al. Acute respiratory distress syndrome caused by Chlamydia psittaci: a case report and literature review. Front Med (Lausanne). 2024;11:1418241. https://doi.org/10.3389/fmed.2024.1418241. eCollection 2024
207. Yang M, Yang D-H, Yang H, et al. Clinical characteristics of Chlamydia psittaci pneumonia infection in central South China. Infect Dis Ther. 2022;11(4):1631–47. https://doi.org/10.1007/s40121-022-00662-4. Epub 2022 Jun 20
208. Schmidt TE, Kazantsev KY, Voskresenskaya ON, et al. Ornithosic myelitis. Neurol J. 2013;5:42–5.
209. Khadka S, Timilsina B, Pangeni RP, et al. Importance of clinical history in the diagnosis of psittacosis: a case report. Ann Med Surg (Lond). 2022;82:104695. https://doi.org/10.1016/j.amsu.2022.104695. eCollection 2022 Oct
210. Deng H, Shi Y, Xie M, et al. Diagnosis and treatment experience of Chlamydia psittaci pneumonia: a multicenter retrospective study in China. BMC Infect Dis. 2024;24(1):1333. https://doi.org/10.1186/s12879-024-10198-2.
211. Nieuwenhuizen AA, Dijkstra F, Notermans DW, van der Hoek W. Laboratory methods for cases of finding psittacosis outbreaks in human: a systematic review. BMC Infect Dis. 2018;18(1):442. https://doi.org/10.1186/s12879-018-3317-0.
212. Li Y, Lin F, Li W, et al. Comparison of clinical, laboratory and radiological characteristics between Chlamydia psittaci and adenovirus pneumonias: a multicenter retrospective study. Int J Infect Dis. 2023;126:114–24. https://doi.org/10.1016/j.ijid.2022.11.029. Epub 2022 Nov 29
213. Yang N, Ou Z, Sun Q, et al. Chlamydia psittaci pneumonia—evolutionary aspects on chest CT. BMC Infect Dis. 2025;25(1):11. https://doi.org/10.1186/s12879-024-10374-4.
214. Chen J, Wang J, Deng Z, et al. Clinical features of 50 cases of chlamydia psittaci pneumonia identified through metagenomic next-generation sequencing. Infect Drug Resist. 2024;17:5775–84. https://doi.org/10.2147/IDR.S493927. eCollection 2024
215. Yan X, Fu H, Deng W, et al. Early and rapid diagnosis of Chlamydia psittaci pneumonia by tNGS in six patients: a case series. Front Med (Lausanne). 2024;11:1491838.
216. Shi Y, Chen J, Shi X, et al. A case of chlamydia psittaci caused severe pneumonia and meningitis diagnosed by metagenome next-generation sequencing and clinical analysis: a case report and literature review. BMC Infect Dis. 2021;21(1):621. https://doi.org/10.1186/s12879-021-06205-5.
217. Dean D, Rothschild J, Ruettger A, et al. Zoonotic Chlamydiaceae species associated with trachoma, Nepal. Emerg Infect Dis. 1948;2013(19):55.
218. Ferreri AJ, Guidoboni M, Ponzoni M, et al. Evidence for an association between Chlamydia psittaci and ocular adnexal lymphomas. J Natl Cancer I. 2004;96(586):94.
219. de Cremoux P, Subtil A, Ferreri AJ, et al. Re: evidence for an association between Chlamydia psittaci and ocular adnexal lymphomas. J Natl Cancer I. 2006;98(365):6.
220. Aigelsreiter A, Gerlza T, Deutsch AJ, et al. Chlamydia psittaci infection in nongastrointestinal extranodal MALT lymphomas and their precursor lesions. Am J Clin Pathol. 2011;135(70):5.
221. Ponzoni M, Ferreri AJ, Guidoboni M, et al. Chlamydia infection and lymphomas: association beyond ocular adnexal lymphomas highlighted by multiple detection methods. Clin Cancer Res. 2008;14(5794):800.
222. Knittler MR, Sachse K. Chlamydia psittaci: update on an underestimated zoonotic agent. Pathog Dis. 2015;73(1):1–15.
223. Balsamo G, Maxted AM, Midla JW, et al. Compendium of measures to control Chlamydia psittaci infection among humans (psittacosis) and pet birds (Avian Chlamydiosis), 2017. J Avian Med Surg. 2017;31(3):262–82. https://doi.org/10.1647/217-265.

224. McGavran MH, Beard CW, Berendt RF, Nakamura RM. The pathogenesis of psittsacosis. Serial studies on rhesus monkeys exposed to small-particle aerosol of Borgstrain. Am J Path. 1962;40(6):653–70.
225. Walton KW. The pathology of fatal case of psittacosis showing intravcytoplasmic inclusions in the meninges. J Path A Bact. 1954;68:565–72.
226. Oberndorfer S. Pathologisch-anatomische Befunded bei Psittakosis (Papageienkrankheit) Münch. Med Wschr. 1930;77:311–2.
227. Carlin E, Marzo-Ortega H, Flew S. British Association of Sexual Health and HIV National Guideline on the management of sexually acquired reactive arthritis. Int J STD AIDS. 2021;32(11):986–97.
228. Rizzo A, Domenico MD, Carratelli CR, Paolillo R. The Role of Chlamydia and Chlamydophila infections in reactive arthritis. Int Med. 2012;51:113–7.
229. Zeidler H, Hudson AP. Chlamydia-induced reactive arthritis: disappearing entity or lack of research? Curr Rheumatol Rep. 2019;21(11):63.
230. Balabanova RM. On the issue of diagnostics and coding of reactive arthropathies. Modern Rheumatol. 2020;2:41–4.
231. Agababova ER. Some unclear and unresolved issues of seronegative spondyloarthropathies. Sci Pract Rheumatol. 2001;4:10–8.
232. Denison HJ, Curtis EM, Clynes MA, et al. The incidence of sexually acquired reactive arthritis: a systematic literature review. Clin Rheumatol. 2016;35(11):2639–48.
233. Bentaleb I, Abdelghani KB, Rostom S, et al. Reactive arthritis: update. Curr Clin Microbiol Rep. 2020;7(4):124–32.
234. Harkness AH. Reiter's disease. Br J Vener Dis. 1949;25(4):185–201.
235. Kuipers JG, Jurgens-Saathoff B, Bialowons A, et al. Detection of Chlamydia trachomatis in peripheral blood leukocytes of reactive arthritis patients by polymerase chain reaction. Arthritis Rheum. 1998;41:1894–5.
236. Rebrov AP, Aleksandrova OL, Ilinykh EV, Statsenko YA. Difficulties in diagnosing reactive arthritis. Sci Pract Rheumatol. 2002;4:55–8.
237. Badokin VV. Reactive arthritis. Urogenital and postenterocolitic. MED Press Inform; 2021. p. 280p.
238. Iglesias-Gammara A, Restrepo JF, Valle R, Matteson EL. A brief history of Stoll-Brodie-Fiessinger-Leroy Syndrome (Reiters Syndrome) and Reactive Arthritis with a Translation of Reiters Original 1916 Article into English. Curr Rheum Rev. 2005;1(1):71–9.
239. Fedotov VP. Reiter's disease (history, etiology, epidemiology, pathogenesis, clinical presentation and course, lesions of the skin, eyes, musculoskeletal system and other organs). Clinical lecture. Dermatovenereol Cosmetol Sexopathol. 2016;1–4:82–107.
240. Panush RS, Wallace DJ, Dorff REN, Engleman EP. Retraction of the suggestion to use the term "Reiter's syndrome" sixty-five years later: the legacy of Reiter, a war criminal, should not be eponymic honor but rather condemnation. Arthritis Rheum. 2007;56(2):693–4.
241. Asner TV, Kalyagin AN. Urogenic reactive arthritis: modern aspects of diagnostics and treatment. Modern Rheumatol. 2010;4:11–5.
242. Pennisi M, Perdue J, Roulston T, Nicholas J, Schmidt E, Rolfs J. An overview of reactive arthritis. J Am Acad Phys Assist. 2019;32(7):25–8.
243. Hamdulay SS, Glynne SJ, Keat A. When is arthritis reactive? Postgrad Med. 2006;82:446–53.
244. Espinoza LR, García-Valladares I. Of bugs and joints: the relationship between infection and joints. Reumatol Clin. 2013;9(4):229–38.
245. Soroka NF, Poleshchuk NN, Duben SA, et al. Algorithm for complex clinical and laboratory diagnostics of reactive chlamydia- induced arthropathies.- BSMU. Minsk; 2007. p. 13p.
246. Goldina IA, Pavlov VV, Prokhorenko VM, Gaidul KV. Proliferative activity of blood mononuclear cells in patients with coxarthrosis associated with persistent Chlamydia infection trachomatis. Int J Appl Basic Res. 2015;8:486–9.
247. Molochkov VA, Petrova MS, Molochkov AV, et al. Persistent chlamydial infection and Reiter's disease, diagnostic and treatment methods. Russian J Skin Venereal Dis. 2011;3:47–52.
248. Villareal C, Whittum-Hudson JA, Hudson AP. Persistent Chlamydiae and chronic arthritis. Arthritis Res. 2002;4(1):5–9.
249. Rihl M, Kohler L, Klos A, Zeidler H. Persistent infection of Chlamydia in reactive arthritis. Ann Rheum Dis. 2006;65(3):281–4.
250. Poluyan OS. Molecular and biological risk factors for Chlamydia dissemination trachomatis from the urogenital tract into the joint cavity in reactive arthritis. Med J. 2017;3(61):128–33.
251. Jubber A, Moorthy A. Reactive arthritis: a clinical review. JR Coll Physic Edinb. 2021;51(3):288–97.
252. Cheeti A, Chakraborty RK, Ramphul K. Reactive Arthritis [Updated 2023]. In: StatPearls [Internet]. Treasure Island, FL: StatPearls Publishing; 2024. https://www.ncbi.nlm.nih.gov/books/NBK499831.
253. Aitken-Saavedra J, Maturana-Ramirez A, Moraga JF. Reactive arthritis: images. Dermatol Online J. 2021;27(7):1–5.
254. Gérard HC, Stanich JA, Whittum-Hudson JA, et al. Patients with Chlamydia-associated arthritis have ocular (trachoma), not genital, serovars of C. trachomatis in synovial tissue. Microb Pathog. 2010;48:62–8.

255. Bojović J, Strelić N, Pavlica L. Reiter's syndrome—disease of young men—analysis of 312 patients. Med Pregl. 2014;67(7–8):222–30. https://doi.org/10.2298/mpns1408222b.
256. Petrova MS, Molochkova YV, Molochkov VA, et al. Reactive arthritis in coinfection Chlamydia trachomatis and chlamydia pneumoniae. Russian J Skin Venereal Dis. 2023;26(2):181–92.
257. Mirakhmedova HT. Remote outcomes of reactive arthritis. Sci Pract Rheumatol. 2016;S1:120.
258. Taniguchi Y, Nishikawa H, Yoshida T, et al. Expanding the spectrum of reactive arthritis (ReA): classic ReA and infection-related arthritis includingpoststreptococcalReA,Poncet'sdisease,and iBCG -induced ReA. Rheumatol. 2021;41:1387–98.
259. Kolkova NI, Rozdin OI, Koroleva EA, et al. Development of a model of chlamydial arthritis in rats. Clin Microbiol Antimicrob Chemother. 2014;16(3):229–37.
260. Tondo-Steeleea K, Rathb K, Niemeierc L. Granulomatous peritonitis secondary to Chlamydia trachomatis: a case report gynecologic. Oncol Rep. 2020;32:100558. PMCID: PMC7078493

Perinatal Chlamydiosis 6

Amongst the most important medical problems, a significant, but often underestimated place is occupied by perinatal infections, which can be caused by a wide range of pathogens, amongst which *Chlamydia* occupies a significant place both in humans and animals. Speaking about perinatal infections, optimally is a systemic approach that includes the mother's body with local and remote inflammatory processes, amniotic fluid, placenta, extraplacental membranes, umbilical cord and the embryo/foetus itself. Obviously, between all components of this system, both in physiological and pathological conditions, there are various complex, not fully understood connections that determine the course of infectious pathology. In the framework of infectology could be discussed: male and female infertility, gestosis of pregnant women, premature birth, congenital malformations of the foetus. We cannot analyse these problems in this publication, but it should be noted that they require a comprehensive study, necessarily including morphological approaches. Some aspects of infectious pathology were described in a relatively complete manner in the manual [1]. Both the literature data and our own long-term experience allow us to present predominantly infectious lesions of the placenta and foetus. Information on other components of the system is fragmentary. A significant gap in our knowledge is the almost complete absence of information on the frequency, clinical and morphological manifestations of mixed infections, although, of course, they are a common occurrence. It is known from general infectology that the simultaneous presence of several pathogens in a patient can have an ambiguous effect on the infectious process [2].

6.1 Lessons of the Afterbirth in *Chlamydia*

Some information about the role of *Chlamydia* in perinatal infectious lesions in animals and humans began to appear in the literature, was summarized by us earlier from the end of the 1960s of the twentieth century. The fundamental possibility of *Chlamydia* affecting trophoblast, leading to both possible infection of the foetus and their functional dysfunction, has been established, but information about the frequency of this phenomenon is contradictory, and the characteristics of the structural changes associated with them are almost never given. However, in many sources devoted to the aetiology of placentitis, *Chlamydia* is not even mentioned.

On our material structural changes typical for chlamydiosis were observed in vascular endothelium, amniocytes, decidual and trophoblastic cells of the basal lamina, smooth and villous chorion in the form of fine vacuolization of the cytoplasm and the presence of small basophilic and pas-positive inclusions and Galberstedter-Provacek bodies in vacuoles. *Chlamydia* antigen could be detected both by IFM and IHC (Fig. 6.1)

V. Zinserling et al., *Chlamydia Infections*, https://doi.org/10.1007/978-3-031-99642-9_6

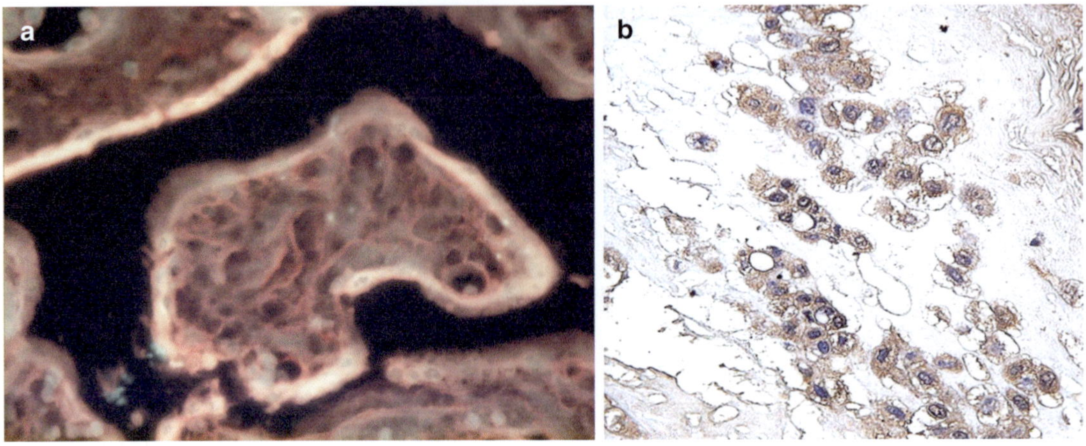

Fig. 6.1 (**a**) *Chlamydia* antigen in stem villus. Immunofluorescent microscopy/×600. (**b**) *Chlamydia* trachomatis antigen in decidua. IHC/×600. (From VZ, AK, SL)

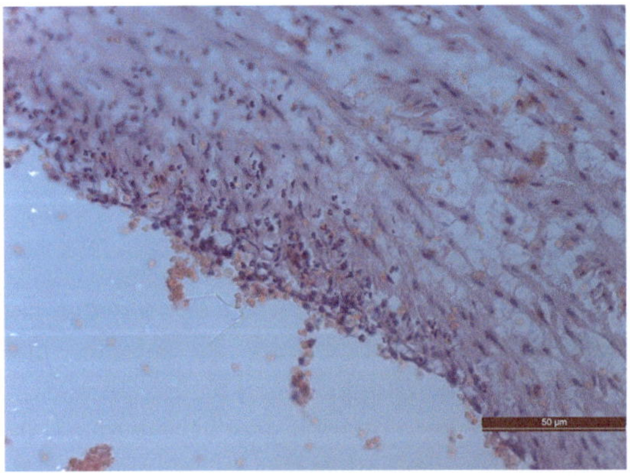

Fig. 6.2 Inflammatory changes in the umbilical artery. Staining haematoxylin and eosin. Magnification 400

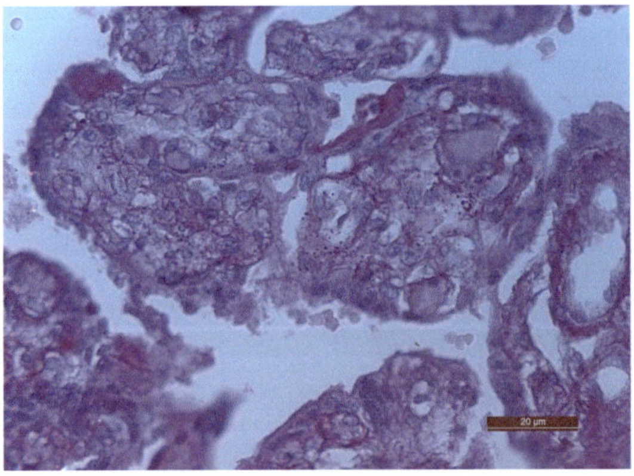

Fig. 6.3 Numerous extra- and intracellular PAS-positive inclusions in stem villi ×600

In addition, vascular disorders of different severity, various variants of pathological immaturity were observed in the afterbirth, which led to placental insufficiency, including acute, chronic compensated, chronic subcompensated. This allowed us to determine the degree of risk for possible pathology of the newborn. Inflammatory changes in umbilical vessels were seen regularly (Fig. 6.2).

Most recently, we conducted a study of the placentas of women suffering from preeclampsia against the background of a new coronavirus infection. Along with immaturity with signs of dissociated maturation, signs of infectious lesions were revealed. Along with the non-constant detection of SARSCOVID-2 s-antigen in all placental membranes, a significant number of extracellular and intracellular pas-positive corpuscles (Fig. 6.3) and a distinct positive immunohistochemical reaction with serum to *Chlamydia trachomatis* (Fig. 6.4) were detected. Many aspects of the revealed phenomenon need further study.

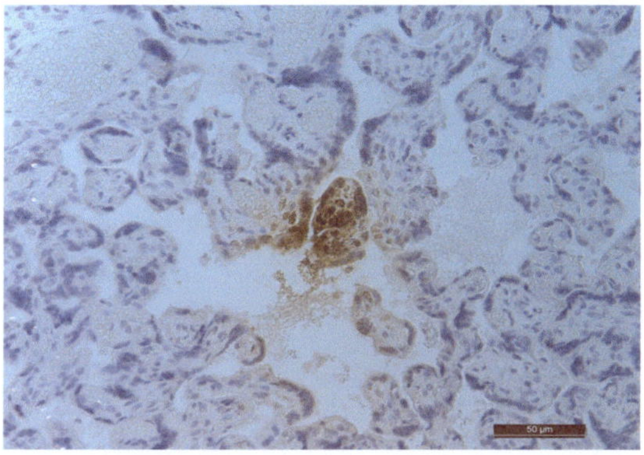

Fig. 6.4 *Chlamydia trachomatis* antigen in villi. IHC ×300. (From VZ, AK, SL)

6.2 Intrauterine Chlamydiosis

The significant frequency and great clinical significance of intrauterine chlamydiosis is currently recognized by all the numerous researchers discussing the issue of perinatal infections. There is evidence that at least 6–7% of children may be infected with *Chlamydia* at birth. In the clinic of intrauterine chlamydiosis, it is customary to distinguish between local (conjunctivitis, gastroenterocolitis, atypical pneumonia) and generalized forms of infection. Amongst the most important manifestations of generalized *Chlamydia* infection, it is customary to consider meningoencephalitis, cardiomyopathy, pneumonia, gastroenteritis, hepatitis, lymphadenitis, often complicated by the development of DIC syndrome. In a significant part of those infected (up to 22%), there are no clinical manifestations of the disease in the early neonatal period, an exacerbation of the process may occur throughout the first year of life and even later, when the connection with intrauterine infection may no longer be traced.

It has to be noted that urogenital and intrauterine chlamydiosis is a very important problem in animal husbandry, especially in cattle (see Chap. 9) Morphological changes in foetal/child tissues are either not discussed at all in the literature, or are considered to be non-specific and described in total without taking into account possible mixed infectious lesions. This served as the basis for the analysis of their own materials.

The results of our long-term studies were partly presented in our previous publication [1].

The diagnosis of *Chlamydia* was made on the basis of a comparison of clinical and anamnestic data (in many cases, the detection of *Chlamydia* in the mother), the results of morphological examination and IF detection of extracellular and intracellular forms of *Chlamydia* in smears from different organs. Intrauterine *Chlamydia* was generalized with damage to a number of internal organs and the central nervous system, which indicates a transplacental infection. In acute placental insufficiency or in chronic compensated placental insufficiency with acute decompensation, accompanied by disorders of uteroplacental circulation, which led to intranatal foetal hypoxia, the manifestations of *Chlamydia* were minimal, mainly with damage to the respiratory organs, which indicates an ascending path of infection. At the same time, the immediate cause of foetal death was asphyxia or related complications. Comparison of the results of histological and immunofluorescence studies in the diagnosis of *Chlamydia* in foetuses and in the study of afterbirth showed a coincidence of the results obtained using these methods.

The morphological manifestations of *Chlamydia* consisted of a peculiar transformation of cells of various origins, which were determined in various affected organs (Figs. 6.5, 6.6, 6.7, 6.8 and 6.9).

The cytoplasm increased quite significantly in size, becoming finely vacuolized. At the same time, fine grain inclusions were determined in it, which are better detected when stained with azur-eosin and according PAS.

During pathomorphological examination, pronounced circulatory disorders (fullness, haemorrhages), distelectases, desquamation of the epithelium, mainly macrophage infiltration with a small admixture of eosinophilic leukocytes, leukocytes and lymphocytes were noted in the lungs. In the liver—fullness, alterative changes, discomplexation of hepatic beams, abundance of islands of extramedullary haema-

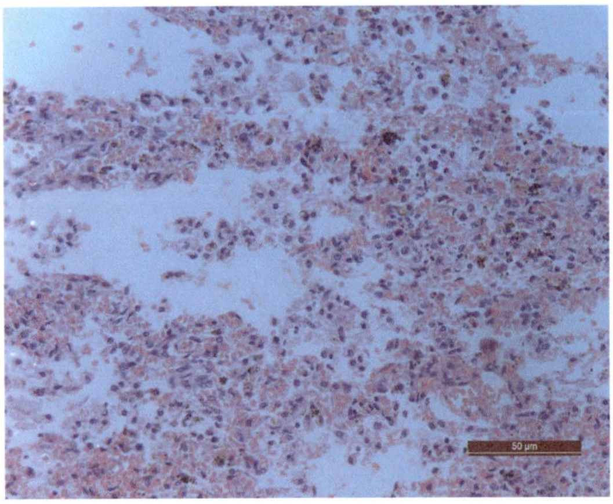

Fig. 6.5 Characteristic changes in the lungs in intrauterine *Chlamydia*. Note macrophages' exudate in alveoli. Haematoxylin and eosin staining. Magnification 360

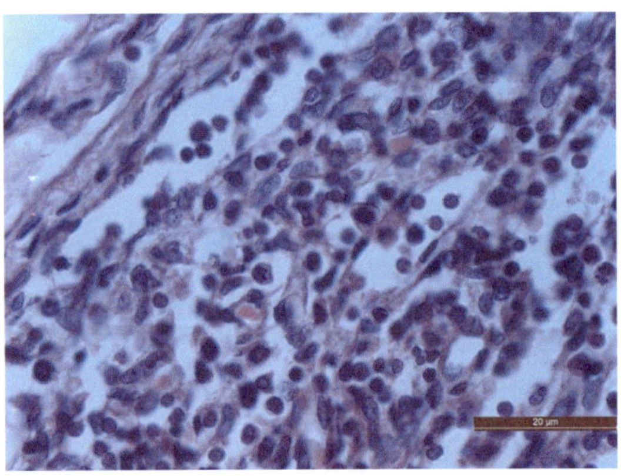

Fig. 6.6 Characteristic changes in the lymph node. Note vacuolized macrophages. Haematoxylin and eosin staining. Magnification 1000

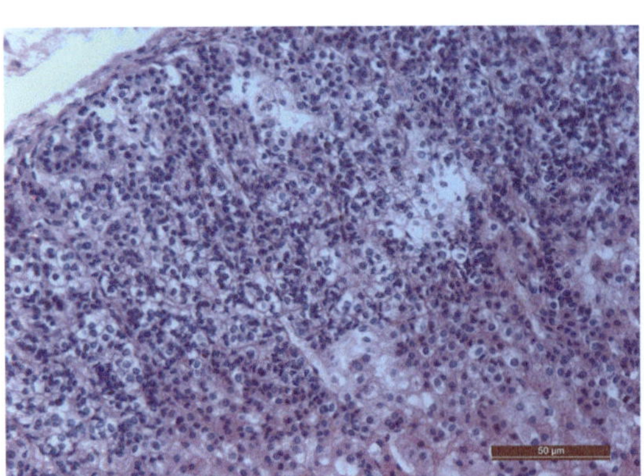

Fig. 6.7 Characteristic changes in the adrenal gland. Note vacuolated cells. Stained by haematoxylin and eosin. Magnification 630

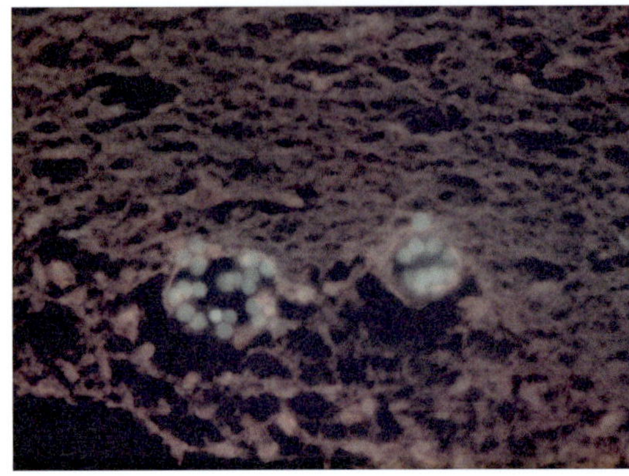

Fig. 6.8 *Chlamydia* antigen in lung. Immunofluorescent microscopy ×600

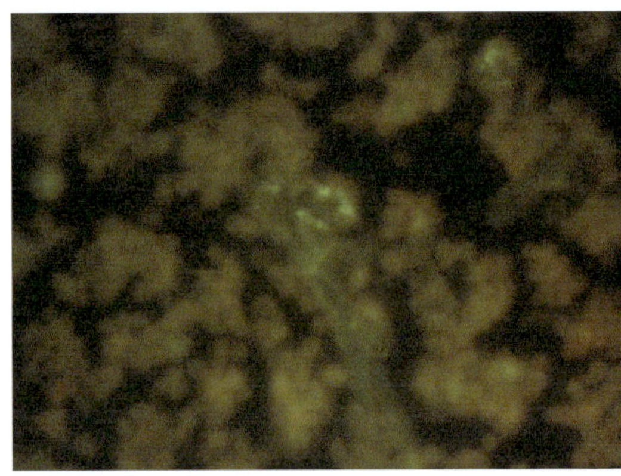

Fig. 6.9 *Chlamydia* antigen in heart. Immunofluorescent microscopy ×600. (From VZ, AK, SL)

topoiesis, lympho-macrophage infiltration around the triads and along the portal tracts, small-scale hepatocyte lipidosis, in cases of stillbirth, hepatocytes with cytoplasm emptying were noted. From the side of the brain tissue—oedema, dystrophic cell changes, fullness of blood, perivascular inflammatory infiltrates and foci of gliosis (Figs. 6.10 and 6.11). It should be noted that in the kidneys, where the glow was noted in all cases, there were no specific morphological changes characterizing the infectious process, but the antigen was revealed by IHC. The processes of circulatory disorders and dystrophic changes in the epithelium of the tubules were determined (Fig. 6.12). There were no significant differences in the morphological picture in all groups.

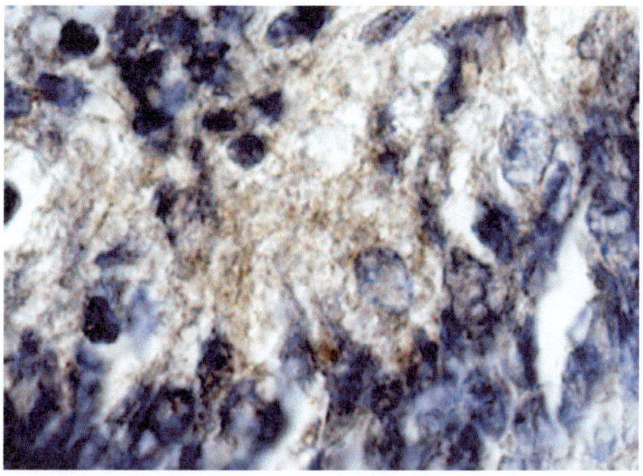

Fig. 6.10 *Chlamydia trachomatis* antigen in ependyma cells. IHC. ×600. (From VZ, AK, SL)

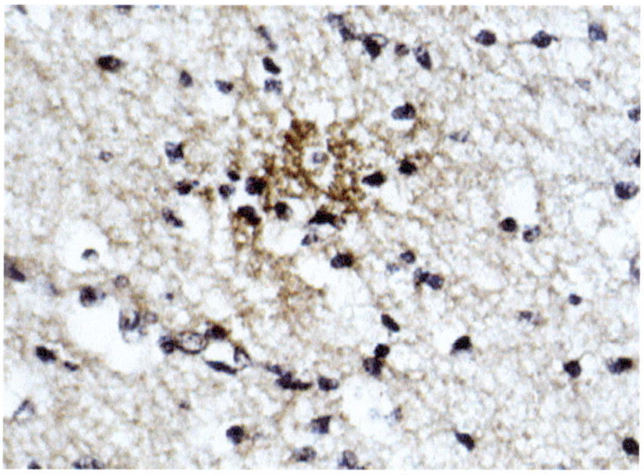

Fig. 6.11 *Chlamydia trachomatis* antigen in brain matter. IHC ×400. (From VZ, AK, SL)

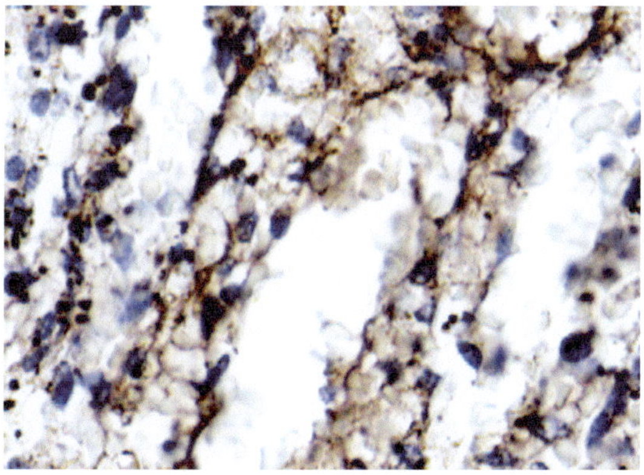

Fig. 6.12 *Chlamydia trachomatis* antigen in kidney. IHC. ×600. (From VZ, AK, SL)

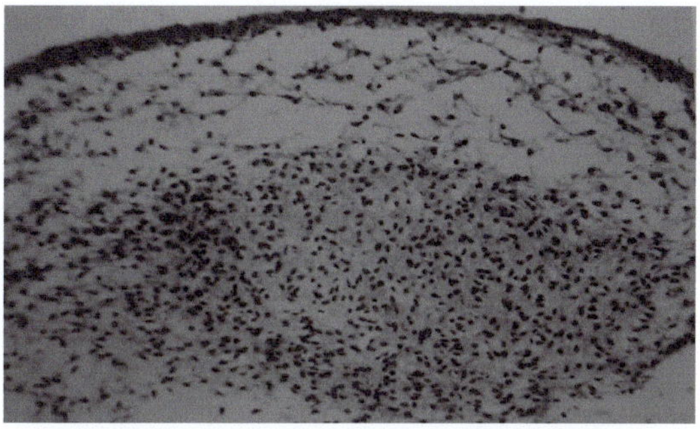

Fig. 6.13 Granuloma in soft meninges. HE. ×50. (Courtesy of SA Zworygin)

Currently, the attention of a number of researchers from the Ural region of Russia (Samokhin PA et al.) in intrauterine *Chlamydia* is attracted by damage to the brain, especially the soft meninges. The authors describe the appearance of peculiar granulomas in them, which are already determined macroscopically on the convex surface of the brain in the form of "cotton-like" formations (Fig. 6.13). Using EM, *Chlamydia* was determined inside the cells of these granulomas (Figs. 6.14 and 6.15). In our material, such pronounced changes in soft meninges are not naturally determined. When studying them purposefully in observations with verified generalized intrauterine *Chlamydia*, we noted a slight increase in the number of fibroblasts in all observations, in about half of the cases with the formation of granuloma-like structures around the vessels. It can be assumed that these differences in soft meninges lesions may be related to differences in the properties of strains circulating in different regions.

We present also our presentation of probably intrauterine chlamydiosis in a child older than 1 year. Originally the observation of VA Zinserling was made in 1983, in 2025 the possibility appeared to review it.

Svetlana M., 1 year 1 month old, was born from the 7th pregnancy, 3 premature births, weighing 2050, length 45 cm, cried after mucus suctioning, Apgar 7/8. On the 6th day of life, due

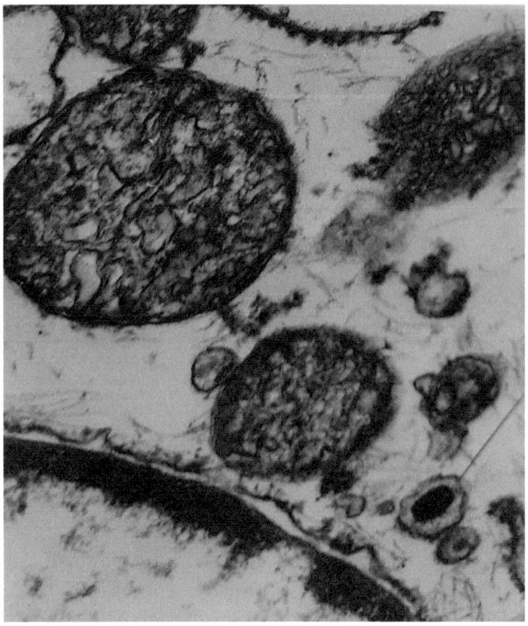

Fig. 6.14 Electron microscopy of brain meninges. Hydropic necrosis of meningocyte with vacuole formation. In cytoplasm numerous elementary and intermediate bodies of Chlamydia. X 12000. (Courtesy of SA Zworygin)

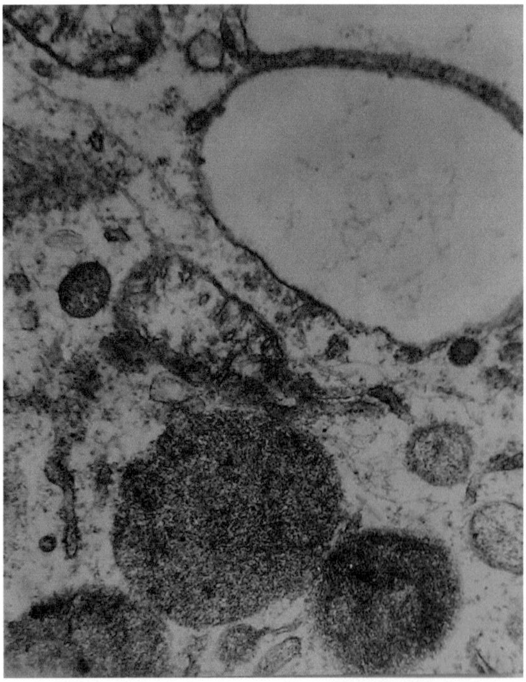

Fig. 6.15 Fragment of macrophage with dividing *Chlamydia*. X 20000. (Courtesy of SA Zworygin)

to prematurity, she was transferred to the children's hospital, where she stayed for a month, where decreased reflexes of newborns, severe jaundice of the skin, catarrhal keratoconjunctivitis, clinical and radiological symptoms of acute viral respiratory infection were detected. Later, she lagged somewhat in psychomotor development—she held her head up from 2 1/2 months; she sat from the 2nd month, at the age of 1 year she did not walk. At the age of 2 months she was re-hospitalized with a diagnosis of moderate acute respiratory viral infection, she was in the hospital for a month. At the age of 7 and 9 months, she was treated twice for anicteric, HBS Ag -negative hepatitis in the children's infectious diseases hospital. The last disease began 10 days before death with a rise in temperature to 39.5°, runny nose, the next day after eating against the background of normal temperature, repeated vomiting was noted. On the 3rd day of the disease, she became very lethargic, drowsy, but periodically very excited. On admission, her condition is extremely serious, unconscious, floating movements of the eyeballs, pupils D = S without reaction to light, eye slits S $\geq$ D, high tendon and periosteal reflexes, clonus of the feet, positive meningeal symptoms. The pharynx is loosened and hyperaemic, shortness of breath and harsh breathing in the lungs. The liver protrudes by 1 cm from under the edge of the costal arch. Blood analysis shows moderate hypochromic anaemia, leukocytosis, neutrophilia with a shift to the left, thrombocytopenia. Biochemical blood test: ALT 5.1, then 14.5; AST 4.4; 7.6: bilirubin 2.56. During her stay in the department, neurological symptoms worsened, coma of the third degree occurred, breathing became of the Kusmaul type. From the 2nd day of her stay in the hospital, she was transferred to artificial ventilation with the Vita- I apparatus.

During her stay in the hospital, the child developed bilateral bronchopneumonia, acute cardiovascular failure stage III and acute renal failure. She received ampicillin, dexazone, cardiotropic, dehydration, detoxification and symptomatic therapy.

Clinical diagnosis: Acute viral encephalitis of unknown aetiology. Complications of the underlying disease: Oedema-swelling of the brain, bilateral bronchopneumonia, respiratory insufficiency II. Acute renal failure. Acute cardiovascular failure.

Associated diseases: Acute respiratory viral infection. Hepatitis of unknown aetiology. Hypotrophy.

At the medical autopsy (V.A. Zinsaerling) phenomena of catarrhal laryngotracheobronchitis were noted. The lungs are of a dense consistency, in the right lower lobe, especially distinct in the region of the 9th and 10th segments, there are multiple small but merging pneumonic foci. Similar changes are also in the region of the 2nd and 6th segments of the upper lobe, as well as in the left lower lobe. The renal cortex has a sharply expressed grayish tint; the cavities of the pelvis and calyces are somewhat expanded. The thymus gland is of a flabby consistency, whitish in colour, weighing 10.0. The liver is significantly enlarged in size (the right lobe is II.5 × 10.5 × 5, the left 7 × 8.5 × 3.5); weighing 420.0 g, it protrudes up to 3 cm from under the costal arch and goes quite far into the left hypochondrium. The organ is of dense consistency, with a slightly rounded edge, brownish-reddish in colour. Its surface is predominantly smooth, only on the upper surface of the left lobe is slight wrinkling observed. On section, a bright yellow pattern of lobules surrounded by a thin bluish-brown rim is observed in all lobes. In the mucosa of the small intestine, moderate plethora and isolated petechial haemorrhages are present. The brain weighs 950.0 g, is of a flabby consistency, its grooves and convolutions are somewhat smoothed out. The pia mater is oedematous. On section, the pattern of the brain in the area of the basal nodes and the thalamus is blurred, the system of the cerebral ventricles is somewhat expanded. The vessels of the white matter are sharply plethoraic. The vascular plexuses are dark cherry in colour.

Cytological examination of smears from the lungs revealed a significant number of neutrophilic leukocytes, as well as desquamated alveolocytes, some of which had vacuolated cytoplasm with small point inclusions, and some had enlarged basophilic stained cytoplasm. Histobacterioscopic examination revealed single small cocci.

Immunofluorescence examination of lung smears revealed positive fluorescence with serum anti-*Chlamydia trachomatis*. The results of the study of smears from the lungs and brain with sera against respiratory viruses and mycoplasmas are negative. Only in the lungs was detected residual luminescence with serum to influenza B.

Bacteriological examination revealed only isolated colonies of *Klebsiella pneumoniae* in the lungs, blood, spleen and ear swab.

During a serological blood test, antibodies to respiratory viruses and mycoplasma pneumoniae could not be detected in the complement binding test; antibodies to influenza B were detected in a titre of 2:80 in the reaction haemagglutination inhibition.

Results of virological cultural examination of the lungs and brain are negative. The results of the comparison of anamnestic, clinical, laboratory and morphological data of those years allowed us to formulate the final pathological diagnosis as follows: generalized infection caused by *Chlamydia trachomatis*: meningoencephalitis, hepatitis, pneumonia, nephritis, pancreatitis, enteritis.

In 2025, it became possible to re-run the PAS reaction on sections made from archival paraffin blocks and conduct a previously unavailable immunohistochemical study with serum to *C. trachomatis* of most internal organs and the brain. The interpretation of the case remained fundamentally the same, but it was possible to show that the severe pneumonia (Fig. 6.16a, b) was caused by *Chlamydia*.

Chlamydia antigen and PAS-positive inclusions were also detected in the kidneys, liver, pancreas, brain and spinal cord, adrenal glands, lymph nodes, spleen and tonsils (Figs. 6.17 and 6.18). It is important to note that *Chlamydia* were detected both in the parenchymatous cells of virtually all organs and in the vascular endothelium. Extracellular forms were comparatively rare (Fig. 6.19).

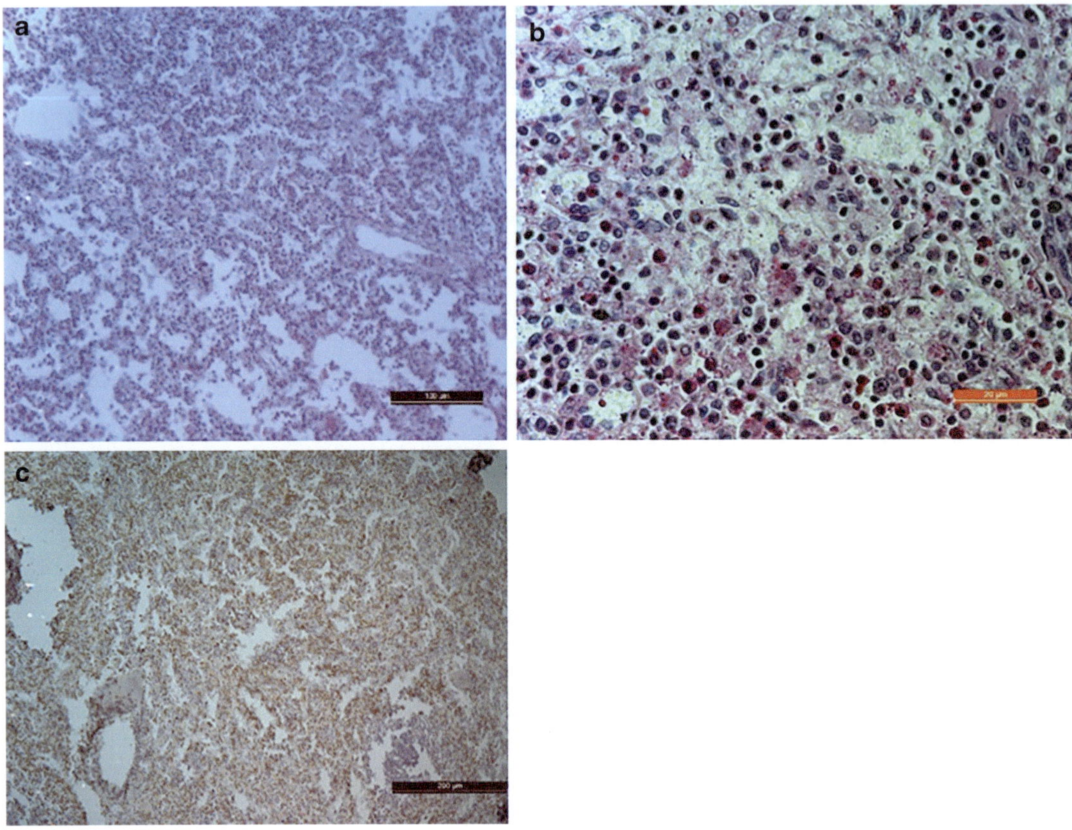

Fig. 6.16 Pneumonia in a girl M.A. (**a**) General appearance with haematoxylin and eosin staining. Magnification 160, (**b**) Numerous PAS-positive extra- and intracellular inclusions. Magnification 640b. (**c**) Significant number of cells positive with serum to *C. trachomatis* IHC, ×100

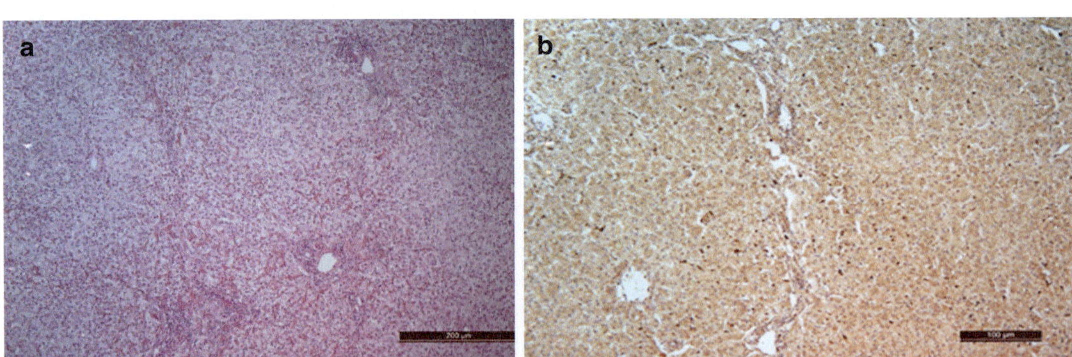

Fig. 6.17 Liver damage in a girl M.A. General appearance. Staining with G-E, UV 100 B A significant number of cells positive with serum to *C. trachomatis* IHC, ×125

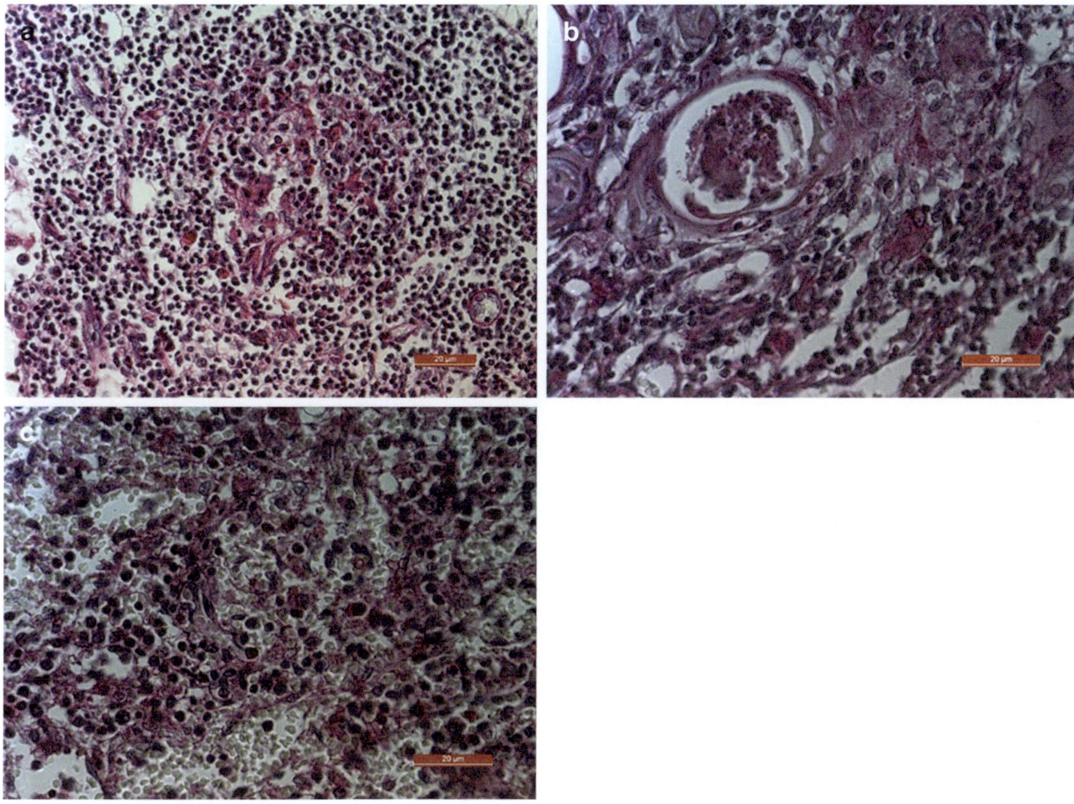

Fig. 6.18 PAS-positive inclusions in lymph node (**a**), thymus (**b**) and spleen (**c**) ×640

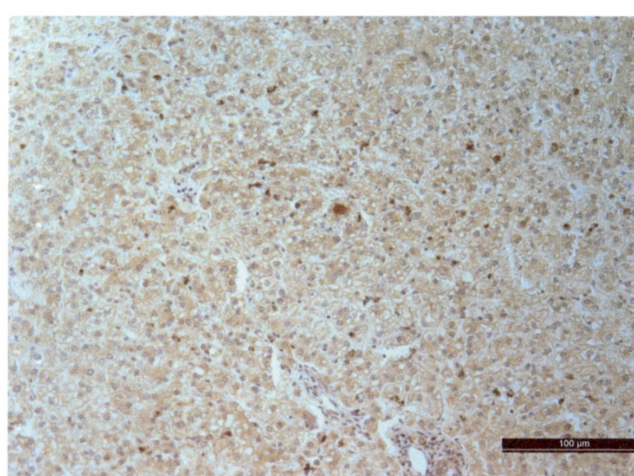

Fig. 6.19 Elementary body of *Chlamydia* in the liver. IHC. Magnification 200

Conclusion

Svetlana M., 1 year old, suffered for a long time from a generalized, probably intrauterine, cyclical infection that caused similar lesions of many internal organs. The nature of the changes revealed during the histological examination and the results of immunofluorescence and immunohistochemical studies make it possible to diagnose chlamydiosis. The child's long stay on artificial ventilation of the lungs and the development of secondary changes in the brain in connection with this significantly complicate the establishment of the causes of the acute development of cerebral coma in the child, which served as the immediate cause of death. Laboratory and morphological comparisons allow us to say that the girl had influenza B within a week. The long course of the underlying disease led to the development of a sharply expressed secondary immunodeficiency state, which undoubtedly contributed to the unfavourable outcome. From a conversation with the child's mother, it became known that her father had suffered from chronic prostatitis for a long time.

6.2.1 Conclusions

- Intrauterine infection with *Chlamydia* can be both intranatal and antenatal.
- Intrauterine *Chlamydia* occurs as a generalized infection with damage to 2 or more organs.

The data provided by our studies of various years, performed using various methods, clearly indicate a significant frequency of perinatal chlamydiosis. Various pathogens from this group can play an aetiological role in the development of pathology of pregnancy, foetus, newborn and older children. The nature of the clinical manifestations of the disease can vary significantly from practically asymptomatic to fatal, with the most characteristic being the chronic course. Morphological changes in *Chlamydia* of different localizations are similar, although they are little known and can be used in diagnosis. Many issues related to the epidemiology, pathogenesis and morphological manifestations of chlamydial infections need further study.

- Given the positive reaction in the kidneys with immunofluorescence and the absence of pronounced morphological manifestations, it can be assumed that the kidney is the organ where the pathogen can persist [1, 3–7].

6.3 Remote Consequences of Intrauterine *Chlamydia* (in Collaboration with YI Vainshenker)

Chlamydia is often not accompanied by obvious symptoms in the neonatal period [1]. In the first few years of life, delayed psychomotor development, respiratory and intestinal infections are diagnosed. At an older age, the infection is masked by other diseases of the central nervous system, aggravating or imitating their course. In some children, the inflammatory process from birth is sluggish in nature, while in others, the onset of clinical manifestations is observed only several years after "recovery" from perinatal encephalopathy, probably under the influence of an intercurrent process or superinfection [8, 9].

During the examination of 42 children (3–15 years) with various non-infectious neurological and psychoneurological diagnoses, who had a diagnosis of perinatal encephalopathy in infancy, 93% (39) of them were found to have (by culture and PCR) pathogens of low-manifest infections (LMIs) in various combinations and in various biological materials, including chlamydial infection was detected in 71% (30) of children.

Etiotropic antibacterial therapy confirmed the involvement of the identified intrauterine infection in the CNS lesion. Retrospectively (based on the regression of neurological symptoms), the clinical manifestations of LMI were identified: asthenia and psychoneurological disorders, brainstem symptoms, extrapyramidal, less often pyramidal and cerebellar syndromes, as well as epileptic, diencephalic syndromes and headache of a meningeal-vascular nature. Taking into account the neuroimaging data, sluggish perinatal encephalitis had features of an inflammatory-degenerative process [9].

Infection with pathogens of intrauterine infections (*C. trachomatis*, *Mycoplasma* spp., *Ureaplasma urealyticum*) was accompanied by a complex of signs of connective tissue dysplasia (arachnoid cysts, dysplasia of the craniovertebral region in combination with dysplasia of the cerebral vessels or internal organs) [9].

References

1. Zinserling VA, Kolobov AV, Lucas S. Placentitis and perinatal infections. Cham: Springer; 2024. p. 119p.
2. Zinserling VA. Infectious pathology of the respiratory tract. Cham: Springer. https://doi.org/10.1007/978-3-030-66325-4. ISBN 978-3-030-66324-7. 259p.
3. Tsinzerling [Zinserling]. AV Chlamydiosis: diagnosis and role in human pathology. Arkh Patol. 1989;51(1):3–9. (in Russian). https://www.elibrary.ru/item.asp?id=25535538.
4. Zinserling VA. School of infectious pathology of AV Zinserling: achievements and perspectives. Arkh Patol. 2014;76(1):3–9. (in Russian)
5. Samokhin PA, Erman BA, Tulakina LG, et al. Morphological characteristics of intrauterine chlamydiosis and its clinical-anatomical characteristics. Arkh Patol. 1997;59(5):27–31. (in Russian)
6. Kacerovsky M, Romero R, Pliskova L, et al. Presence of Chlamydia trachomatis DNA in the amniotic fluid in women with preterm prelabor rupture of membranes. J Matern Fetal Neonatal Med. 2021;34(10):1586–97. https://doi.org/10.1080/14767058.2019.1640676.
7. Gorbunov EF, Zinserling VA, Semenov NV. Characteristics of internal organ lesions in perinatal chlamydiosis. Arkh Patol. 2007;69(3):33–6. (in Russian)
8. Vainshenker YI, Kalinina OV, Nuralova IV, et al. Low-manifest infections in children and adolescents with consequences of perinatal damage to the nervous system. J Microbiol Epidemiol Immunobiol. 2012;5:77–80. (in Russian)
9. Vainshenker YI, Kalinina OV, Nuralova IV, et al. Low-manifest infections of the perinatal period and their clinical and neurological manifestations in children and adolescents. Infect Dis. 2013;11(1):44–9. (in Russian)

7 Problems of Mixed Chlamydial Infections

Mixed infections are of significant importance in the development of pathological processes in various organs [1–3], although there are very few studies devoted to them. The number of pathogens detected in one patient can be quite significant, and in the case of HIV infection, exceed 10. Obviously, all of them cannot but interact with various consequences, which in most cases remain unknown. *Chlamydia* is also a frequent participant in the "collective."

Thus, as is known, more than half of the world's population is simultaneously seropositive, for example, to *C. pneumoniae*, *Helicobacter pylori* and cytomegalovirus [4]. With the proven increased risk of atherosclerosis in association with *C. pneumonia* (as well as other bacterial and/or viral pathogens), the idea of a vascular microbiome involved in the development of atherosclerosis has recently been put forward: microbiota originating from the oral cavity and/or intestine have been found in the atherosclerotic plaque [4] (see Sect. 8.1 for more details).

7.1 *Chlamydia* and Influenza

Influenza is one of the infections that attracts close attention of researchers in different fields, the population, the media and various administrative structures. Amongst the relatively rarely discussed issues is the role of the influenza virus in mixed infections, as its role in preparing a platform for the development of bacterial pneumonia [1] and its role in the development of severe meningococcaemia [2] has been shown. Given the ability of this virus to suppress the immune response and reduce local defence reactions, it is logical to predict its ability to activate chronic and latent infectious processes, amongst the pathogens of which *Chlamydia* occupies a prominent place.

One of the studied cases is of particular interest.

A 31-year-old male patient IV with obesity got ill acutely, with fever up to 39 °C. Three days later, he was hospitalized in the intensive care unit with severe respiratory insufficiency. Intubation and, later on, tracheostomy were performed. The clinical diagnosis of "swine influenza" was supported by RT PCR and serology (increase of antibody level 0–640). In spite of intensive treatment including antibiotics and antiviral drugs, the patient died on the 35th day of the illness.

At the autopsy, remarkable changes were found only in the lungs: necrotic posttracheostomic tracheitis, large abscesses in the lower lobes of the lungs in the stage of organization, bilateral fibrinous pleuritis. The rest of lung tissue was dark red, firm. During the histological examination in the lungs, changes typical for rather old abscesses, late stages of respiratory distress syndrome were noted. The changes that we consider to be typical for influenza (virus-induced transformation of epithelial cells) were expressed only in the moderate number of the cells. We notified

V. Zinserling et al., *Chlamydia Infections*, https://doi.org/10.1007/978-3-031-99642-9_7

numerous intra-alveolar macrophages, partly with vacuolated cytoplasm (Fig. 7.1), and PAS-positive inclusions (Fig. 7.2).

Some cells had slightly enlarged hyperchromic nuclei. Similar changes were noted in other organs as well. Postmortem RT-PCR of lung and spleen specimens for influenza A/H1N1sw was negative. During the bacteriological investigation of lung specimens, cultures of *E. coli*, non-pathogenic *Corynebacteria*, *Enterococcus*, *S. viridans* and *S. epidermiditis* were isolated.

In lungs, strong positive reaction in IHC with serum against *Chlamydia spp*. Fig. 7.3), moderate against *Adenovirus* and weak against influenza H1N1 were obtained.

The reactions with sera against HSV1/2, CMV, EBV, RS, entero- and parvoviruses, as well as *Mycoplasma pneumoniae* were negative. During the electron microscopic investigation of lungs, we succeeded in evaluating numerous elementary and reticular bodies of *Chlamydia* (Fig. 7.4), in brain only reticular bodies, predominantly in cytoplasm of endothelial cells (Fig. 7.5).

In their nuclei, several PML-nuclear bodies (small intranucleolar inclusions containing promyelocytic leukaemia protein) were found.

Death of young healthy man occurred on the 35th day of illness clinically regarded as influenza with bacterial superinfection. The results of postmortem morphological and laboratory investigation proved that clinically diagnosed infections were expressed rather weakly, but provoked the

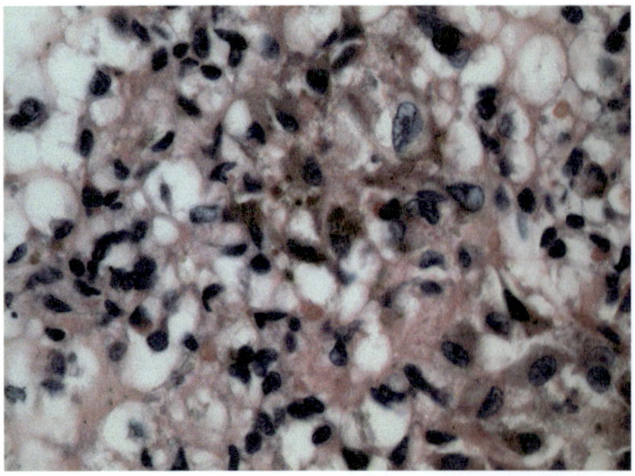

Fig. 7.1 Numerous cells with vacuolated cytoplasm. HE. ×640

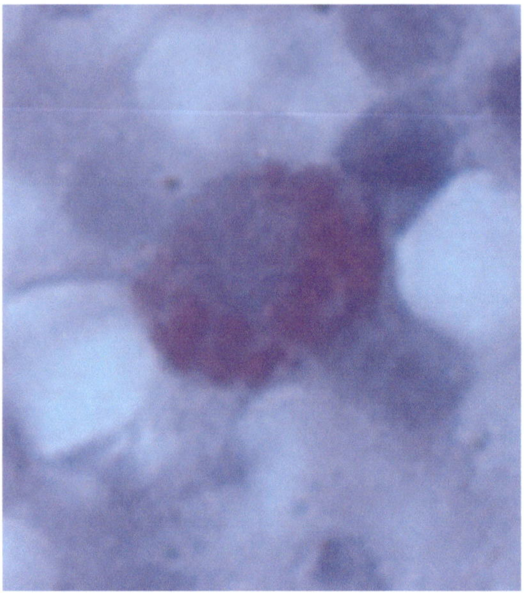

Fig. 7.2 Intracellular PAS-positive inclusions

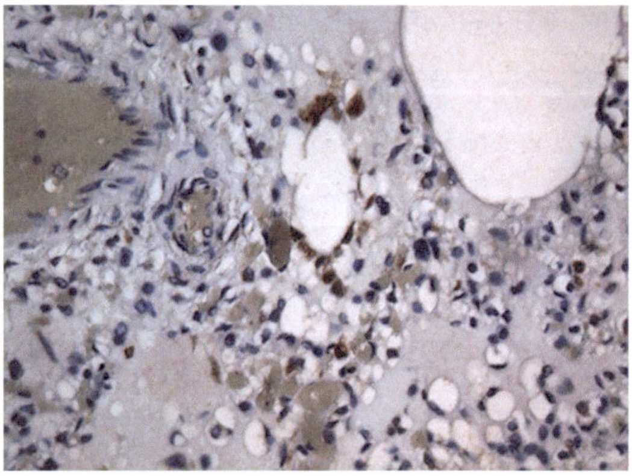

Fig. 7.3 Antigen of *Chlamydia* in lung macrophages. IHC ×640

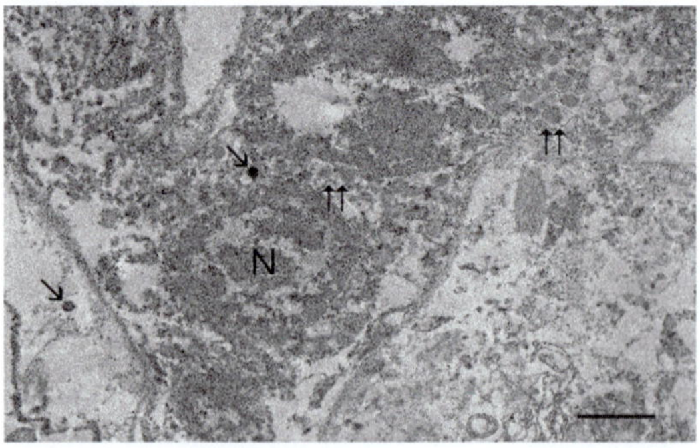

Fig. 7.4 Lungs. Single arrows indicate mature elementary bodies of *Chlamydia*. Double arrows indicate clusters of maturing elementary bodies surrounded by a loosely adhering membrane. *N* nucleus of macrophage/large-scale mark (ruler) 2 microns

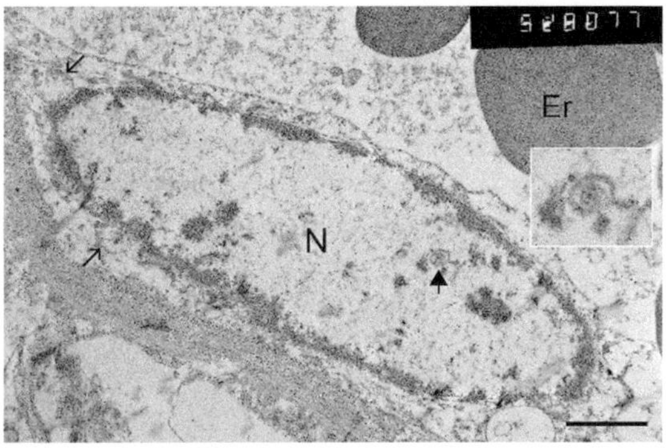

Fig. 7.5 Reticular bodies of *Chlamydia* (on arrows) in cytoplasm of brain endothelium

activation and severe course of respiratory chlamydiosis (with probable generalization) and adenoviral infection.

7.2 Chlamydiosis and Covid

It is now obvious that the extremely severe course of the new coronavirus infection is associated with a variety of pathogenetic mechanisms. The virus has tropism for many organs that have the ACE-2 receptor, the ability to damage the endothelium of vessels of various sizes and disrupt the blood coagulation system, which leads to a variety of thrombotic complications (from pulmonary embolism to microthrombosis in the capillaries of the renal glomeruli). Its ability to cause damage to the immune system (from signs of immunodeficiency to the initiation of autoimmune reactions) has been shown.

It can be assumed that coronavirus can contribute to the activation of chronic low-manifest infectious lesions of the respiratory organs. It is currently known that a number of pathogens, primarily *Chlamydia*, can often cause both "primary atypical pneumonia," characterized by a long low-manifest course, and remain inside the cells of the respiratory organs for a long time, practically without causing clinical symptoms.

When studying microscopic preparations from 36 observations of fatal outcomes from COVID-19 in April–May 2020, 5 were identified in which, along with the previously described changes in the lungs, as well as in the lymph node (2 observations) and meninges (1 observation), characteristic of the new coronavirus infection, a peculiar vacuolization of the cytoplasm was detected, which makes one suspect the presence of infections caused by mycoplasmas or *Chlamydia*. To clarify the emerging assumption, the corresponding preparations were stained using the PAS method, which is recommended for diagnosing these infections. In all observations, extra- and intracellular bodies were detected, which made it possible to speak with a high degree of probability about the chlamydial aetiology of the process.

7.2.1 Description of a Clinical Case

A 39-year-old female patient was hospitalized on an emergency basis on January 19, 2023, with complaints of shortness of breath with minimal physical exertion, weakness and cough with scanty sputum.

She has been ill for 4 months; at the onset of the disease, shortness of breath appeared during short walks, cough with expectoration. The diagnosis of new coronavirus infection was established based on clinical data and isolation of SARS-CoV-2 by PCR. Radiologically (09/14/2022), areas of decreased pneumatization were noted in the middle-lower sections on both sides and an increase in the pulmonary pattern. She received antibacterial and antiviral therapy on an outpatient basis (she does not know the names of the drugs) without improvement: shortness of breath and cough persisted.

In December 2022, she was consulted by a TB specialist. Sputum microscopy for acid-fast mycobacteria and a Diaskin test were performed with negative results. The patient refused the proposed hospitalization.

According to the computed tomography of the chest organs performed immediately before hospitalization, signs of interstitial lung damage with the involvement of 80% of the parenchyma (CT-4), enlargement of the lower paratracheal, axillary and subclavian lymph nodes, minimal left-sided hydrothorax and hydropericardium were noted.

It is known from the anamnesis that HIV infection was detected in 2005, the route of transmission is sexual. In 2005–2019, she took effective ART regimens (the last one: 3TC, TDF, ATV/r), she interrupted the treatment on her own. Concomitant diseases: chronic pyelonephritis, chronic tonsillitis, gastritis. There is no penitentiary history, there were no tuberculosis contacts, no bad habits.

Laboratory examination in December 2022: HIV viral load 1.9×10^6 cop/ml, CD4 < 100 cells/µl. Due to the persistent clinical picture of new coronavirus infection, ART was resumed on an outpatient basis.

Objectively upon admission: the condition is moderate, the skin is pale, without signs of cyanosis, auscultation in the lungs reveals harsh breathing, no wheezing, respiratory rate is 18–20 per minute, saturation from 90% to 93% (in atmospheric air).

Laboratory examination data upon admission: complete blood count: leukocytes 4.14×10^9/l, lymphocytes 31.1%/1.29×10^9/l, haemoglobin 109 g/l, platelets 224×10^9/l. Biochemical analysis: ALT 67.2 U /l, AST 71.9 U/l, creatinine 51 µmol /l, LDH 581 U /l, C-reactive protein 5.59 mg/l, ferritin 459 µg/l; according to coagulogram: fibrinogen 5.04 g/l, INR 1.06, D- dimer 193 ng /ml. CD4 lymphocyte level: 1.7%—23 cells/µl; HIV viral load—7.2×10^3 cop/ml. Viral hepatitis markers (HBsAg, HCV Ab)—negative. SARS-CoV-2 virus RNA PCR—positive result.

In the department, she received complex therapy, including continuation of ART, a course of molnupiravir (1600 mg/day for 5 days), pathogenetic therapy: low-molecular heparins parenterally, oxygen therapy. Due to the phenomena of respiratory failure of 1–2 stage, dexamethasone was used at a maximum dosage of 12 mg/day.

Given the profound immunodeficiency in the patient with diffuse interstitial lung tissue damage, the diagnostic examination was expanded to exclude HIV-associated lung tissue lesions. Despite the negative results of PCR analysis of sputum and bronchial washings for nucleic acids (NA) of *P .jirovecii* and NA of CMV, persistent dyspnoea and decreased blood oxygen saturation with minimal physical exertion did not allow us to exclude opportunistic infections of the lungs. Consecutive courses of treatment for *Pneumocystis pneumonia* (trimethoprim/sulfamethoxazole, 1440 mg × 4 times a day, 5 weeks) and cytomegalovirus infection (ganciclovir 500 mg/day, 3 weeks) were administered without significant clinical and radiological effect. Bacterioscopy, molecular genetic and cultural examination methods excluded pulmonary tuberculosis and mycobacteriosis caused by non-tuberculous mycobacteria. Based on the results of the analysis of bronchial washings for fungi (microscopy and culture), no data were obtained for invasive pulmonary mycosis.

Repeated SARS-CoV-2 PCR tests (10.02., 20.03., 02.04.) showed a positive result. ELISA determination of the titre of specific IgG to SARS-Cov-2 (22.03.2023) showed a negative result (0 BAU/ml). ELISA IgM and IgG to *Chl. pneumoniae* showed a negative result. Blood test from 09.03.2023 showed a CD4 lymphocyte level of 0.6%/4.3 cells/µl; HIV VL—1.1×10^3 cop/ml.

Due to the appearance of purulent sputum and the obtained cultures of pathogenic microorganisms, she received targeted courses of antibacterial drugs (*K. pneumoniae* 10^5, sensitive to amoxicillin/ clavulanic acid, meropenem and amikacin were isolated; and *Burkholderia lata* 10^4 sensitive to ceftazidime, meropenem and trimethoprim-sulfamethoxazole).

According to the control CT scan of the chest organs (03/16/2023), a multidirectional process was noted, which included an active viral interstitial lesion (CT-4) and the presence of pneumofibrosis patterns. The clinical picture was assessed as manifestations of a protracted course of new coronavirus infection with persistent viral replication. Due to the early threshold number of the SARS-CoV-2 NC detection cycle in PCR of a nasopharyngeal swab (Ct = 19.0) in the sixth month from the onset of the disease, by decision of the medical commission, after obtaining informed consent from the patient, a repeated course of antiviral therapy with remdesivir was administered for 10 days in combination with an anti-COVID plasma transfusion in the "off-label" mode (outside the instructions). The multicom-

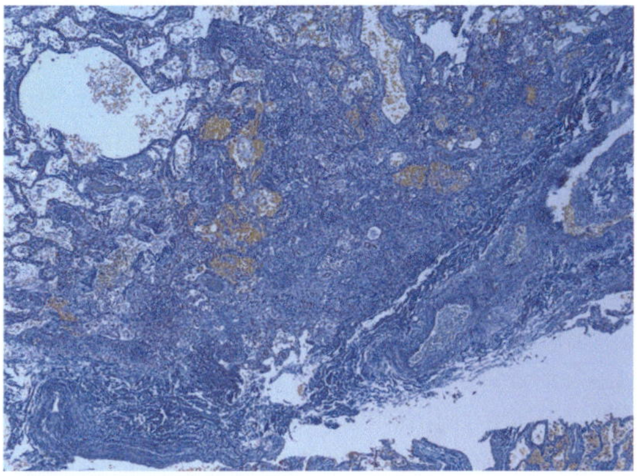

Fig. 7.6 Severe pulmonary fibrosis. Mallory stain. Magnification 50

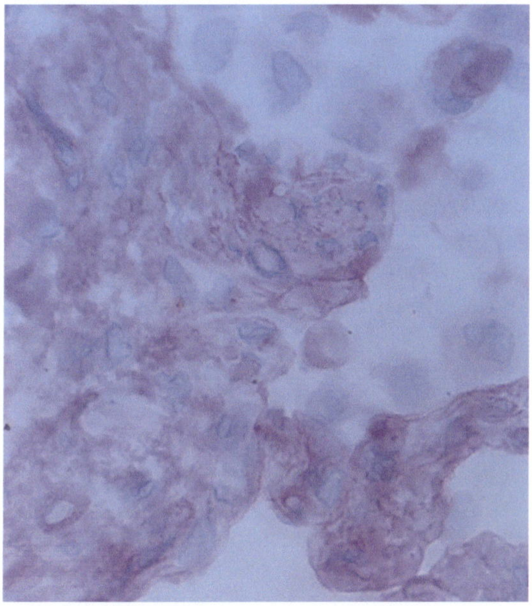

Fig. 7.7 Numerous extra- and intracellular PAS-positive inclusions. PAS reaction. Magn. 600

ponent therapy did not provide a clinical effect. Due to progressive respiratory failure and lack of effect from oxygen therapy, the patient was connected to a ventilator on 04/04/2023. A fatal outcome was recorded on 05/04/2023 (on the 77th day of hospital stay).

Pathomorphological examination revealed significant pneumofibrosis (Fig. 7.6).

In the lung tissue, there are a significant number of vacuolated macrophages containing PAS -positive inclusions (Fig. 7.7), the nature of

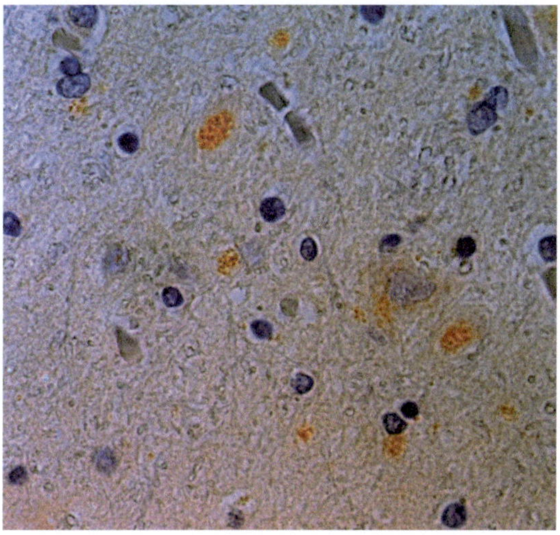

Fig. 7.8 *C. trachomatis* antigen in brain tissue. IHC magnification 600

which was established by immunohistochemical examination, which gave a positive reaction with serum to *C. trachomatis*. The same antigen was also detected in brain tissue (Fig. 7.8).

Amongst the exfoliated cells of the ciliated epithelium, there were multinucleated ones, the formation of which can presumably be associated with a new coronavirus infection. No signs of pneumocystosis were detected.

Discussion Long-term excretion of the SARS-CoV-2 virus in a patient with immunodeficiency significantly complicates the diagnosis of the activity of the pathological process. Laboratory parameters routinely used in hospitals to determine signs of the development of a cytokine storm and acute respiratory distress syndrome are not relevant for a protracted course of the disease. In addition, HIV infection per se is characterized by chronic inflammatory response syndrome, which creates additional difficulties in adequately assessing the level of acute phase blood parameters.

An unexpected finding during the morphological study was the detection of chlamydial infection of the lungs and brain. The most likely is the activation of its latent form during the current new coronavirus infection. It is possible that one of the factors that determined the protracted course of new coronavirus infection in the presented observation is precisely the presence of a mixed infection [5–10].

7.3 Combined Brain Lesions in Severe Non-infectious Lesions (Jointly with Yu.I. Vainshenker)

In chronic non-infectious pathology of the central nervous system, the detection of various microorganisms, such as *Chlamydia* spp., *Mycoplasma* spp., *Ureaplasma* spp., VEB, CMV, HHV-6, HSV-1, HSV-2, VZV, pathogenic (capsular) forms of *Bacteroides fragilis*, and in different biomaterials (cerebrospinal fluid, blood, nasopharyngeal scrapings, conjunctiva) is presented in Fig. 7.1 and 7.2. The data were obtained during the examination of patients with chronic disorders of consciousness,(CDC) (n = 68) and with other various neurological diseases (VNDs): children, n = 57 and adults, n = 104. As follows from the figure, *Chlamydia* had a direct tropism for the central nervous system (Fig. 7.2). The same study showed that different types of *Chlamydia* could be found in patients both in different and in the same biomaterial, and they often had different sensitivities to antimicrobial drugs. Thus, with CDC, *Chlamydia* spp. in the cerebrospinal fluid/intrathecally (n = 18) represented the ratio *Ch. trachomatis: Ch. pneumoniae: Ch. psittaci* equal to 10:9:4 (3:2:1). In this case, a false-negative diagnostic result *Chlamydia* spp. in the cerebrospinal fluid (culture method), *along* with other reasons, correlated with the presence of two or more different genera of intracellular bacteria in the CNS ($p < 0.01$, RR =35).

As established in the work of Vainshenker (2020), the vast majority of the examined microorganisms (Figs. 7.1 and 7.2) were not only directly but also inversely related to immunopathological processes. Moreover, the effect caused by the microorganism could vary depending on the conditions, biomaterial (cerebrospinal fluid or blood), be variable in relation to different immune indicators (e.g. *Chlamydia* spp. are directly related to the indices of inflammatory demyelination, but are inversely related to the antinuclear factor; *HHV -6*—vice versa), the combination could potentiate (e.g. *Chlamydia* spp. + other intracellular bacteria) or, conversely, suppress (e.g. *Chlamydia* spp. + *HHV -6)* immunopathological effect of individual pathogens, or the microorganism could have an indirect effect through the effect of another pathogen *(B. fragilis).* No analogues of this study were found in the literature. It is likely that mutual "compensation" of the immunopathological effects of a complex of pathogens may be one of the reasons for the absence of manifestation of the infectious process, as well as the absence of reliable relationships between pathogens and immune parameters. Given the presence of many pathogens and their combinations, it is not possible to predict the "final effector immune picture"; however, it is possible that different diseases/conditions have their own typical combination of key microorganisms, which makes sense to diagnose. For example in patients with CNS, combinations of microorganisms differed depending on the level of consciousness and the duration of its impairment, which was proposed to be used to determine the prognosis of recovery of consciousness (Figs. 7.9 and 7.10).

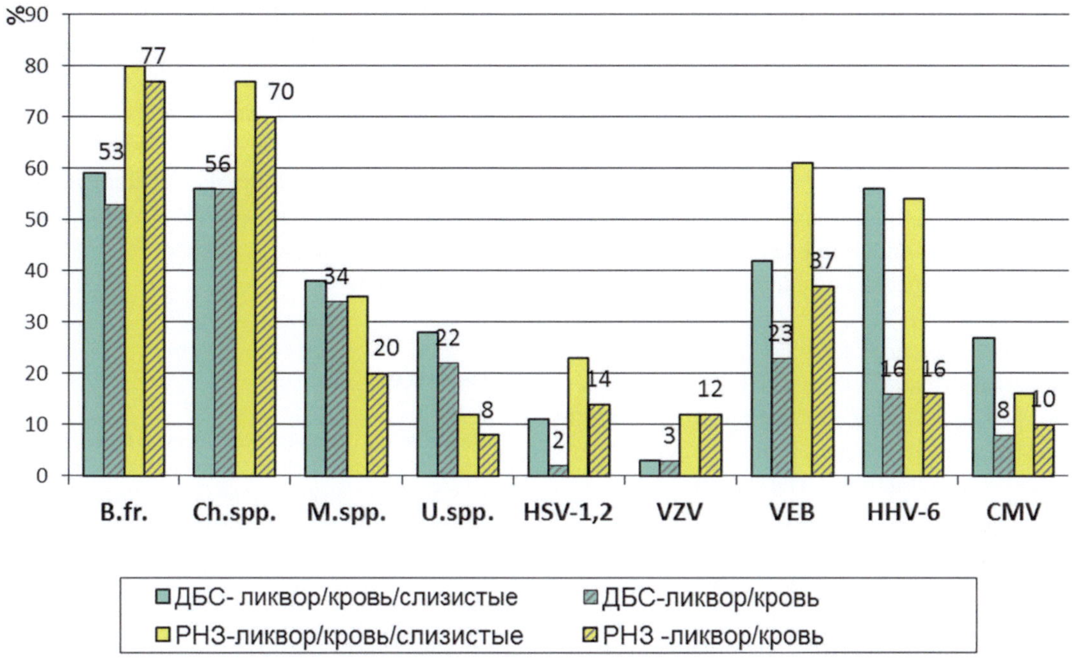

Fig. 7.9 Occurrence (%) of pathogens according to the study of cerebrospinal fluid, blood and mucous membranes of the nasopharynx, conjunctiva (cases of infection) and according to the data of cerebrospinal fluid and/or blood in patients with chronic respiratory failure (n = 68) and in patients with VND (children and adults, n = 161)

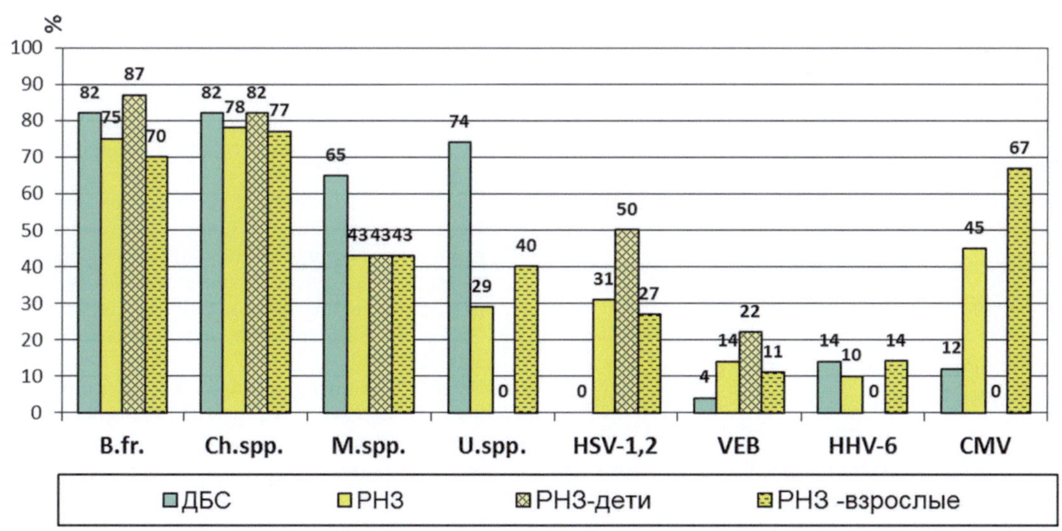

Fig. 7.10 Prevalence (%) of microorganisms in cerebrospinal fluid in case of infection (cerebrospinal fluid, blood, mucous membranes): comparison of CDC *(n = 68)* and VND taking into account the age of patients (children, n = 57, and adults, n = 104) [4, 11–13]

7.4 *Chlamydia* and Other Urogenital Infections

Chlamydia is known to be highly prevalent in patients with other sexually transmitted infections (STIs). The contribution of *Chlamydia* to the clinical manifestations of the underlying disease is usually not established; its diagnosis may require some special considerations (see Chap. 4; Sect. 3.1 and 5.1).

STI is a broader term compared to the term "venereal diseases." In practical dermatovenereology, it is customary to distinguish a group of classical (venereal diseases) and a group of "new-generation" infections. The group of classical STIs includes diseases such as syphilis, gonorrhoea, chancroid, venereal lymphogranuloma, donovanosis, and "new STIs" include *Chlamydia*, mycoplasmosis, trichomoniasis, candidiasis, gardnerellosis, HSV, HPV, HIV infection, etc. .

The "new generation of STIs" has been known for a long time, but the causative pathogens responsible for many of them were discovered relatively recently.

These pathogens differ in their biological properties, but in general, they cause approximately similar lesions of the UGT, which allows us to combine them into one group according to their clinical characteristics and study the role of these pathogens in the aetiology and pathogenesis of diseases.

The above infections do not leave behind stable immunity; therefore, repeated infections and relapses are observed, which occur both in clinically expressed (with manifestations) and, which is much more common, in latent (inapparent) forms. According to the literature, there are a lot of information reflecting the aetiological role of infectious agents combined with UGH in the occurrence of chronic processes of the genitourinary organs. The clinical similarity of inflammatory diseases of the UGT does not allow for a timely establishment of their aetiological diagnosis and, thus, excludes the possibility of timely effective therapy. Due to the ability of each of the STIs, as well as their associations, to cause similar inflammatory diseases, the main role should be given to laboratory diagnostics.

Mixed infections are a complex process of interaction between two or more pathogens and the patient's body. In this case, the clinical features characteristic of monoinfection may be absent, which leads to a change in the ratio of individual signs of the disease, prolongation of the course of the disease and the development of genital and extragenital complications of varying severity [14–21].

References

1. Zinserling VA. Infectious pathology of the respiratory tract. Springer. https://doi.org/10.1007/978-3-030-66325-4. ISBN 978-3-030-66324-7, 259p.
2. Zinserling VA. Infectious lesions of the Central nervous system. Springer. ((978-3-030-96259-3). https://doi.org/10.1007/978-3-030-96260-9.
3. Zinserling VA, Kolobov AV, Lucas S. Placentitis and perinatal infections. Springer; 2024. p. 119p.
4. Di Pietro M, Filardo S, Romano S, Sessa R. Chlamydia trachomatis and chlamydia pneumoniae interaction with the host: latest advances and future prospective. Microorganisms. 2019;7(5):140. https://doi.org/10.3390/microorganisms7050140.
5. Contini C, Seraceni S, Cultrera R, Castellazzi M, Granieri E, Fainardi E. Chlamydophila pneumoniae infection and its role in neurological disorders. Interdiscip Perspect Infect Dis. 2010;2010:273573.
6. Contini C, Fainardi E, Seraceni S, Granieri E, Castellazzi M, Cultrera R. Molecular identification and antibody testing of Chlamydophila pneumoniae in a subgroup of patients with HIV-associated dementia complex. Preliminary results. J Neuroimmunol. 2003;136(1–2):172–7.
7. Vainshenker YI, Tsinzerling VA, Leonova ON, Ivchenko IM, Vetrova MN, Korotkov AD, et al. On the participation of minor infections in the development of central nervous system damage in immunodeficiency. HIV Infect Immunosuppress. 2010;2(4):100–1.
8. Gartner S. HIV infection and dementia. Science 2000;287.
9. Uzun N. Chlamydia infection's role in neurological diseases. In: Sarier M, editor. Chlamydia—secret enemy from past to present. https://doi.org/10.5772/intechopen.110842.
10. Chacko A, Delbaz A, Walkden H, Basu S, Armitage CW, Eindorf T, Trim LK, Miller E, West NP, St John JA, Beagley KW, Ekberg JAK. Chlamydia pneumoniae can infect the central nervous system via the olfactory and trigeminal nerves and contributes to Alzheimer's disease risk. Sci Rep. 2022;12:2759. https://doi.org/10.1038/s41598-022-06749-9.
11. Telyatnikova N, Hill Gaston JS. Prior exposure to infection with chlamydia pneumoniae can influence

the T-cell-mediated response to chlamydia trachomatis. FEMS Immunol Med Microbiol. 2006;47:190–8.
12. Bojović J, Strelić N, Pavlica L. Reiter's syndrome—disease of young men—analysis of 312 patients. Med Pregl. 2014;67:222–30.
13. Hu J, Zhao H, Lou D, et al. Human cytomegalovirus and Epstein-Barr virus infections, risk factors, and their influence on the liver function of patients with acute-on-chronic liver failure. BMC Infect Dis. 2018;18(1):577.
14. Kozlova, V.I. Viral, chlamydial and mycoplasmal diseases of the genitals: manual for doctors. V.I. Kozlova, A.F. Pukhner. - M: triada-X, 2003. -440 p.
15. Khvorik DF. Chlamydial -associated infections: diagnostics and treatment: monograph. D.F. Khvorik. – Grodno: GrSMU; 2011. 328 p.
16. Poznyak AL. Common forms of urogenital chlamydia in young people: diagnostics, clinical picture, treatment Abstract of dissertation for a PhD in medicine. St. Petersburg, 2003 (scientific director Lobzin Yu.V.).
17. Lobzin YV, Poznyak AL, Sidorchuk SN. Chlamydial infections: diagnostics, clinical picture, treatment, rehabilitation: manual for doctors. St. Petersburg: Foliant; 2010. 484 p
18. Djoba Siawaya JF. Chlamydia trachomatis, Human Immunodeficiency Virus (HIV) distribution and sexual behaviors across gender and age group in an African setting. PLoS One. 2014;9(3):e90174. https://doi.org/10.1371/journal.pone.0090174.
19. Jansen K, Steffen G, Potthoff A, et al. STI in times of PrEP: high prevalence of chlamydia, gonorrhea, and mycoplasma at different anatomic sites in men who have sex with men in Germany. BMC Infect Dis. 2020;20:110. https://doi.org/10.1186/s12879-020-4831-4.
20. da Silva Góes S, de Souza Fonseca RR, de Sousa Avelino ME, et al. Exposure to Chlamydia trachomatis infection in individuals who are newly diagnosed with HIV and antiretroviral-Naïve from Belém, Northern Brazil. Vaccines (Basel). 2022;10(10):1719. https://doi.org/10.3390/vaccines10101719.
21. Ghasemian E, Harding-Esch E, Mabey D, Holland MJ. When bacteria and viruses collide: a tale of chlamydia trachomatis and sexually transmitted viruses. Rev Viruses. 2023;15(9):1954. https://doi.org/10.3390/v15091954.

Chlamydia and Non-infectious Diseases

8

Due to high frequency of chlamydiosis, it can be diagnosed in patients with different pathologies. Several authors try to find pathogenic connections between them. It is pertinent to note that the association between *Chlamydia* and some of these diseases is tenuous, with minimal data to support the association. Not only has a causal relationship not been demonstrated in a subset of these studies, the infection is difficult to eradicate with antibiotic treatment, and no statistically significant improvement in symptoms of any disease associated with *C. pneumoniae* infection, except respiratory disease, has been demonstrated following antibiotic treatment [1–3]. In this chapter, we discuss several diseases with possible participation of *Chlamydia* in their pathogenesis.

8.1 *Chlamydia pneumonia* and Atherosclerosis (Jointly with Yu.I. Vainshenker)

In recent decades, there is increasing evidence that commonly encountered bacteria and viruses are linked to the development of accelerated atherosclerosis. One of the extensively studied bacteria, which has been linked to atherosclerosis, is *Chlamydia pneumoniae* (see Chap. 1). The scientific interest in the role of *Chlamydia pneumoniae* in triggering chronic ongoing inflammatory processes cumulated in significant factual evidence on the role of chlamydia in the aetiology and pathogenesis of atherosclerosis.

Convincing evidence of the involvement of *Chlamydia pneumoniae* in the pathogenesis of atherosclerosis has been obtained experimentally. As one of the earliest reports, a link between *Chlamydia pneumoniae* and atherosclerotic cardiovascular disease was suggested by Saikku et al. [4] Since then, an abundance of animal and human studies using a wide variety of approaches have been published on this topic. This includes amongst others seroimmunological investigations. The monograph by A. Shor represents a compendium of the initial studies [5].

The development of atherosclerosis is thought to be triggered by dysfunction and/ or induction of a chronic inflammatory process by cells infected with *Chlamydia pneumoniae*. In particular, it has been established that *Chlamydia pneumoniae* promotes endothelial dysfunction in normolipidic and hyperlipidic animal models. Furthermore, it has been demonstrated that acceleration of the progression of atherosclerotic lesions in hyperlipidemic animals is linked to *Chlamydia pneumoniae* infection [6].

Herein, the inflammatory and immune mechanisms activated by *Chlamydia pneumoniae* contribute to dyslipidaemia. For example the ability of *Chlamydia pneumoniae* to activate Nod-like receptor family pyrin domain-containing 3 (NLRP3) inflammasome has been shown, leading to subsequent increase of IL-1β in macrophages, resulting in accumulation of intracellular cholesterol and foam cell formation [7]. It appears that *Chlamydia pneumoniae* and lipids

V. Zinserling et al., *Chlamydia Infections*, https://doi.org/10.1007/978-3-031-99642-9_8

engage the same innate immune signalling pathways (Toll Like receptor-4/myeloid differentiation primary response 88), accelerating the atherosclerotic process [8].

On subcellular level, endothelial cell damage was studied in aortic endothelial using electron microscopy from deceased patients with underlying cardiovascular pathology by AI Lysenko and NA Solovieva [9, 10]. Within this context, two types of bacterial inclusions were demonstrated: typical and atypical forms. This finding was interpreted as indication to the presence of a productive cycle of development of *C. pneumoniae* and a persistent form of infection.

Further to the pathogenesis of the ongoing chronic inflammatory process in *Chlamydia* infection, studies have shown that the bacterium infects a variety of cell types other than endothelial cells, including vascular smooth muscle cells and monocytes/macrophages [11], as demonstrated using, amongst others, immunohistochemical studies .

It was demonstrated that *Chlamydia pneumoniae* induces in macrophages, platelets, endothelial cells and vascular smooth muscle cells increased production of pro-inflammatory cytokines and adhesion molecules such as IL-6, IFN-γ, TNF- α, intercellular adhesion molecule-1, and vascular cell adhesion molecule-1. These pro-inflammatory cytokines and adhesion molecules are responsible for the initiation, progression and destabilization of atherosclerotic plaques [6, 12].

Further, molecular mechanisms linking oxidative stress (contribute to the early as well as the late stages of the atherosclerotic process by promoting endothelial dysfunction) and inflammation with *Chlamydia pneumoniae*-mediated atherosclerosis have been identified [5].

Nevertheless, till present, unambiguous conclusions about prevention by antibiotic treatment of this widespread disease cannot be drawn.

It is commonly accepted and has been demonstrated that in atherosclerosis (including in atherosclerotic plaques), other widespread bacterial and viral microorganisms are detected (other *Chlamydia* species as well), including translocated oral and intestinal microbiota [5]. Although the pathogenetic significance of mixed microbiota cannot be excluded, there are no published studies focusing on this finding .

In conclusion, taking into account the available clinical and experimental data, chlamydial infection (adjusted for other risk factors) looks very attractive as an etiopathogenetic factor of atherosclerosis. However, despite the above-outlined evidence, prospective multicentre studies of the effect of antibiotic use in connection with *C. pneumoniae* on the course of atherosclerosis, including the development of atherogenic cerebral stroke and coronary pathology, did not produce the expected result [13–15]. The failure of clinical antibiotic trials to demonstrate an effect on development and progression of atherosclerotic burden warrants further evaluation of the role of *C. pneumoniae* in the etiopathogenesis of atherosclerosis [5–7, 11, 12, 14–37].

8.2 Role of *Chlamydia pneumoniae* in the Pathogenesis of Multiple Sclerosis

Studies of a possible connection between *C. pneumoniae* and multiple sclerosis (MS) began after the identification of *C. pneumoniae* in the cerebrospinal fluid of patients with rapidly progressive MS and the reduction of symptoms after antibacterial therapy by S. Sriram et al. According to their data, *C. pneumoniae* were detected in cerebrospinal fluid samples by the culture method in 65% (24 of 37) of MS patients and in 11% (3 of 27) of patients with other neurological diagnoses, while by the PCR method using primers corresponding to the gene of the major outer membrane protein (MOMP)—in 97% (36 of 37) and in 18% (5 of 27), respectively. In the cerebrospinal fluid, IgG antibodies to *C. pneumoniae* were present in 86% (32 of 37) of MS patients and were absent in the control group (27 patients) [38]. In a pathological examination of brain samples from MS patients, *C. pneumoniae* was detected in the ependyma and periventricular region [39]. According to other data, in MS patients, *C. pneumoniae* were determined in the cerebrospinal fluid in 2.9–69% of cases [12], and the frequency of detection of *C. pneumoniae* in patients with MS was always higher than in the control group. However, in a number of studies, *C. pneumoniae* was not diagnosed in patients with MS [14]. The frequency of detection of IgG to *C. pneumoniae* differed from the results obtained in PCR diagnostics in patients with MS and when compared with the control group [14].

There is a concept that *C. pneumoniae* is associated with the activity of the immune response in the CNS. When MOMP, 16S rRNA and HSP-70 were simultaneously determined by PCR in three groups of patients (MS, other inflammatory diseases of the CNS and the control group), MOMP and 16S rRNA were diagnosed with the same frequency in all groups. However, amongst patients with MS, they were encountered more often in the remitting than in the progressive course of the disease, and more often in clinically and MRI-active forms than in the stable course of the disease. HSP-70 was detected only in three patients with a remitting course in the exacerbation phase. A higher frequency of *C. pneumoniae* detection also corresponded to an increase in the lesion according to MRI data [40].

However, according to the antibody specificity index (ASI), IgG to *C. pneumoniae* were more prevalent in patients with MS (16.9%) and inflammatory diseases of the central nervous system (21.6%) compared to other patients (1.9%). Moreover, amongst the group of patients with MS, they were more prevalent in patients with a progressive form of the disease [41]. A similar result was noted when identifying specific high-affinity antibodies: in seropositive cerebrospinal fluid samples, they were more often detected in progressive MS. Reports of clinical studies on the effect of antichlamydial therapy on MS are contradictory and poorly comparable, including due to the lack of standards. According to some data, the treatment did not affect the number of active foci diagnosed by MRI; according to others, it contributed to MRI remission. The results of a retrospective analysis of 26 studies in which *C. pneumoniae* was detected by various methods (1332 patients with MS and 1464 controls), obtained by statistical processing with adjustment for gender and other differences, were insufficient to establish an aetiological link between infection with *C. pneumoniae* and morbidity MS [13, 38, 41–53].

8.3 *Chlamydia* and Neurodegenerative Diseases

8.3.1 Link Between *Chlamydia* Infection and Alzheimer's and Parkinson's Diseases

The involvement of infection in the development of degenerative diseases is rarely discussed. However, the presence of proinflammatory cytokines, activation of microglial cells and the formation of microglial nodules in the area of neuronal death in the brain have prompted the search for possible microorganisms—cofactors in the development of genetically non-determined Alzheimer's disease (AD) [13]. Only a few studies have been published (since 1998) that have detected *C. pneumoniae* in the brain of AD patients. Most of them were conducted by BJ Balin et al. and only two comparable results were obtained by independent researchers. In other studies, attempts to identify *C. pneumoniae* in the brain in AD were unsuccessful.

C. pneumoniae was first identified by BJ Balin et al. by the PCR method in patients with AD in various areas of the brain (hippocampus, cerebellum, temporal cortex and prefrontal cortex) inside neurons, neuroglia, endothelial and paraendothelial cells and extracellularly [54–57]. *C. pneumoniae* were located near amyloid deposits and neurofibrillary tangles, but did not directly contact amyloid plaques [56–58].

In 58% (11 of 19) of patients with AD, an association of the APOE-ε4 gene with *C. pneumoniae was detected* in brain tissue. Since the APOE-ε4 allele of the gene affects the deposition of the β-A4 amyloid component (present in senile plaques, neurofibrillary tangles and cerebral vessel walls in AD), it is suggested that the identified symbiosis is involved in the pathobiology of AD [55].

In the experiment, intranasal infection *with C. pneumoniae* non-transgenic young female BALB/c mice directly promoted the production of amyloid (A β1–42) in the mouse brain, which may be a model of the primary trigger for the development of the AD pathological process in sporadic cases of the disease [59].

In intranasal infection of mice, *C. pneumoniae* was detected in the olfactory bulbs, which correlated with the results of pathological studies in AD [60]. In a randomized, placebo-controlled, multicentre clinical trial to determine the effectiveness of antichlamydial therapy (doxycycline and rifampicin) on the clinical course of the disease, it was found that the progressive decline in cognitive function in patients receiving antibiotics was less intense than in the control group [57, 58, 61].

Data on the role of *C. pneumoniae* in the development of Parkinson's disease (PD) are less extensive than in AD. It is assumed that chlamydia can enhance the aggregation of α-synuclein through microglial activation and oxidative stress. However, direct objective evidence of the association of *C. pneumoniae* with PD is currently insufficient and most studies focus on indirect indicators of the inflammatory process caused by *C. pneumoniae*. A number of studies have found that chronic inflammation caused by *C. pneumoniae infection* can contribute to the death of dopaminergic neurons in patients with PD.

The role *of C. pneumoniae* in the development of PD remains hypothetical. Long-term studies and more precise experimental designs are needed to confirm these associations.

8.3.2 The Role of *Chlamydia* in the Development of Schizophrenia (Jointly with V.A. Orlova)

Fellerhoff et al. [62] hypothesized that chlamydial infection is one of the pathogenetic factors in the development of schizophrenia. In a study (PCR) of blood samples, *Chlamydia* spp. were detected in 50% (9 of 18) of patients with schizophrenia, and in the control group only in 6.97% (8 of 115). Treatment (immunocorrection and antibiotics) showed a stable improvement in mental status in patients with schizophrenia [62]. The data were confirmed in a larger group of patients. A reliable relationship was found between the incidence of schizophrenia and infection with *Chlamydia*, in particular *C. psittaci*. Schizophrenia in combination with the HLA-A genotype was also more often observed in chlamydial infection caused by *C. psittaci* [63]. Using the PCR method, Chlamydiaceae was detected in samples of the frontal lobes of the brain in patients suffering from schizophrenia significantly more often (23.5% of 34) than in control samples (5.7% of 35). It is assumed that the development of mental disorders is caused by changes in the functional activity of infected microglial cells and neurons with disruption of interneuronal connections [64].

At the same time, published data cannot be considered as final evidence of the role of chlamydial infection in the origin of schizophrenia in general, as some researchers in this field relied more on extensive material. There is view that this brain infection is possible only as a comorbid pathology, the presence of which, however, affect the course of the underlying disease. This requires both representative samples of pathological observations and informative clinical descriptions of these observations, which are insufficient in the cases presented.

However, according to other data, the relationship between schizophrenia and other mental disorders with *C. trachomatis* and other IUIs has not been determined [65]. It has been suggested that infections may participate in the formation of autistic syndrome, including by modulating the immunopathological state of the central nervous system. In all examined patients with autism, elevated titres of antibodies to various neurospecific peptides were detected in the blood serum (ELISA), indicating an immunopathological process in the central nervous system with a violation of the BBB, and antibodies to *C. pneumoniae* and *Streptococcus* [66].

The above allowed us to present two of our own observations with a special assessment of the pathomorphology of chlamydial lesions of the central nervous system with the use of an external psychiatric assessment of cases based on clinical data available at the time of autopsy.

We present these observations.

Observation 1

Patient E., 37, was transferred to the Botkin Clinical and Infectious Diseases Hospital from City Public Health Hospital No. 3, where she had been staying from 08.02 to 18.02.22. She had suffered from a mental illness since 1995. At the onset, she experienced autistic love, which was later accompanied by pseudo-hallucinatory auditory deceptions of perception and delusional ideas of persecution by her brother. She exhibited signs of Kandinsky-Clerambault syndrome: she felt an influence on herself, it seemed that her brother was completely controlling her—he was reading her thoughts, controlling her tongue. She heard the voice of the prophet Elijah in her head. She believed that she could read the thoughts of others. She was repeatedly treated in psychiatric hospitals (City Public Health Hospital No. 3, Bekhterev Research Institute). Remissions were poor, with pseudo-hallucinatory symptoms persisting. Over time, an emotional-volitional defect developed. She was diagnosed with paranoid schizophrenia. From 12.11.2009 to 03.03.2010, she was treated at City Hospital No. 3 due to the development of catatonic-hebephrenic symptoms. She had an elevated mood with a silly tint and made faces. Her speech was accelerated, and she giggled awkwardly. She claimed that she had 8 husbands and had recently given birth to 9 children. She claimed that she had met Dima Bilan, whom she was going to marry. She immediately called herself a vampire, a sorceress. She heard voices in her head. At times, she ran to the window and shouted the name "Ilya." She swore obscenely, put on other people's clothes. She was aggressive towards the doctor. She froze in awkward poses, made pretentious stereotypical movements. Impulsive actions were noted, when she suddenly jumped out of bed, began to squat, do push-ups from the floor, screamed hysterically. After intensive pharmacotherapy in the hospital, she was not hospitalized for the next almost 12 years, until 2022, but was treated as an outpatient. There are no descriptions of the patient's mental status during this period. It is only possible to state the fact that against the background of multiple hospitalizations in psychiatric hospitals, a period appeared when she "held on" to outpatient therapy, which suggests a relative stabilization of the condition with the absence of gross behavioural disorders.

From 02.01.2022 to 04.01.2022, she was in City Hospital No. 3 in the gynaecological department due to curettage of the uterine cavity caused by menstrual cycle disorders. Immediately after discharge, from 06.01.2022 onwards— she suffered from a steady deterioration of mental health. According to the available very brief information from the medical history, she became excited, her speech became incoherent, she screamed that she heard voices. She was hospitalized at City Hospital No. 3, where she received specialized treatment from 07.01.22 to 04.02.22, but there was no effect of psychotropic therapy. In this regard, on 04.02.22, she was transferred for examination to the Dzhanelidze Research Institute of Emergency Medicine, where no data on neurosurgical pathology were found, but a new coronavirus infection was diagnosed (rapid test). The patient's mental state remained unstable, and on 02/07/22, the patient was returned to City Hospital No. 3, and a few days later, due to hypotension and increasing respiratory failure, she was transferred to the intensive care unit (ICU). From 02/17/22 onwards, the condition worsened with impaired consciousness, and on 02/18/22, the RCH team delivered the patient to Botkin Clinical Hospital, to ICU-2.

The patient was admitted to ICU-2 in an extremely serious condition: deep stupor, unstable haemodynamics, vasopressor support with norepinephrine 0.4 mcg/kg/min, BP against this background 90/65 mm Hg, heart rate 93 per minute. Despite the intensive care provided in full, the patient's condition progressively worsened and on 20.02.2022, she died due to progressive multiple organ failure.

The autopsy revealed the body of a middle-aged woman, of normal build, normosthenic constitutional type and adequate nutrition.

The convolutions of the brain are somewhat flattened in the region of the gyrus postcentralis, the sulci are narrowed. The brain tissue is dull, with a clear boundary between the gray and white matter. The cerebral cortex is thinned in places to 0.3 cm. The cerebral ventricles are of regular configuration: the ependyma is smooth, contains transparent cerebrospinal fluid, the vascular plexuses of the ventricles are red-pink, anaemic. The pineal gland is 1.3 cm in diameter—on section, there is a smooth-walled cyst of 1.0 cm with transparent contents.

The mucous membrane of the larynx, trachea and bronchi is shiny, red-pink, and a small amount of viscous gray-yellow mucus is found in the lumen of the trachea and large bronchi. The lungs are compacted in all lobes, bluish-pink. The walls of the bronchi are slightly thickened, grayish, and yellowish mucus flows from the lumen of the bronchi in the lower lobes of both lungs when they intersect. The peribronchial lymph nodes are oval, up to 0.5 × 0.5 × 0.5 cm in size, bluish-gray and elastic on sections. Other macroscopically changes were unremarkable.

Results of histological examination. Lungs. Foci of acute emphysema, small zones of subpleural atelectasis. Small vessels are mostly dilated and full-blooded, zones of diapedetic haemorrhages. In the lumen of some bronchi—leukocyte-mucous masses. In the lumen of some alveoli, there is a large number of exfoliated alveolocytes and macrophages, focal interstitial fibrosis of the lung tissue and weakly expressed monocytic infiltration of the septa. Oedema fields, in the lumen of the alveoli, there are fibrin threads in places, some cells are vacuolated and contain PAS-positive inclusions.

Kidneys. Glomeruli are of normal size, some reduced in size, in the lumen of some glomerular capsules there are small clusters of fresh erythrocytes. The total number of glomeruli is reduced. Coagulation necrosis of the epithelium of the proximal tubules; some cells are vacuolated and contain PAS-positive inclusions.

Brain. The pia mater is moderately sclerotic, with uneven blood filling. Many neurocytes of the cortex are enlarged, swollen, some cells are vacuolated and contain PAS-positive inclusions. Moderately expressed depletion of pyramidal cells in the cortex. The number of Purkinje cells in the cerebellum is significantly reduced, preserved with severe dystrophic changes. Expressed oedema of the white matter, extracellular PAS-positive inclusions are determined. Uneven focal-diffuse proliferation, gliosis.

Immunohistochemical examination revealed chlamydia antigen in the kidneys, lungs, nerve cells and white matter of the brain, liver and spleen.

Final Pathological Diagnosis:

Main disease: New coronavirus infection COVID-19, the virus has been identified (PCR (+) from 02/07/2022, from 02/19/2022, posthumously from 02/23/2022 not detected).

Competing: (1) Schizophrenia, paranoid form. Catatonic-hebephrenic syndrome with hallucinatory-delusional inclusions (according to clinical data). (2) Generalized chlamydial infection with damage to the white and gray matter of the brain, lungs, kidneys.

Complications: Acute respiratory failure, VPO since admission, mechanical ventilation since 02/20/2022 (according to medical records). Antibiotic-associated colitis. Serous-fibrinous peritonitis (1500 ml). Hyperplasia of mesenteric lymph nodes, paretic dilation of the intestine. Pulmonary oedema. Acute cardiovascular failure.

Associated diseases: Multiple subserous and submucous uterine leiomyomas. Menstrual irregularities, curettage of the uterine cavity. Cerebrospinal fluid cyst of the pineal gland.

Observation 2

Patient B., 47 years old, was transferred to the Botkin Infectious Hospital from another, where he was treated from 23.06 22 to 01.09.22 with a diagnosis of simple schizophrenia, stabilization of the condition (F20.6). There is no psychopathological description of the condition. According to the extract from the medical history, he suffered from a mental illness since 1995, he is a permanently disabled person of the 2nd group. The presented documentation does not contain any other data on the patient's illness. In 1995, he suffered from a traumatic brain injury

(TBI). Against the background of an increase in temperature and X-ray data with a diagnosis of pneumonia, he was transferred to the Botkin Clinical Infectious Diseases Hospital, where he died 12 h after admission.

Pathological diagnosis:

Main disease: Cholelithiasis, exacerbation with bedsores in the fundus area and perforation of the wall and penetration into the cardiac region of the stomach.

Complications of the underlying disease: massive erosive gastric bleeding.

Associated diseases: Simple schizophrenia, continuous course. Chronic pyelonephritis. Hypertension with eccentric myocardial hypertrophy. Moderate atherosclerosis of the aorta and vessels of the base of the brain. Osteochondrosis of the spine, spondyloarthrosis at the level of Th 8–Th 10, condition after surgery on 17.06.22. Obesity 3.

Along with the macro- and microscopic changes that characterized the unrecognized underlying disease during life, changes in the brain were of particular interest given the objectives of this study. Small cysts 0.1–0.2 cm in diameter, significant lumen narrowing (up to 50%) due to atherosclerotic plaques of the brain base vessels were detected in the thalamus area. Microscopic examination revealed foci of demyelination, calcification and microglial nodules in addition to the picture of atherosclerotic encephalopathy. Focal clusters of intracellular PAS-positive formations were also detected, which corresponded to a positive IHC reaction with serum to *C. trachomatis*.

The lungs showed marked oedema, diffuse alveolar damage with the appearance of hyaline membranes and microthrombosis. No clear signs of chlamydial lesions were detected.

Discussion. The death of patient E. was associated with a new coronavirus infection, the manifestations of which were moderate at the time of death, as well as with antibiotic-associated colitis. Despite the postmortem culture of a number of microorganisms, no signs of a generalized bacterial infection were detected. Of significant importance in the genesis of death, of course, was the generalized chlamydial infection, diagnosed only postmortem. It is impossible to reliably judge its duration, but based on our experience in studying chlamydial infection, it seems highly likely that it was chronic. Based also on literary data on the relationship of persistent chlamydial infection in the central nervous system with various factors, including schizophrenia-like psychopathological symptoms, one can raise the question of its chronic nature in the patient and its importance in the pathogenesis of brain damage.

In the second observation (patient B.), acute surgical pathology was missed against the background of mental disorder and multiple somatic diseases. Brain lesions are caused by atherosclerosis, consequences of TBI and other pathologies. Atherosclerotic changes can be associated with chlamydial infection, and TBI can contribute to the activation of this infection [67–69]. This is very likely, since it was chlamydial infection that was proven during postmortem pathomorphological examination, and isolated in the brain. Noteworthy is the almost exclusively intracellular localization of the pathogen, characteristic of chronic persistent forms of the disease.

It should be noted that in the cases considered, no clearly expressed psychopathological signs were noted that would indicate their connection with an infectious lesion of the brain. In particular, in the first case (patient E.), where there was a psychiatric history of the disease, no general cerebral and meningeal phenomena were noted, even short-term disorders of consciousness in the form of stunning, delirious, twilight and other states, movement disorders in the form of hyperkinesis and paralysis, neurological symptoms, as well as psychoorganic personality changes, which are considered classic for differentiating symptomatic infectious psychoses and, in general, exogenous types of reactions, including endoform ones, from psychoses associated with schizophrenia. However, can we expect a classic infectious psychosis if what initially occurs is not an acutely developed encephalitic reaction, but an exacerbation of a chronic, including asymptomatic or asymptomatic, brain infection?

Thus, the discussion of the presented cases in the traditional key leaves open the question: is it possible to define the mental disorder of patients, the clinical signs of which, in the opinion of specialists, corresponded to the criteria of schizophrenia, as schizophrenia or as chronic infectious encephalitis with schizophrenia-like symptoms and classify it in the first case under the heading "organic delusional (schizophrenia-like) disorder" (F 06.2), in the second, possibly under the headings "organic affective disorder" (F 06.3) or "personality and behaviour disorders due to disease, damage and dysfunction of the brain" (F 07) with dominant manifestations of apathoabulia. According to the ICD-10 criteria, only the identification of an infectious disease by laboratory tests and a somatic examination and monitoring the correspondence of its dynamics and the dynamics of psychopathological manifestations allows for an accurate differentiation of the indicated diseases from clinically similar syndromes within schizophrenia. In the cases indicated, such work was not carried out.

Thus, the analysis of the presented cases shows the limitations of psychopathological diagnostics and routine somatic examination in psychiatry, and once again raises the question of the likelihood of an etiopathogenetic commonality between schizophrenia and cerebral infection that occurs atypically, without the classic signs of acute encephalitis.

8.4 Brain Lesions in *HIV*-Infected Patients Associated with *C. pneumoniae* (in Collaboration with Y.I. Vainshenker)

Despite the widespread prevalence *of Chlamydia* spp., the similarity of target cells for HIV and *Chlamydia* spp., neurochlamydia and neuroAIDS are hardly considered together.

It is assumed that *C. pneumoniae* is involved in the progression of primary neurological disorders [70]. In AIDS-dementia complex, *C. pneumoniae* was detected (PCR using primers of the MOMP and 16 S rRNA genes) in the cerebrospinal fluid and brain tissue samples in 17.4% (4 of 23) of patients; in addition, a high level of specific antibodies was determined in the cerebrospinal fluid [12]. In two patients with HIV in the AIDS stage examined during their lifetime, *Chlamydia* spp. were detected in the cerebrospinal fluid (by culture), as well as antibodies: in AIDS-dementia complex to *C. trachomatis* and *C. pneumoniae*, in aseptic meningitis to *C. pneumoniae*, other opportunistic infections were not detected. During targeted morphological examination of the brain of patients with HIV, different types *of Chlamydia spp* were detected [70–73].

In HIV, the factors that determine the course, progression and prognosis of primary (HIV-related) neurological disorders have not been established [74–77].

8.5 Different Neurological Pathology Associated with *Chlamydia* (in Collaboration with Y.I. Vainshenker)

Autistic syndrome is considered as an important rather frequent neurological pathology of unclear origin. Amongst different views on its aetiology, infections are considered as well. In autistic syndrome *Mycoplasma* spp. was detected (PCR) more often than other microorganisms—in 58.3% (28 of 48) compared to the control group of the same age—in 4.7% (2 of 45); however, *C. pneumoniae* and HHV-6 were also probable cofactors of the disease. In autism, a reliable predominance *of C. pneumoniae* was determined [78].

In children and adolescents with psychoneurological diagnoses and identified "asymptomatic" infections with *Chlamydia* spp., *Mycoplasma* spp., *Ureaplasma* spp., as a result of etiotropic treatment (selection of antimicrobial drugs according sensitivity on cell culture), improvement was noted in 94% (17 of 18) cases. In cerebral palsy with intellectual-mnestic and speech disorders (in 3 of 5 patients), in autistic syndrome (in 4 of 5), improvement in learning ability, speech, social response and contact with others was noted. In attention-deficit hyperactivity disorder, all (8 patients) showed a significant improvement in attention, emotional background and behaviour [79].

Taking into account the biological properties of the pathogens, causing subclinical infections, these data are consistent with modern ideas that the disruption of intersynaptic connections in autism may be the result of an activated state of microglia in different areas of the brain [80].

The role of *Chlamydia* spp. was demonstrated in post-comatose vegetative states (VS). During examination (culture, PCR, ELISA of samples of cerebrospinal fluid, blood, scrapings from the mucous membranes of the nasopharynx and conjunctiva) of 32 patients in VS (a consequence of traumatic brain injury and hypoxia), pathogens low manifest infections (LMI) were detected in all of them, amongst which *Chlamydia* species predominated—in 72% (23 of 32) of patients in the CSF and in 81% (26 of 32) in the blood [81]. Antichlamydial antibodies in the cerebrospinal fluid and blood serum were detected in 84% (27 of 32) of patients: 25% of them had antibodies to *C. psittaci*, the rest had antibodies to *C. trachomatis* and *C. pneumoniae* and half of the cases had antibodies to 2–3 types of *Chlamydia* spp. There were no inflammatory changes in the cerebrospinal fluid or specific inflammatory changes in MRI in patients with chlamydial (and other pathogens of LMI) CNS lesions. Pathological examination of 4 patients confirmed the presence of intra- and extracellular forms of *Chlamydia* spp., glial proliferation, demyelination and vasculitis [81]. *Chlamydia* spp. in most cases were associated with pathogenic capsular forms *of Bacteroides fragilis, HHV -6, VEB* and *Cytomegalovirus* (CMV). A reliable connection *of Chlamydia* spp. with the demyelinating process and a tendency towards an association with vasculitis were revealed [82].

Similar data were found in patients with chronic CNS diseases (epilepsy, vascular, degenerative diseases), in whom *Chlamydia* spp. was detected in the cerebrospinal fluid and blood [34, 83].

During treatment of LMI (primarily caused by *Chlamydia* spp.) in patients in the VS, a reliable improvement in the psychoneurological status and brain metabolism (PET), as well as better long-term results were observed compared to the control group, in which LMI treatment was not performed. This indicates the clinical significance of the detected, primarily chlamydial, CNS damage in patients in the VS [82].

LMI (primarily those caused by *Chlamydia* spp.) probably contributes significantly to the progressive brain atrophy and Wallerian degeneration observed in VS.

The association of chlamydia with cerebral palsy is most often considered through the prism of intrauterine infections and chorioamnionitis, which cause inflammation and damage to the developing foetal brain. Studies from the USA, Australia and Europe provide the most convincing data, while studies from Asia (China, India, Iran, Turkey) and Canada often confirm this association, but with less specificity for *Chlamydia*. Pathogenetic mechanisms include direct infection of the CNS, molecular mimicry and systemic inflammation. However, a causal relationship remains unproven, and further studies using PCR, serology and histology on larger samples are needed [83–87].

It should be noted that chlamydial encephalitis may manifest as acute psychosis. In one case, acute psychosis developed after an episode of headache with fever and remained the only clinical manifestation of encephalitis caused by *C. pneumoniae* for 3 weeks. There were no neurological symptoms or inflammatory changes in the cerebrospinal fluid [77]. In another case, psychosis caused by *C. psittaci was* accompanied by minimal neurological symptoms and occurred against the background of pneumonia [87].

The lack of standardization of laboratory diagnostic methods and sometimes an insufficient number of studies do not allow us to finally judge the role of various types of chlamydia. In the development of demyelinating, degenerative, vascular diseases of the central nervous system, schizophrenia, autism and AIDS-dementia complex. The role of chlamydia as a cofactor is probable, but not proven. The role of other infectious agents in the diseases under consideration is also not specified.

8.6 Other Diseases Probably Associated with Chlamydiosis

Reactive arthritis. Presence of *C. trachomatis* and *C. pneumonia* DNA, antigens, elementary bodies in synovial fluid; elevated levels of antibodies to chlamydia in the blood serum of patients with (see Chap. 5). Probable mechanism of pathogenesis: *Chlamydiae* use monocytic cells as their "Trojan horses" to reach the synovium, where hypoxic stress suppresses indoleamine 2,3-dioxygenase (IDO) activity and nutrient deprivation promotes bacterial persistence.

Molecular mimicry between host and chlamydial HSP60 proteins and the presence of other chlamydial antigens induces potent secretion of inflammatory cytokines.

Asthma. Supporting data: *C. pneumoniae*-specific antibodies IgA, IgE, IgG and IgM were detected in patients with asthma; IgE showed a positive linear relationship with asthma severity. Children who reported multiple episodes of bronchial asthma were found to have a positive *C. pneumoniae* PCR result (See Chap. 1).

Primary biliary cirrhosis (PBC). C. pneumoniae antigens and 16S rRNA were detected in explanted liver tissue or biopsy; elevated levels of anti-chlamydial antibodies in patients with PBC or anti-mitochondrial antibody (AMA)-positive patients with PBC. But, absence of bacteria or bacterial DNA in liver tissue; absence of significant serum anti-*C. pneumoniae* IgG in patients with PBC makes such liaison not very veritable (See Chap. 1).

References

1. Sutherland ER, et al. A trial of clarithromycin for the treatment of suboptimally controlled asthma. J Allergy Clin Immunol. 2010;126:747–53.
2. Deniset JF. Pierce GN possibilities for therapeutic interventions in disrupting Chlamydophila pneumoniae involvement in atherosclerosis. Fundam Clin Pharmacol. 2010;24:607–17.
3. Cannon CP, et al. Antibiotic treatment of chlamydia pneumoniae after acute coronary syndrome N. Engl J Med. 2005;352:1646–54.
4. Saikku P, Leinonen M, Mattila K, Ekman MR, Nieminen MS, Mäkelä PH, Huttunen JK, Valtonen V. Serological evidence of an association of a novel chlamydia, TWAR, with chronic coronary heart disease and acute myocardial infarction. Lancet. 1988;2:983–6.
5. Shor A. Chlamydia atherosclerosis lesion: discovery, diagnosis and treatment. London: Springer; 2007. ISBN: 978-1-84628-809
6. Di Pietro M, Filardo S, Romano S, Sessa R. Chlamydia trachomatis and chlamydia pneumoniae interaction with the host: latest advances and future prospective. Microorganisms. 2019;7(5):140. https://doi.org/10.3390/microorganisms7050140.
7. Tumurkhuu G, Dagvadorj J, Porritt RA, Crother TR, Shimada K, Tarling EJ, Erbay E, Arditi M, Chen S. Chlamydia pneumoniae hijacks a host autoregulatory IL-1 β loop to drive foam cell formation and accelerate atherosclerosis. Cell Metab. 2018;28:432–448.e4.
8. Chen S, Shimada K, Crother TR, et al. Chlamydia and lipids engage a common signaling pathway that promotes Atherogenesis. J Am Coll Cardiol. 2018;71(14):1553–70. https://doi.org/10.1016/j.jacc.2018.01.072.
9. Lysenko AI. Solovieva NA the role of chlamydia pneumoniae in damage to human aortic endothelial cells in atherosclerosis. Arch Pathol. 2010;72(2):21–5. (in Russian)
10. Lysenko AI, Solovieva NA. Morphological factors of chlamydia pneumoniae during productive and persistent cycles of development in human endothelial cells of coronary arteries and aorta in atherosclerosis. Arch Pathol. 2012;74(1):26–32. (in Russian)
11. Nurgul U. Chlamydia infection's role in neurological diseases. In: Sarier M, editor. Chlamydia—Secret enemy from past to present. https://doi.org/10.5772/intechopen.110842.
12. Gaydos CA. Growth in vascular cells and cytokine production by chlamydia pneumoniae. J Infect Dis. 2000;181:S473–8.
13. Contini C, Seraceni S, Cultrera R, Castellazzi M, Granieri E, Fainardi E. Chlamydophila pneumoniae infection and its role in neurological disorders. Interdiscip Perspect Infect Dis. 2010;2010:273573.
14. Yucesan C, Sriram S. Chlamydia pneumoniae infection of the central nervous system.//. Curr Opin Neurol. 2001;14(3):355–9.
15. Campbell LA, Rosenfeld ME, Persistent C. Pneumoniae infection in atherosclerotic lesions: rethinking the clinical trials. Front Cell Infect Microbiol. 2014;4:34. [Google Scholar] [CrossRef] [PubMed]
16. Espinola-Klein C, Ruprecht HJ, Blankenberg S, Bickel C, Kopp H, Victor A, et al. Impact of infectious burden on progression of carotid atherosclerosis. Stroke. 2002;33(11):2581–6.
17. Elkind MSV, Tondella MLC, Feikin DR, Fields BS, Homma S, Di Tullio MR. Seropositivity to chlamydia

pneumoniae is associated with risk of first ischemic stroke. Stroke. 2006;37(3):790–5.
18. Cochrane M, Pospischil A, Walker P, Gibbs H, Timms P. Distribution of chlamydia pneumoniae DNA in atherosclerotic carotid arteries: significance for sampling procedures. J Clin Microbiol. 2003;41(4):1454–7.
19. LaBiche R, Koziol D, Quinn TC, Gaydos C, Azhar S, Ketron G, et al. Presence of Chlamydia pneumoniae in human symptomatic and asymptomatic carotid atherosclerosis plaque. Stroke. 2001;32(4):855–60.
20. Piechowski-Jóźwiak B, Mickielewicz A, Gaciong Z, Berent H, Kwieciński H. Elevated levels of anti-chlamydia pneumoniae IgA and IgG antibodies in young adults with ischemic stroke. Acta Neurol Scand. 2007;116(3):144–9.
21. Di Pietro M, Filardo S, de Santis F, Mastromarino P, Sessa R. Chlamydia pneumoniae and oxidative stress in cardiovascular disease: state of the art and prevention strategies. Int J Mol Sci. 2014;16:724–35.
22. Mueller KE. Wolf, KC pneumoniae disrupts eNOS trafficking and impairs NO production in human aortic endothelial cells. Cell Microbiol. 2015;17:119–30.
23. Filardo S, Di Pietro M, Farcomeni A, Schiavoni G, Sessa R. Chlamydia pneumoniae-mediated inflammation in atherosclerosis: a metaanalysis. Mediat Inflamm. 2015;2015:378658. [Google Scholar] [CrossRef] [PubMed]
24. Ljungström L, Franzen C, Schlaug M, Elowson S, Viidas U. Reinfection with chlamydia pneumoniae may induce isolated and systemic vasculitis in small and large vessels. Scand J Infect Dis Suppl. 1997;104:37–40.
25. Rimenti G, Blasi F, Consentini R, Moling O, Pristerà R, Tarsia P, et al. Temporal arteritis associated with Chlamidya pneumoniae DNA detected in an artery specimen. J Rheumatol. 2000;27(11):2718–20.
26. Bonnet F, Morlat P, Delevaux I, Gavinet AM, Parrens M, Bernard N, et al. A possible association between Chlamydiae psittacci infection and temporal arteritis. Joint Bone Spine. 2000;67(6):550–2.
27. Wagner AD, Gerard HC, Fresemann T, Schmidt WA, Gromnica-Ihle E, Hudson AP, Zeidler H. Detection of chlamydia pneumoniae in giant cell vasculitis and correlation with the topographic arrangement of tissue-infiltrating dendritic cells. Arthritis Rheum. 2000;43(7):1543–51.
28. Wagner AD, Wittkop U, Prahst A, Schmidt WA, Gromnica-Ihle E, Vorpahl K, et al. Dendritic cells co-localize with activated CD4+ T cells in giant cell arteritis. Clin Exp Rheumatol. 2003;21(2):185–92.
29. Helweg-Larsen J, Tarp B, Obel N, Baslund B. No evidence of parvovirus B19, chlamydia pneumoniae or human herpes virus infection in temporal artery biopsies in patients with giant cell arteritis. Rheumatology. 2002;41(4):445–9.
30. Regan MJ, Wood BJ, Hsieh YH, Theodore ML, Quinn TC, Hellmann DB, et al. Temporal arteritis and chlamydia pneumoniae: failure to detect the organism by polymerase chain reaction in ninety cases and ninety controls. Arthritis Rheum. 2002;46(4):1056–60.
31. Boyko EV, Poznyak AL, Nuralova IV, Maltsev DS, Suetov AA, Ageyev VS, et al. On the development of multiorgan chlamydial lesions in primary local infection of the eye in an experiment. Arch Pathol. 2011;6:15–8.
32. Odinak MM, Mikhailenko AA, Onishchenko LS, Nuralova IV, Seropegin AD. Pathology of the nervous system in experimental chlamydial infection. Bull Russian Milit Med Acad. 2006;1(15):42–8. (in Russian)
33. Vainshenker YI, Nuralova IV, Onishchenko LS. Chlamydia of the central nervous system. Laboratory diagnostics and clinical and morphological features. Arch Pathol. 2014;76(1):57–62. (in Russian)
34. Zinserling VA, Orlova VA, Mikhailova II. Chapter 20.1: Some non-communicable diseases of the central nervous system with a possible infectious etiology. Schizophrenia and schizoaffective psychosis. Possible etiopathogenetic role of infection. In: Zinserling VA, editor. Infectious lesions of the central nervous system. Springer; 2022. p. 299–324. https://doi.org/10.1007/978-3-030-96260-9.
35. Mitra S, Drautz-Moses DI, Alhede M, Maw MT, Liu Y, Purbojati RW, Yap ZH, Kushwaha KK, Gheorghe AG, Bjarnsholt T, et al. In silico analyzes of metagenomes from human atherosclerotic plaque samples. Microbiome. 2015;3:38.
36. Lindskog Jonsson A, Hållenius FF, Akrami R, Johansson E, Wester P, Arnerlov C, Bäckhed F, Bergström G. Bacterial profile in human atherosclerotic plaques. Atherosclerosis. 2017;263:177–83.
37. Ascher S, Reinhardt C. The gut microbiota: an emerging risk factor for cardiovascular and cerebrovascular disease. Eur J Immunol. 2018;48:564–75.
38. Sriram S, Stratton CW, Yao S, et al. Chlamydia pneumoniae infection of the central nervous system in multiple sclerosis. Ann Neurol. 1999;46(1):6–14.
39. Sriram S, Ljunggren-Rose A, Yao S-Y, Whetsell WO Jr. Detection of chlamydial bodies and antigens in the central nervous system of patients with multiple sclerosis. J Infect Dis. 2005;192(7):1219–28.
40. Contini C, Cultrera R, Seraceni S, et al. Cerebrospinal fluid molecular demonstration of chlamydia pneumoniae DNA is associated to clinical and brain magnetic resonance imaging activity in a subset of patients with relapsing-remitting multiple sclerosis. Mult Scler. 2004;10(4):360–9.
41. Fainardi E, Castellazzi M, Casetta I, Cultrera R, Vaghi L, Granieri E, Contini C. Intrathecal production of chlamydia pneumoniae-specific high-affinity antibodies is significantly associated to a subset of multiple sclerosis patients with progressive forms. J Neurol Sci. 2004;217(2):181–8.
42. Fainardi E, et al. Intrathecal synthesis of anti-chlamydia pneumoniae antibodies in patients with multiple sclerosis. J Neuroimmunol. 2008;197(1):137–42.

43. Hudson AP, et al. Detection of chlamydia pneumoniae in the central nervous system of patients with multiple sclerosis. Ann Neurol. 2000;48(2):270–9.
44. Munger KL, DeLorenze GN, Levin LI. Infectious causes of multiple sclerosis: focus on chlamydia pneumoniae and Epstein-Barr virus. Curr Neurol Neurosci Rep. 2004;4(5):385–91.
45. Diniz JAF, et al. The role of infectious agents in multiple sclerosis: a review. Mult Scler. 2003;9(5):531–42.
46. Marrie RA. Environmental risk factors in multiple sclerosis aetiology. Lancet Neurol. 2004;3(12):709–18.
47. Layh-Schmitt G, Bredt W, Weber B, Dorries R. Chlamydia pneumoniae DNA in cerebrospinal fluid of multiple sclerosis patients. Clin Diagn Lab Immunol. 2000;7(6):881–8. https://pubmed.ncbi.nlm.nih.gov/10805338/
48. Zhang Y, Xu Y, Zhao M. Chlamydia pneumoniae infection and the risk of multiple sclerosis: a meta-analysis. Eur J Neurol. 2006;13(1):90–5. https://pubmed.ncbi.nlm.nih.gov/16900753/
49. Zhang L, Yang Z, Huang Q, et al. Association between chlamydia pneumoniae infection and multiple sclerosis: a meta-analysis. Mult Scler Relat Disord. 2023;71:104525. https://pubmed.ncbi.nlm.nih.gov/37442074/
50. Sotgiu S, Pugliatti M, Fois ML, et al. Chlamydia pneumoniae infection and multiple sclerosis: the Sardinian experience. J Neurol. 2001;248(10):877–81. https://pubmed.ncbi.nlm.nih.gov/11795458/
51. Furrows SJ, Rees J, Boggild M, et al. Chlamydia pneumoniae infection in the central nervous system of patients with multiple sclerosis. J Neurol Neurosurg Psychiatry. 2004;75(5):752–4. https://www.ncbi.nlm.nih.gov/pmc/articles/PMC1757474/
52. Russian Congress on Multiple Sclerosis. Moscow. Conference proceedings. (in Russian); 2018.
53. Stratton CW. Subramaniam Sriram Association of chlamydia pneumoniae with central nervous system disease. Microbes Infect. 2003;5:1249–53. https://doi.org/10.1016/j.micinf.2003.09.004.
54. Balin BJ, Appelt DM. Role of infection in Alzheimer's disease. J Am Osteopath Assoc. 2001;101(12, Suppl. 1):S1–6.
55. Balin BJ, Gérard HC, Arking EJ, Appelt DM, Branigan PJ, Abrams JT, et al. Identification and localization of chlamydia pneumoniae in the Alzheimer's brain. Med Microbiol Immunol. 1998;187(1):23–42.
56. Gérard HC, Dreses-Werringloer U, Wildt KS, Deka S, Oszust C, Balin BJ, et al. Chlamydophila (chlamydia) pneumoniae in the Alzheimer's brain. FEMS Immunol Med Microbiol. 2006;48(3):355–66.
57. Hammond CJ, Hallock LR, Howanski RJ, Appelt DM, Little CS, Balin BJ. Immunohistological detection of chlamydia pneumoniae in the Alzheimer's disease brain. BMC Neurosci. 2010;11:121.
58. Dreses-Werringloer U, et al. Initial characterization of Chlamydophila (chlamydia) pneumoniae cultured from the late-onset Alzheimer brain. Int J Med Microbiol. 2009;299:187–201.
59. Little CS, Hammond CJ, MacIntyre A, Balin BJ. Appelt DM chlamydia pneumoniae induces Alzheimer-like amyloid plaques in the brains of BALB/c mice. Neurobiol Aging. 2004;25(4):419–29.
60. Little CS, Bowe A, Lin R, Litsky J, Fogel RM, Balin BJ, Fresa-Dillon KL. Age alterations in extent and severity of experimental intranasal infection with Chlamydophila pneumoniae in BALB/c mice. Infect Immun. 2005;73(3):1723–34. PMID: 15731073 PMCID: PMC1064908. https://doi.org/10.1128/IAI.73.3.1723-1734.2005.
61. Loeb MB, Molloy DW, Smieja M, Standish T, Goldsmith CH, Mahony J, et al. A randomized, controlled trial of doxycycline and rifampin for patients with Alzheimer's disease. J Am Geriatr Soc. 2004;52(3):381–7.
62. Fellerhoff B, Laumbacher B, Wank R. High risk of schizophrenia and other mental disorders associated with chlamydial infections: hypothesis to combine drug treatment and adoptive immunotherapy. Med Hypotheses. 2005;65(2):243–52.
63. Fellerhoff B, Laumbacher B, Mueller N, Gu S, Wank R. Associations between Chlamydophila infections, schizophrenia and risk of HLA-A10. Mol Psychiatry. 2007;12(3):264–72.
64. Fellerhoff B, Wank R. Increased prevalence of Chlamydophila DNA in post-mortem brain frontal cortex from patients with schizophrenia. Schizophr Res. 2011;129(2–3):191–5.
65. Buka SL, Tsuang MT, Torrey EF, Klebanoff MA, Bernstein D, Yolken RH. Maternal infections and subsequent psychosis among offspring. Arch Gen Psychiatry. 2001;58(11):1032–7.
66. Vojdani A, Campbell AW, Anyanwu E, Kashanian A, Bock K, Vojdani E. Antibodies to neuron-specific antigens in children with autism: possible cross-reaction with encephalitogenic proteins from milk, Chlamydia pneumoniae and Streptococcus group A. J Neuroimmunol. 2002;129(1–2):168–77.
67. Benitez AJ, et al. Comparison of real-time PCR and a microimmunofluorescence serological assay for detection of Chlamydophila pneumoniae infection in an outbreak investigation. J Clin Microbiol. 2012;50:151–3.
68. Deniset JF, et al. Chlamydophila pneumonia infection leads to smooth muscle cell proliferation and thickening in the coronary artery without contributions from a host immune response. Am J Pathol. 2010;176:1028–37.
69. Zhan P, et al. Chlamydia pneumoniae infection and lung cancer risk: a meta-analysis. Eur J Cancer. 2011;47:742–7.
70. Contini C, Fainardi E, Seraceni S, Granieri E, Castellazzi M, Cultrera R. Molecular identification and antibody testing of Chlamydophila pneumoniae in a subgroup of patients with HIV-associated dementia complex. Preliminary results. J Neuroimmunol. 2003;136(1–2):172–7.
71. Vainshenker YI, Tsinzerling VA, Leonova ON, et al. On the participation of low-manifest infections in the

development of CNS damage in immunodeficiency. HIV Infect Immunosuppress. 2010;2(4):100–1. (in Russian)
72. Clifford DB, Ances BM. HIV-associated neurocognitive disorder. Neurology. 2013;81(4):1–8.
73. Shrestha S, et al. Chlamydia pneumoniae seropositivity in HIV patients with cognitive impairment. J Neurovirol. 2017;23(4):512–8.
74. Zinserling V. Infectious lesions of the central nervous system. Springer; 2022. ISBN 978-3-030-96259-3
75. Torrey EF, et al. Chlamydia pneumoniae and schizophrenia: a possible link? Schizophr Bull. 2006;32(3):547–52.
76. Fellerhoff B, et al. High prevalence of chlamydia pneumoniae in psychiatric patients. Med Microbiol Immunol. 2007;196(2):87–93.
77. Xavier M, Correa B, Coromina M, Canas N, Guimarães J. Sudden psychotic episode probably due to meningoencephalitis and chlamydia pneumoniae acute infection. Clin Pract Epidemiol Ment Health. 2005;1:15. https://doi.org/10.1186/1745-0179-1-15.
78. Nicolson GL, Gan R, Nicolson NL, Haier J. Evidence for Mycoplasma ssp., Chlamydia pneunomiae, and human herpes virus-6 coinfections in the blood of patients with autistic spectrum disorders. J Neurosci Res. 2007;85(5):1143–8.
79. Vainshenker YI, Kalinina OV, Nuralova IV, Ivchenko IM, Melyucheva LA, Tsinzerling VA. Low-manifest infections of the perinatal period and their clinical and neurological manifestations in children and adolescents. Infect Dis. 2013;11(1):44–9. (in Russian)
80. Rodriguez JI, Kern JK. Evidence of microglial activation in autism and its possible role in brain underconnectivity. Neuron Glia Biol. 2011;7(2–4):205–13.
81. Vainshenker YI, Ivchenko IM, Tsinzerling VA, Nuralova IV, Khlopunova OV, Berezina LA, et al. Low-manifest infections with CNS damage in patients with prolonged unconscious states of non-inflammatory etiology. J Microbiol Epidemiol Immunobiol. 2011;6:85–9. (in Russian)
82. Medvedev SV, Vainshenker YI, Ivchenko IM, et al. Latent infectious and inflammatory processes in the central nervous system in patients in a vegetative state (prolonged coma) as a nonspecific factor that consolidates a stable pathological condition. In: Fundamental sciences—medicine: abstracts of reports at conferences and seminars on scientific directions of the program in 2010. Moscow; 2010. p. 163–84. (in Russian).
83. Miller JE, Pedersen LH, Streja E, et al. Maternal infections during pregnancy and cerebral palsy: a population-based study. Paediatr Perinatal Epidemiol. 2013;27(6):542–52. https://doi.org/10.1111/ppe.12082.
84. Grether JK, Nelson KB. Maternal infection and cerebral palsy in infants of normal birth weight. JAMA. 1997;278:207–11.
85. Polivka BJ, Nickel JT. Wilkins JR urinary tract infection during pregnancy: a risk factor for cerebral palsy? J Obstet Gynecol Neonatal Nurs. 1997;26:405–13.
86. Shatrov JG, Birch KM, Lam LT, et al. Chorioamnionitis and cerebral palsy: a meta-analysis. Obstet Gynecol. 2010;116(2, part 1):387–92. https://doi.org/10.1097/AOG.0b013e3181e90046.
87. Saeki S, Hirata I, Fukusako T, Negoro K, Nogaki H, Morimatsu M. A case of psittacosis with psychiatric symptoms, abnormal EEG, and abnormal SPECT. No to Shinkei = Brain Nerve. 1996;48(12):1141–5.

Chlamydiosis in Animals 9

Modern achievements in the epidemiology, pathology and immunology of veterinary chlamydia are described in numerous works by N. Borel, S. Martinov, V.A. Fedorova and others [1–3].

Veterinary chlamydiae include all currently known organisms of the family *Chlamydiaceae*, with the exception of *Chlamydia trachomatis* (see Chap. 1). However, there are several publications on detection *of Chlamydia trachomatis* in birds. Almost all of them are capable of causing diseases in their primary host.

C. abortus is an economically significant infection in sheep and goats, causing abortions, stillbirths and prematurity. Furthermore, it is a zoonotic pathogen, well known for its ability to be transmitted from animals to humans, and poses a risk to pregnant women.

C. psittaci, which causes chlamydiosis in birds, is the most important veterinary chlamydial agent in terms of economic impact and human health. Recently, avian chlamydiosis has been supplemented by new species: *C. avium*, *C. gallinacea, C.ibidis*, *C.buteonis*.

In addition, zoonotic species include *C. felis*, which causes conjunctivitis in cats, and *C. caviae*, a pathogen of guinea pigs. The latter is widely used in experimental animal models. Similarly, mouse models of *C. muridarum infection* have been used for decades to study human genital chlamydial diseases.

C. pecorum has a wide host range, including livestock and wild ruminants, as well as marsupials such as the koala in Australia.

C. pneumoniae, originally thought to be specific to humans, has a wide host range, including horses, koalas, reptiles and amphibians.

C. suis, a pathogen of pigs, is the only chlamydial species that is currently capable of maintaining stable resistance to tetracycline.

A rapidly growing number of culture-independent studies demonstrate the high diversity of chlamydiae across a wide range of habitats and hosts, and it is expected that various new chlamydial species will be described in the near future. Recent studies leading to the description of new species or *Candidatus* species of the family Chlamydiaceae have focused on birds and reptiles, but this may represent only the "tip of the iceberg" of new chlamydial species found in animal hosts.

In the previous chapters, it was shown that chlamydia can affect almost all animals, including farm animals. In world veterinary science and practice, this issue has been studied in detail [4–6]. In Russian veterinary science, it is impossible not to refer to the long-term research of P.M. Mitrofanov [7, 8] who gave the most complete information on diseases of cattle, sheep and pigs. An essential feature of chlamydia is the long-term persistence of the pathogen in the body of the host who has suffered this infection.

V. Zinserling et al., *Chlamydia Infections*, https://doi.org/10.1007/978-3-031-99642-9_9

The main organs of long-term habitation of chlamydia are the gastrointestinal and genital tracts.

In chronic course of the disease, direct tissue damage can be caused by immune complexes. Manifestations of immunopathological processes are glomerulonephritis, vasculitis and endocarditis.

9.1 Chlamydia in Cattle

Pathogens: *C. pecorum, psittaci.*

Depending on the serotype, virulence of the strain, the dose of chlamydia administered, the route of infection, species, age, sex, physiological and immune state, livestock farming practices and other factors, chlamydia in cattle has various clinical and morphological forms: in cows—inflammation of the genitals and abortions, in bulls—inflammation of the genital tract and testicles, in newborn calves—intestinal and respiratory infection, polyarthritis, polyserositis, conjunctivokeratitis.

9.1.1 Chlamydia in Calves

In sick calves, chlamydia manifests itself as gastroenterocolitis, keratoconjunctivitis, polyarthritis and bronchopneumonia. In bulls, cows and heifers infected with chlamydia, the disease often proceeds latently or subclinically, but during pregnancy, the infection process is activated, chlamydia multiply intensively. Microcolonies of chlamydia are determined in the cytoplasm of placental cells, which leads to intrauterine infection of the foetus. Chlamydia causes both miscarriages and stillbirths. Some intrauterinely infected foetuses are born alive, but they have poor development, in the first few days of life—diarrhoea, polyarthritis and signs of damage to the nervous system associated with the development of meningoencephalitis.

In natural conditions, newborn calves are infected mainly by the oral and aerogenic route or through the conjunctiva. During the process of reproduction in the epithelial cells of the abomasum, small and large intestines, chlamydia cause alterative changes, which leads to their sloughing, disruption of permeability and absorption processes and the development of diarrhoea.

The pathogen from the gastrointestinal tract enters the regional lymph nodes, liver, lungs, spleen, thymus, kidneys and other organs by hematogenous or lymphogenous routes, causing their lesions. Chlamydia, multiplying directly in the lymphoid organs (including the thymus), causes a secondary immunodeficiency state in some young animals, which is the cause of activation of polymicrobial autoinfection. Various stress factors, as well as loose housing of cattle, lead to a more severe course of the disease and its rapid spread.

In permanently unfavourable farms, calves may not have diarrhoea or it may be mild, which is associated with the presence of anti-chlamydial antibodies in colostrum.

Experiments on one-day-old calves deprived of colostrum and infected with chlamydia culture orally have established that these microorganisms multiply in the epithelial cells of the abomasum and small intestine, causing their alterative changes. This leads to their sloughing, disruption of the permeability process, absorption and the development of diarrhoea. Against this background, a shift in the bacterial population occurs: *E. coli* from the large intestine moves to the small intestine and abomasum. In patients, along with diarrhoea, subfebrile fever and leucocytosis are observed.

In calves that died in the first few days of life, the morphological picture of the disease is characterized by acute catarrhal gastroenteritis. The mucous membrane of the abomasum is oedematous, hyperaemic; in the fundus and pyloric part, it is dotted with pinpoint haemorrhages. Erosions and ulcers of irregular shape are often visible on it. The inflammatory process occurs in the entire small intestine, but it is more pronounced in the ileum, where there are numerous haemorrhages. The mesenteric lymph nodes are enlarged in volume, oedematous and haemorrhages are observed in the sinuses. Severe alterative changes are determined in the liver; it is unevenly coloured. Pinpoint haemorrhages are also found in the thymus and on the epicardium.

Pathognomonic for chlamydial intestinal infection is the microscopic detection of the pathogen in the cytoplasm of goblet enterocytes, intestinal epithelial cells and in the macrophages of the stroma of the villi.

Against the background of diarrhoea, some animals develop polyarthritis involving mainly the hock, wrist and less often the elbow and other joints. Chlamydial polyarthritis is observed, as a rule, in the winter-spring period, when 2–15% of calves become ill. The pathological process in the joints of calves with chlamydia can develop both in utero and in the postnatal period.

In case of intrauterine infection of animals, pathological processes develop in many joints involving adjacent tendon sheaths, bursae, and the functions of the central nervous system are disrupted. Such calves show depression, adynamia, weakening of tactile and pain sensitivity, apathy, and animals cannot hold their heads. The affected joints are enlarged, painful, the periarticular tissue is tense, and the synovial fluid is turbid. The number of cellular elements in it reaches $3{,}2 \times 10^3/mm^3$.

The synoviocytogram shows an increase in the number of neutrophils, synoviocytes and macrophages. Animals with the described clinical picture of the disease die at the age of 3–11 days or develop bedsores and fistulas in the area of the affected joints. Later, the inflammatory process becomes purulent-fibrinous, which leads to destructive changes in the joint capsule and cartilage. Such animals are culled.

Morphological examination of forcibly killed and dead calves reveals changes characteristic of serous-fibrinous or serous-haemorrhagic polyarthritis and tendovaginitis. The synovial membrane is usually hyperaemic, dotted with multiple point haemorrhages. The periarticular tissue is oedematous, infiltrated with serous-haemorrhagic exudate.

In the postnatal period, clinical signs of arthritis are observed mainly in calves aged 10–78 days. The carpal and hock joints are most often affected. Local inflammatory phenomena in the joint area are less pronounced and are characterized by their swelling, soreness, increased local temperature and moderate lameness. In some animals, clinical signs of arthritis are absent, although synoviocytogram analysis shows the presence of arthritis and synovitis.

The chronic course of the disease is characterized by the attenuation of local inflammatory processes and the formation of a slight dense painless swelling in the area of the affected joints. Morphological examination of the material taken from calves with the postnatal form of chlamydia reveals serous-fibrinous arthritis, chronic gastroenterocolitis, focal interstitial pneumonia and interstitial nephritis. In calves with the postnatal mechanism of arthritis development, lesions of the central nervous system are usually absent and pathological changes in the parenchymatous organs are less pronounced.

In calves with chlamydiosis, symptoms of respiratory system damage are second only to the digestive tract. The disease is enzootic and develops in animals aged 20 days and older, when they are weaned off their mother's milk and transferred to a common calf barn.

The most favourable conditions for the spread of chlamydial pneumonia are created in large farms, complexes for growing and fattening young animals, where susceptible cattle are constantly brought from various supplier farms. It can also be caused by loose housing of animals, overcrowding, drafts and other factors that reduce natural resistance and immunity. Chlamydial bronchopneumonia often occurs in association with other respiratory infections.

Symptoms of respiratory disease in calves caused by chlamydia are expressed to varying degrees and range from mild catarrh of the airways to severe pneumonia. Apparently, in addition to the above factors, the course of the disease is greatly influenced by the age of the animals and the virulence of the pathogen.

At first, the disease manifests itself by an increase in body temperature to 40.5 °C, loss of appetite and serous-mucous discharge from the nasal cavities. On the 3rd–5th day, a rare dry cough appears and wheezing is heard in the lungs.

During rhinocytoscopic examination in the first 7–9 days of the disease, colonies of chlamydia are found in the cytoplasm of ciliated epithelial cells of the nasal cavity. The course of the disease becomes chronic; sometimes, under the influence of unfavourable factors, there are exacerbations. Sick calves lag behind in growth and development, and with untimely and incorrect treatment, the fatal outcome reaches 20–30% of the number of ill animals.

The autopsy picture of animals killed with uncomplicated chlamydial bronchopneumonia is characterized by catarrhal inflammation of the mucous membrane of the airways; the presence of small foci of compaction in the cranial lobes of the lungs and hyperplasia of the retropharyngeal, bronchial and mediastinal lymph nodes.

Histological examination reveals catarrhal rhinitis, tracheitis and bronchitis with severe infiltration of the mucosal layer by lymphoid-histiocytic cells, intralobular, interstitial and focal pneumonia, productive peribronchitis and perivasculitis. In addition, micronecrosis and lymphoid-histiocytic infiltrates in the liver, reduction of lymphatic follicles and proliferation of cells of the monocyte-macrophage system of the spleen, proliferative glomerulonephritis and endocarditis are constantly observed.

In calves that are killed and die as a result of complications of secondary polymicrobial auto-infection, purulent-catarrhal inflammation of the mucous membrane of the airways, lobular-confluent or lobar catarrhal-purulent broncho-pneumonia are observed, often with the formation of focal necrosis and abscesses reaching the size of a walnut or more. In chronic cases, in the lungs, along with the above-described changes, bronchiectasis, sclerotic processes, foci of carnification and atelectasis are observed.

Typical for chlamydiosis in calves with intestinal, respiratory and systemic infection is development of polyarthritis, conjunctivitis and keratitis. The frequency and severity of eye damage vary greatly, which probably largely depends on the chlamydia strain and the immunity of sick animals. In some farms, conjunctivitis is observed in 30% of calves, and cases of keratitis are rare; in others, chlamydial eye infection occurs in the form of enzootics, affecting up to 90% of the livestock and is often accompanied by severe complications leading to blindness.

In the initial stage of the disease, lacrimation, photophobia, vascular hyperaemia, oedema and swelling of the conjunctiva are observed. In smears-prints taken from the affected eyes, polymorphonuclear leukocytes (up to 68%), exfoliated epithelial cells (up to 25%) and macrophages predominate, in the cytoplasm of which chlamydia are found. Subsequently, discharge from the eyes gradually disappears, multiple greyish-white nodules up to 10 mm in diameter appear on the conjunctiva. In the cytological picture of smears from the eyes, a decrease in the number of neutrophils is observed and lymphoid and plasmacytic cells appear.

As the inflammatory process progresses, pathological changes are also observed in the cornea. Superficial keratitis predominates, often catarrhal and vascular (87%), less often phlyctenular and purulent. The cornea becomes cloudy and spots appear on it, the size of which depends on the intensity of the inflammatory process. Clouding can be limited or diffuse and usually begins with the peripheral parts of the cornea, gradually spreading to the centre.

Later, the cornea may become vascularized due to the ingrowth of blood vessels. In severe cases, erosions and even ulcers form on the cornea; corneal perforation, lens loss and eye atrophy are possible. In the absence of complications and with proper treatment, the opacity disappears. After vascular and phlyctenular keratitis, scars form. Neutrophilic-histiocytic infiltration, hyperaemia of blood vessels and oedema are microscopically observed in the conjunctiva. Starting from the 10th to 12th day of the disease, hyperplastic lymphatic follicles with expanded reactive centres appear. Follicular conjunctivitis with severe infiltration of the connective tissue base of the mucous membrane of the eye with lymphoid and plasmacytic cells is characteristic of the subacute and chronic course.

9.1.2 Genital Chlamydia in Cows

One of the clear signs of chlamydiosis is abortions in cows. The abortogenicity of chlamydia has been proven by intravenous, intramuscular, subcutaneous and intradermal administration of chlamydia cultures to experimental cows that are 3–8 months pregnant. It has been established that cows infected with chlamydia intravenously abort after 5–36 days, whereas when infected by other routes, they abort in the second half of pregnancy or give birth to weak calves.

Under natural conditions, chlamydial abortions are also observed in the second half of pregnancy (at 7–9 months). In the case of primary introduction of chlamydia, their percentage in unfavourable herds can reach 30–60%, especially among first-calf heifers and those newly introduced into the herd. In stationary foci, abortions and stillbirths do not exceed 5–7%, although in many infected cows, pathogens are found in postpartum discharge from the genital tract. This is due to the fact that most animals become immune after an abortion and repeated abortions are very rare. Before a miscarriage, they do not show any special clinical signs. In a significant number of aborted animals, separation of the placenta is delayed, which causes the development of endometritis, endosalpingitis, vaginitis and, ultimately, infertility.

Macroscopic changes in the genitals of cows with chlamydia are not typical. After an abortion, catarrhal endometritis, cervicitis and vaginitis with multiple haemorrhages on the mucous membrane occur. Haemorrhages are also noted in the regional (uterine, pelvic) lymph nodes. The inflammatory process in the genital tract is often aggravated by the activation of a secondary bacterial infection. In this case, purulent-catarrhal, fibrinous or ichorous exudate accumulates in the uterine cavity. Microscopically, abundant mononuclear infiltration is detected in the proper layer of the mucous membrane of the uterus and vagina. Chlamydia is detected in the epithelial cells of the genital tract.

Chronic chlamydial endometritis is often accompanied by epithelial metaplasia, fibrosis of the connective tissue base of the mucosa and glandular atrophy. Sometimes the oviducts are involved in the pathological process (catarrhal and catarrhal-purulent endosalpingitis).

In cows, in addition to damage to the genitals, small scars in the lungs and synechiae between the lobes may be detected. In areas of former pneumonia, papillomatous growths of the bronchial epithelium, cellular infiltration and fibrosis of the connective tissue base of the mucosa, as well as a violation of the alveolar architectonics are microscopically visible. Signs of chronic gastroenteritis (folding and thickening of the mucous membrane, abundant cellular infiltration of the proper plate), often endocarditis and glomerulonephritis, perihepatitis and perisplenitis are also detected. When examining the foetal membranes of aborted cows, oedema and gelatinous infiltration of the intercotyledon chorion are detected. There are many small necrotic foci of a greyish-yellow colour in the cotyledons. Microscopic examination reveals changes characteristic of placentitis: necrosis of the trophoblastic epithelium, leukocyte infiltration and vasculitis in the chorion, accumulation of fibrinous-purulent exudate between the surface of the chorion and the uterus, focal necrosis of the uterine epithelium, especially pronounced between caruncles. Chlamydia is detected in the epithelial cells of the trophoblast.

Characteristic structural changes are found in the organs of aborted foetuses, which are used in diagnostics. The foetuses themselves are usually well developed, with a pronounced coat. Oedema of the subcutaneous tissue and accumulation of a large amount of fluid in the abdominal and thoracic cavities are noteworthy. Multiple point haemorrhages are often detected in the mucous membrane of the abomasum, larynx, trachea, tongue, eyes, costal and pulmonary pleura, endo- and epicardium, thymus and in the portal lymph nodes. The liver is enlarged in volume, brittle, unevenly coloured, in the kidneys—alterative changes. The mucous membrane of the abomasum, small and large intestines is swollen, hyperaemic, dotted with haemorrhages. Regional lymph nodes are enlarged and hemorrhagically infiltrated.

Hydropic and focal necrotic changes in the parenchyma, lymphohistiocytic infiltrates of the stroma are observed in the liver. Chlamydial hepatitis is characterized by the accumulation of brown pigment granules in liver cells and macrophages. The epithelium of the convoluted tubules of the kidneys is in a state of vacuolar dystrophy and necrosis, the mucous membrane of the abomasum and small intestine is in a state of mucous dystrophy, sometimes desquamated. The proper plate is loosened, infiltrated with cellular elements. Chlamydia is detected in the cytoplasm of affected epithelial cells when stained with special methods. In 60–70% of cases, changes in the brain (productive perivasculitis, focal non-purulent meningoencephalitis) are found. In some foetuses (especially from experimentally infected cows), granular decay and lysis of muscle fibres, loosening and cellular infiltration of the connective tissue of the myocardium are observed.

9.1.3 Genital Chlamydiosis in Bulls

The causative agent of bovine chlamydiosis is transmitted by sick breeding bulls and sperm infected with chlamydia. In bulls, genital chlamydiosis is usually preceded by chlamydial lesions of the gastrointestinal and respiratory tract, eyes, lungs, joints and (less often) other organs, observed in the first days or weeks of life. As immunity develops in sick bulls, inflammatory changes in the above organs subside, although chlamydia continues to persist for a long time.

With the appearance of sex cells of different generations in the seminiferous tubules and the beginning of spermatogenesis, chlamydia are localized in the genitals, causing their damage. The testicles are slightly enlarged in volume, are slightly mobile and painful. Many animals have discharge from the prepuce, some have symptoms of colic, anxiety when urinating (bending of the spine, shifting from one foot to the other). In such animals, rectal examination reveals enlargement and soreness of the vesicular glands, the head of the prostate and, less often, the bulbourethral gland.

Clinical signs of chlamydia in yearling bulls and older are weakly expressed. In breeding bulls, it proceeds mostly asymptomatically, but a characteristic sign is a change in the quality of sperm (in 80% of patients). In particular, a decrease in the concentration and motility of sperm, aspermia and necrospermia are noted. Due to the low concentration of spermatozoa, up to 17% of ejaculates are rejected, low sperm activity (less than 7 points)—up to 40%.

In sperm smears from bulls with chlamydi, a large number of cellular elements with a predominance of neutrophils (56–78%) are found, but lymphocytes (2–7%), macrophages (up to 12%), exfoliated cells of the spermatogenic epithelium (3–20%) and the urethra (2–13%) are also detected. Chlamydia is detected in the cytoplasm of some macrophages and epithelial cells. An increased number of neutrophils are also noted in smears—imprints taken from the urethra.

During postmortem examination at the initial stage of the disease, a turbid fluid with an admixture of fibrin was found in the cavity of the vaginal membrane. The testicles were slightly swollen. On a section with a bulging parenchyma, small greyish-white or greyish-yellow foci in the form of cords are visible, often located closer to the protein membrane or mediastinum of the organ. Subsequently, the serous exudate is absorbed and small deposits of fibrin are noted on the surface of the serous layer of the vaginal membranes. In the chronic course of the disease, connective tissue growths (synechiae) are visible between the layers of the vaginal membrane, especially numerous in the area of the tail of the appendage.

Histological examination of the testicles revealed changes characteristic of focal intratubular orchitis. In the initial stage of the disease, a significant number of convoluted seminiferous tubules with dystrophic and necrotic changes were noted.

As the disease progresses, their number increases. Sperm cells in the tubules change shape and are then displaced by connective tissue cells. Subsequently, sclerosis, calcification of the seminiferous tubules, proliferation of intertubular connective tissue and disappearance of glandulocytes lead to a sharp decrease and even cessation of spermatogenesis in the affected areas of the testicle.

In genital chlamydiosis of bulls, the urethra, accessory sex glands and prepuce are also involved in the pathological process. Catarrhal urethritis and posthitis are chronic and are accompanied by infiltration of the subepithelial connective tissue by mononuclear cells.

Prostatitis occurs in 20% of cases, seminal vesiculitis—in 16.7%; couperitis is observed less frequently.

In bulls aged 10 months and older, sick with chlamydiosis, balanoposthitis, serous-fibrinous pleurisy, peritonitis, perihepatitis, perisplenitis and periorchitis are often observed; in breeding bulls—chronic gastroenteritis with hyperplasia of solitary follicles and Peyer's patches, distelectasis, productive peribronchitis, reticular sclerosis, adhesions between the lobes of the lungs, fibroplastic glomerulonephritis and endocarditis.

Clinically, epizootological and pathomorphological data serve as the basis for making a preliminary diagnosis. The final diagnosis is made based on the results of laboratory tests, which include detection of chlamydia in smears taken from affected organs using light microscopy or immunofluorescence, isolation of chlamydia in chicken embryos or laboratory animals with subsequent identification and detection of specific antibodies in the blood serum. In modern conditions, PCR is of paramount importance.

Of great diagnostic significance is the detection of chlamydia in smears-prints taken from the mucous membrane of the genital tract of sick cows, and in addition, in the semen of bulls. In calves, smears are taken from the mucous membrane of the nasal cavity, eyes, and after death—from the mucous membrane of the trachea, abomasum, ileum, synovial membrane of the affected joints.

Differential diagnostics. Chlamydiosis should be distinguished from other infectious diseases: brucellosis, leptospirosis, pustular vulvovaginitis, genital mycoplasmosis, vibriosis, trichomoniasis. It should also be remembered that mixed infections exist.

9.2 Chlamydia in Sheep

Chlamydiosis manifests by abortions, stillbirths of weak, non-viable lambs and inflammatory changes in the genital tract, in lambs—gastroenteritis, bronchopneumonia, polyarthritis and keratoconjunctivitis. The causative agents are *C. pecorum*, abortus, psittaci.

The pathogenesis of chlamydial abortion in sheep is largely determined by the high tropism of the pathogen to the tissues of the placenta and genitals. In pregnant sheep, during the period of chlamydemia, it enters the chorion and cotyledon villi through the bloodstream from the sites of primary localization (gastrointestinal, respiratory and genital tract), and then into the internal organs of the foetus. The infection is accompanied by inflammation of both cotyledons and caruncles, which leads to the separation of the chorionic villi from the maternal tissue. During the period of increased reproduction of chlamydia, toxic substances are released that have both local and general effects. With combined damage to the placenta and fetus, abortion occurs.

Some lambs infected in utero are born alive. But they are usually weak, non-viable and die within the first day. If they survive, they develop gastroenteritis and then bronchopneumonia.

The main primary site of reproduction of chlamydia in lambs is the digestive tract, from where they are carried into the general bloodstream by hematogenous and lymphogenous routes, resulting in the development of chlamydemia. Then they enter various internal organs, primarily the liver, spleen, thymus, and lungs. Chlamydia reproduce mainly in the macrophages of these organs. Expansion of the localization area and their accumulation in cells lead to the development of secondary chlamydemia when they overcome the hemo- and lymphosynovial barrier of the joints. Reproduction of chlamydia in synoviocytes and their subsequent release into the synovial fluid cause joint inflammation. Chlamydial arthritis is characterized by predominant damage to the superficial layers of the synovial membrane and in most cases ends with complete restoration of joint function even after a long illness.

During puberty, many rams experience relapses of arthritis associated with repeated chlamydemia due to the accumulation of pathogens in the genitals. But even in such cases, residual arthritis is characterized by small connective tissue growths on the synovial membrane, and only in isolated cases is it possible to observe limited mobility in the joints due to fibrous ankylosis.

The incubation period of chlamydial abortion in sheep under natural conditions can last several months, after experimental infection of pregnant sheep—45–60 days. Its duration depends on the route of infection, virulence and dose of the pathogen, time of pregnancy and other factors. With a typical form of the disease, ewes have abortions, stillbirths and the birth of weak lambs. During the first outbreak of the disease, up to 60% of sheep or more abort, and in permanently unfavourable farms—5–10%. Sick sheep abort only once and become immune in subsequent years. Abortions are usually observed in the last days of pregnancy and proceed without significant changes in the general condition of the sheep. In some animals, vaginal discharge and an increase in body temperature appear several days before an abortion or premature birth. These signs can also be observed in the first days after an abortion or lambing. Many aborted ewes show retention of the placenta and clinical signs of vaginitis, endometritis, and in 30–38% of animals, follicular conjunctivitis.

In the latent course of the disease, lambing in sheep occurs normally, but the young animals are born weak, non-viable and die within the first day. In permanently unfavourable farms, abortions are observed mainly in ewes.

In farms with unfavourable conditions for chlamydial polyarthritis of lambs, abortions and stillbirths are also frequent. In different flocks, the incidence of lambs can vary from 10% to 80%. They limp, often lie down or take an unusual pose. They experience depression, decreased appetite, subfebrile fever, swelling and soreness of the carpal, tarsal and other joints, often diarrhoea and dehydration. Almost every second or third lamb with joint damage shows signs of bilateral conjunctivitis, but pathological changes in the eyes can be observed without signs of arthritis. In severe cases, profuse discharge from the eyes, eyelid oedema, photophobia and corneal opacity are common.

Chlamydial polyarthritis in lambs is chronic. Sick animals are significantly retarded in growth and development. Signs of urethritis and balanoposthitis are observed in rams. In adult rams, chlamydia does not manifest itself clinically, but microscopic examination of sperm reveals changes in its quality, cellular elements of both hematogenous (neutrophils, lymphocytes) and tissue (sloughed epithelial cells, macrophages) origin.

The most pronounced structural changes in chlamydial abortion of sheep are found in the foetal membranes, parenchymatous organs of stillborn and living but non-viable lambs, and in the genitals of aborted animals. Placentas taken from ewes with early abortions show signs of pronounced autolysis. In ewes that aborted in the last days of pregnancy, the placenta is oedematous, the surface of the intercotyledonous chorion is infiltrated in some places with gelatinous or hemorrhagic infiltration, covered with greyish-white flakes. The cotyledons are hyperaemic, chocolate-coloured, and multiple necrotic foci of greyish-yellow colour are visible on their open surface.

Autopsy of aborted foetuses and lambs that died immediately after birth reveals oedema of the subcutaneous tissue, accumulation of bloody fluid in the body cavities, pronounced dystrophic changes in the kidneys and myocardium, foci of atelectasis in the lungs, pinpoint haemorrhages on the pulmonary pleura, capsule of the spleen, under the epicardium, in the thymus, on the mucous membrane of the oesophagus, abomasum and small intestine. The liver is enlarged in volume, clay-coloured with pale grey stripes.

During post-mortem examination of aborted sheep, accumulation of catarrhal-purulent exudate in the uterine cavity, haemorrhages on the mucous membrane of the genital tract, hyperaemia and swelling of regional lymph nodes are noted and, in some, catarrhal-purulent endosalpingitis.

Structural changes in chlamydial polyarthritis of lambs depend on the stage and severity of the disease. At the initial stage of the process, in the cavity of the affected joints (mainly wrist, tarsal, knee, less often—others), there is an increase in the amount of turbid synovial fluid with an admixture of greyish-yellow films of fibrin. The synovial membrane is oedematous, hyperaemic, in places dotted with haemorrhages. Along the course of nearby tendon sheaths, gelatinous infiltrates are noted.

In chronic disease, the joint capsule is thickened, and connective tissue growths are visible on it in some places. In severe forms of the disease, ankylosis of the joints is observed. Sometimes the articular cartilage is involved in the pathological process, on which small erosions are formed. The digestive organs are most often affected. At the onset of the disease, catarrhal gastroenteritis is observed; in the late stage, the inflammatory process is accompanied by thickening, increased folding of the mucous membrane, hyperplasia of the lymphoid tissue of the small intestine and mesenteric lymph nodes. In most cases, greyish-white nodules are found on the abomasal mucosa.

In breeding rams that test positive for chlamydia, serous-fibrinous or adhesive periorchitis, focal necrotic orchitis and catarrhal urethritis, often with involvement of the accessory sex glands in the pathological process, occur. In the early stage of the disease in sheep, the epithelial cells of the chorion are enlarged; in their cytoplasm, clusters of elementary bodies of chlamydia are visible. The connective tissue base of the chorionic villi is oedematous, in places infiltrated by neutrophils, macrophages and plasma cells. Further, necrosis of the epithelium of the villi of the cotyledons, fibrinoid necrosis, thrombosis of blood vessels and cellular infiltration of the mucous membrane of the uterus occur.

In the uterus of aborted sheep, an inflammatory process of a catarrhal-purulent nature is detected, with diffuse cellular infiltration of the proper layer. In some cases, metaplasia of the epithelium of the uterine mucosa and catarrhal-purulent endosalpingitis are observed. In sheep with conjunctivitis, hyperplasia of lymphoid follicles and abundant infiltration of the proper plate of the mucosa with mononuclear cells are characteristic features.

In aborted foetuses and lambs that died in the first days of life, haemodynamic disturbances are characteristic of chlamydiosis, manifested by haemorrhages, oedema and loosening of the connective tissue stroma in various organs, severe alterative and necrotic processes in the parenchyma of the liver and kidneys, accumulations of lymphoid-histiocytic cells in the interstitial tissue of the lungs, liver, kidneys and myocardium, morphological signs of suppression of embryonic haematopoiesis and thymus hypoplasia. In addition, leptomeningitis is often detected.

Lambs with articular chlamydiosis develop serous or serous-fibrinous polyarthritis and tendovaginitis. The synovial membrane is oedematous, infiltrated with leukocytes and macrophages. Chlamydia is found in the cytoplasm of altered synoviocytes and macrophages. In some sick lambs, lysis of the capsule wall and formation of fistulas occur on the 7th to 10th day of the disease under the influence of proteolytic enzymes of neutrophils. The penetration of bacteria into the joint cavity through fistulas aggravates pathological processes. At the same time, strongly expressed reactive changes occur in the periarticular connective tissue (oedema, haemorrhage), nearby muscles (myositis) and tendon sheaths.

In uncomplicated disease, after 1.5–2 months, lymphoid and plasma cells predominate in the cellular infiltrates of the capsule. Unresorbed fibrin undergoes organization. Hyperplasia and hypertrophy of the integumentary cells of the synovial membrane are locally observed.

Since chlamydial polyarthritis is a systemic infection, changes are also observed in other organs. Among them, chronic gastroenteritis with hyperplasia of the lymphoid tissue of the small intestine, lymphoid-histiocytic infiltrates in the liver, lungs and other organs are characteristic features.

Chlamydia in sheep is diagnosed based on the analysis of epizootological data; clinical, pathological signs and laboratory test results. Characteristic pathological changes are placenta and foetal organs. The final diagnosis is made upon detection of chlamydia in pathological material by light microscopy or immunofluorescence, detection of specific antibodies in the blood serum of sick and recovered animals or isolation of chlamydia in chicken embryos, as well as laboratory animals with their subsequent identification; PCR has recently acquired key importance. The microscopic method of diagnosing chlamydia in sheep is fast, accessible and effective. After an abortion, chlamydia is easily detected within 7–10 days, sometimes 20–30 days.

Pathognomonic for chlamydia in lambs is the detection of chlamydia in the cytoplasm of synoviocytes, intestinal epithelial cells and conjunctiva.

Chlamydial abortion of sheep is differentiated primarily from other infectious abortions, in particular those of brucellosis aetiology, as well as from campylobacteriosis, toxoplasmosis and leptospirosis. It should be taken into account that mixed forms of infection can occur in natural conditions: chlamydia and salmonellosis, chlamydia and brucellosis. Chlamydial polyarthritis should be distinguished from infectious diseases that also involve joints (infectious agalactia of sheep, colibacillosis, erysipelas, diplococcal septicaemia, streptococcal polyarthritis).

9.3 Chlamydiosis in Pigs

Chlamydiosis is a chronic infectious disease characterized in sows by abortions, stillbirths and non-viable piglets, inflammatory changes in the genital tract, in boars by urethritis, orchitis and balanoposthitis, in young animals by mass enteritis, pneumonia, polyserositis, dermatitis and focal skin necrosis.

In permanently unhealthy farms, the disease often proceeds latently, periodically worsening when the resistance of the animals' bodies decreases.

Chlamydia enters the body of healthy pigs mainly through the alimentary, airborne and sexual routes, first on the mucous membranes of the gastrointestinal, respiratory and genital tracts, and then into the epithelial cells and macrophages, where their primary reproduction occurs. Subsequently, from the sites of primary localization, they enter the regional lymph nodes and into the blood lymphogenously (primary chlamydemia), from which they are carried to the parenchymatous organs. Subsequently, in piglets, chlamydia intensively reproduces in the macrophages of the spleen, liver, lungs, hepatocytes, in the epithelial cells of the convoluted tubules and synoviocytes.

Circulating in the blood, chlamydia penetrates endothelial cells, causing their alterative changes, which leads to impaired vascular permeability and, consequently, inflammatory oedema and haemorrhage. Long-term persistence of chlamydia in the body of animals causes the development of immunopathological processes, the consequence of which are vasculitis, glomerulonephritis and endocarditis.

In the pathogenesis of chlamydiosis, the ability of the pathogen to overcome the haematoplacental barrier in pregnant sows and the hematotesticular barrier in boars is of particular importance. This leads to abortions, stillbirths and postpartum gynaecological diseases, and in males—to the appearance of orchitis and a decrease in spermatogenesis, which can cause infertility.

In the pathogenesis of chlamydial infection, a direct damaging effect of chlamydia on the body of pigs is also noted, especially in piglets in the first days of life.

The main signs of the disease in sows are abortions and the birth of stillborn and non-viable piglets. Abortions predominate in the initial occurrence of the disease on the farm. In permanently unfavourable farms, stillborn (8–10%), underdeveloped and non-viable (20–25%) piglets predominate in the litters of sows, of which up to 30–50% die in the first 3–5 days of life. Abortions usually occur in the last weeks of pregnancy, and most of the foetuses are full-term, covered with bristles. After birth, the sows lie for a long time, reluctantly eating feed. Some of them develop endometritis and mastitis, leading to agalactia.

In newborn piglets, the skin is stagnantly hyperaemic, with a bluish tint, the sucking reflex is poorly developed. Later, they experience lethargy, drowsiness, massive debilitating diarrhoea, body temperature often rises to 41–41.5 °C, after weaning, bronchopneumonia develops, often pericarditis, arthritis and keratoconjunctivitis. Moreover, in some farms, weaned piglets show predominantly signs of bronchopneumonia, in others—arthritis and keratoconjunctivitis. Approximately 7–10% of young animals show signs of eye damage, eyelid oedema, which often stick together, as a result of which they cannot open their eyes. In fattening piglets, the disease is clinically manifested mainly by bronchopneumonia.

During the period of attenuation of the disease, 30–85% of sick piglets develop dark red areas of skin on the skin of the ears, body and at the base of the tail, which become necrotic and are rejected; in some animals, signs of meningoencephalitis are observed.

Most adult boars have no symptoms of chlamydiosis. They lose weight, their sexual activity decreases and sometimes, blood is found in their semen.

Autopsy of aborted foetuses and piglets that died in the first days of life reveals oedema of the subcutaneous tissue, in places in the form of gelatinous infiltrates, in the chest and abdominal cavities—a large amount of bloody fluid. Serous-fibrinous pericarditis, pleurisy and peritonitis are often observed. The spleen is without visible changes. The lungs of aborted foetuses are congested, in newborn piglets—with foci of atelectasis and emphysema, the liver—with alterative changes, enlarged, unevenly coloured—from dark cherry to greyish-red with a yellowish tint. Pinpoint haemorrhages are visible on the epicardium, in the cortex of the kidneys, liver, thymus, on the mucous membrane of the gastrointestinal tract and under the pulmonary pleura.

In weaned piglets, the most common are subacute gastroenteritis, catarrhal pneumonia localized mainly in the apical lobes, hyperplasia and oedema of the regional lymph nodes.

In sows killed in the first day after parturition or abortion, the mucous membrane of the uterine horns is oedematous, unevenly hyperaemic, with haemorrhages, where bubbles the size of a pea or smaller, filled with a thick greyish-white secretion, are visible on it. Residual effects of pneumonia are found in the lungs: cicatricial contractions and synechiae between the lobes.

In boars, changes in the internal organs are minor and similar to those in sows. The most pronounced macroscopic abnormalities are found in the genitals: compaction of the testicles due to the proliferation of interlobular connective tissue, adhesions between the vaginal membranes. Regional lymph nodes are enlarged by 1.5–2 times due to hyperplasia of lymphoid tissue. Multiple greyish-white nodules are visible on the mucous membrane of the penis and prepuce.

Pathohistological examinations of organs of aborted foetuses and newborn piglets that died from chlamydia show severe alterative and necrotic lesions of parenchymatous organs. In the liver, many hepatocytes are vacuolated. In sections stained with Romanovsky Giemsa, colonies of chlamydia are visible in the cytoplasm of liver and Kupffer cells. Small foci of active necrosis are formed from small groups of necrotic hepatocytes. As the disease progresses, small lymphoid-histiocytic infiltrates are formed in the parenchyma and interlobular connective tissue.

In the initial stage of the disease, vacuolization of the epithelium of the convoluted tubules is determined in the kidneys. In subsequent stages, the main changes are noted in the glomeruli of the renal corpuscle: proliferation of endothelial and mesangial cells, focal thickening of the basement membrane of the capillaries.

In piglets aged 20–30 days and older, respiratory diseases predominate in the form of catarrh of the airways, interstitial and focal catarrhal pneumonia, productive peribronchitis and perivasculitis.

In aborted sows, endometritis with cystic-dilated uterine glands, catarrhal inflammation of the vaginal mucosa and cervix with cellular infiltration of the proper layer of the mucosa are microscopically visible. Many sows also have membranous proliferative and fibroplastic glomerulonephritis, chronic gastroenteritis and signs of previous bronchopneumonia.

In breeding boars, characteristic histopathological changes are detected in the testicles, where the cells of the spermatogenic epithelium undergo severe alterative changes, sometimes leading to the complete disappearance of the epithelium and sclerosis of the seminiferous tubules. Along with this, proliferation of intertubular connective tissue with atrophy of interstitial cells, focal chronic urethritis and, less often, inflammation in the accessory sex glands are noted.

The diagnosis is established on the basis of clinical, epizootological and pathomorphological data, the results of laboratory tests, including microscopic detection of the pathogen in the affected organs, isolation and identification of chlamydia, serological indicators.

When diagnosing chlamydia in pigs, it is necessary to exclude brucellosis, leptospirosis, parvovirus infection, porcine reproductive and respiratory syndrome and hypovitaminosis A.

9.4 Conclusion

In reviews [4, 5] are presented also brief characteristics of lesions in several birds, horses and fishes. For other farm animals, birds and reptiles, detailed clinical and morphological data are lacking.

In conclusion, we can summarize:

- Clinical and morphological changes in different animals and humans have significant similarities.
- Despite recent advances, both surveillance and documentation of zoonotic cases need to be improved to understand the extent and impact of chlamydial zoonotic infections.
- New data on the pathogenesis of chlamydial infections in animals will provide insight into the specific strategies used by pathogens. Future projects should focus on chlamydial latency, differences in strain virulence and variability in host immune responses.
- A thorough investigation of tetracycline-resistant and tetracycline-susceptible *C. suis strains* isolated from pigs is critical to better understand chlamydial antibiotic resistance and its transmission through recombination events.
- Now that genome sequence analysis has been performed for the major chlamydial pathogens, the focus should shift to transcriptome analysis to provide comprehensive studies of pathogen–host interactions.
- Coinfections *Chlamydia* spp. and/or other pathogens, have emerged as an important research topic that should be further developed.

References

1. Borel N, Polkinghorne A, Pospischil A. A review on chlamydial diseases in animals: still a challenge for pathologists? Vet Pathol. 2018;55(3):374–90.
2. Fedorova VA, Lyapina AM, Khizhnyakova MA, et al. Chlamydia of animals and humans. Moscow: Federal State Unitary Enterprise. Academic Scientific Publishing, Production, Printing and Book Distribution Center “Nauka”; 2019. 135 p. (in Russian).
3. Martinov S. Chlamydiae and chlamydial infections. New York: River Publishers; 2018. 504p
4. Tan M, Hegemann JH, Caister CS, editors. Chlamydia biology: From genome to disease. Academic; 2020.
5. Everett KD, Hornung LJ, Andersen AA. Rapid detection of the Chlamydiaceae and other families in the order Chlamydiales: three PCR tests. J Clin Microbiol. 1999;37(3):575–80. https://doi.org/10.1128/JCM.37.3.575-580.1999. PMID: 9986815; PMCID: PMC84475
6. Corsaro D, Greub G. Pathogenic potential of novel Chlamydiae and diagnostic approaches to infections due to these obligate intracellular bacteria. Clin Microbiol Rev. 2006;19(2):283–97. https://doi.org/10.1128/CMR.19.2.283-297.2006. PMID: 16614250; PMCID: PMC1471994
7. Mitrofanov PM. Pathomorphology in chlamydial- parainfluenzal infection in calves. Veterinaria. 1979;7:35–8. (in Russian)
8. Mitrofanov PM. Pathological diagnostics of less known infections of farm animals. Saransk: Edition of Mordov University; 1997. 107 p. (in Russian).

10 Experimental Chlamydiosis

10.1 Review of Existing Models of Chlamydial Infections

Animals infected with *Chlamydia*, both naturally and artificially, are used. In practice, laboratory mice and guinea pigs are most often selected as surrogate models for studying urogenital *Chlamydia* and trachoma, infecting them with *C. muridarum* and *C. caviae*, respectively [1].

Over the past few decades, various clinical variants of *Chlamydia* have been reproduced experimentally on numerous occasions, primarily to study the pathogenesis of urogenital infections and develop approaches to their treatment [2–7].

10.2 Review of Existing Experimental Models of Chlamydial Infection of the Nervous System

Modelling of neurochlamydiosis in an experiment showed the tropism of the pathogen to the nervous system, and the morphological manifestations of the infectious process in the central nervous system or peripheral nervous system did not differ fundamentally depending on the route of infection and the type of pathogen [8, 9]. In the membranes of the brain, ependyma of the ventricles and brain matter, the pathogen was determined predominantly paravasal, which was accompanied by inflammatory changes of a lymphocytic-macrophage nature [8–10].

The fact that *Chlamydia* and *Chlamydophila* pass through the blood-brain barrier (BBB) and the blood-neural barrier, and the ability of pathogens to persist and reproduce in the cells of the nervous system have also been shown in other experimental studies [9–13].

Recent research demonstrated that *Chlamydia muridarum*, a bacterium often used to model chlamydial infections in humans, was able to rapidly enter the brain of mice via the olfactory and trigeminal nerves.

This study has important implications for understanding the pathogenesis of chlamydial CNS infections:

- It provides experimental evidence for rapid penetration of *Chlamydia* into the brain via neural pathways, something previously only suspected for *C. pneumoniae.*
- Finding that *C. muridarum* can infect glial cells explains how the bacteria can evade the immune response and invade nerves.
- Differences in the response of olfactory and trigeminal glial cells to infection may have implications for understanding the spread of infection in the CNS.
- The study provides a model for studying the link between chlamydial infections and neurodegenerative diseases such as late-onset dementia.

V. Zinserling et al., *Chlamydia Infections*, https://doi.org/10.1007/978-3-031-99642-9_10

This study demonstrates that *C. muridarum* is able to rapidly penetrate the CNS via the olfactory and trigeminal nerves, infecting glial cells. These results have important implications for understanding the pathogenesis of chlamydial CNS infections and may facilitate the development of new strategies for the prevention and treatment of associated neurological complications [14–24].

10.3 Ultrastructural Changes in Experimental Chlamydial Meningoencephalitis (L. S. Onischenko, Partly in Collaboration with M. M. Odinak, M. M. Mikhailenko, I. V. Nuralova)

The neurotropism of *Chlamydia* has been known for a long time, but many questions of the pathogenesis and pathomorphology of the lesions of the central and peripheral nervous system caused by them cannot be resolved on clinical material. Electron microscopic studies of the central and peripheral nervous system were carried out during infection with *Chlamydia* in an experiment. And intracerebral, intraperitoneal and intranasal methods of infecting mice with *Chlamydia* were used. Ba1b/ c *Chlamydia* (*C. trachomatis, psittaci* and *C. pneumonia*).

For all types of infection, mice were dissected under aseptic conditions on the 4th–5th day at the height of clinical manifestations of the disease. For morphological examination, pieces of the brain and lumbar spinal cord, roots of the equine tail and sciatic nerve were taken from 4 animals for each type of infection and from 4 mice in the control group.

In all types of infection, examination of pia mater (PMM) imprints using fluorescence microscopy showed the presence of chlamydial antigen in its cells.

For light microscopy, materials taken from the CNS and PNS were fixed in 9 6° alcohol and 10% neutral formalin and, after dehydration, embedded in celloidin or paraffin. Then, 5–7 μm thick sections were made, which were stained using known neurohistological methods and studied under a light microscope.

10.3.1 Material and Methods

For electron microscopic examination, the material taken from different parts of the brain and sciatic nerves was immediately filled with a 2.5% solution of glutaraldehyde cooled to +4°C in 0.1 M phosphate buffer (pH 7.2–7.4). Then thin (1–2 mm) frontal incisions were made across the entire brain from the frontal lobes to the brainstem, including the cerebellum. The fixation time in this solution was generally about a day until the final cutting of pieces of the required size. The next day, additional fixation was carried out in a 2% osmium solution on the same phosphate buffer.

Intracerebral Infection (ICI) For infection, mice weighing 14–16 g were taken. For challenge a 10% suspension of *Chlamydia* (chlamydophila)-infected yolk sac membranes of chicken embryos or mouse brain, prepared in sterile saline 0.01 M phosphate buffer (pH 7.2–7.4) was used. The infection dose was 0.03 ml of suspension diluted to 1:20–1:40 (depending on the degree of pathogen accumulation in the original material). Infected animals were constantly monitored to detect the first signs of infection (ruffled fur, low mobility, convulsions of the hind limbs, etc.). Mice were dissected on the 4th–5th day at the height of clinical manifestations of the disease.

Intact animals, yolk sacs of chicken embryos, and specially treated L-929 and LL-mk cell cultures served as controls in all experiments.

Intranasal Infection (INI) Suspensions of yolk sacs of chicken embryos infected with *C. pneumonia* (strain "TWAR") were used as infectious material.

Mice Balb/c weighing (18–20 g) under ether rausch anaesthesia were injected into each nostril with a thin needle of a tuberculin syringe with

0.02 ml (2–3 drops) of a suspension of infectious material *C. pneumonia* from the membranes of the yolk sacs of chicken embryos in doses of 10-3—10-5 (LD /50) to form a persistent chlamydial infection. In this experimental group, there were a total of 50 animals.

Intra-abdominal Infection (IAI) 2–4 h before infection with *Chlamydia*, mice weighing 18–20 g were given 5 mg of hydrocortisone intramuscularly to reduce resistance beforehand, and then 0.5 ml of a 10% suspension of *Chlamydia*-infected yolk sac membranes of chicken embryos were given intraperitoneally.

In the case of intraperitoneal infection, sections of the pia mater and various parts of the brain, the lumbar segment of the spinal cord, the roots of the equine tail and the sciatic nerves were taken as material for light and electron microscopic examination at the preterminal stage of infection development. Material was also taken on the 4th–5th day after infection of mice from 4 control and 4 experimental animals immediately after their dissection and processed according to standard methods.

For all types of infection of mice, semi-thin sections were first made from the material embedded in araldite, which were stained on glass with toludine blue and viewed in a light microscope. Then, ultra-thin sections (300–500 nm thick) were made from the same blocks, which were placed on grids, contrasted with lead citrate and an aqueous solution of uranyl acetate, and then studied by transmission electron microscopy in JEM -100 C (Japan), Tesla (Czech Republic) and LEO -910 (Germany) electron microscopes with a microscope magnification of 2000 to 40,000–70,000 times.

10.4 Results

The results of electron microscopic examination of chlamydial infection can be systematized into three groups of morphological indicators:

- The presence of *Chlamydia* in the vessels of the microcirculatory bed, as well as in the cells and fibres of the central and peripheral nervous systems
- Changes in the ultrastructure of nerve and glial cells of the central and peripheral nervous system, endothelial cells and perivascular space
- Changes in myelinated and non-myelinated nerve fibres of the central and peripheral nervous systems, as well as changes in synaptocomplexes

In all types of infections, *Chlamydia* in the CNS and PNS were found in the form of elementary bodies and, less frequently, reticular bodies. Elementary bodies of *Chlamydia* were found everywhere in the lumen and endothelium of vessels and perivascular space, in cells and fibres of the pia mater of the brain, ependymal cells of the cerebral ventricles, neurogliocytes, myelin and non-myelinated fibres.

10.4.1 Intracerebral Infection (ICI)

Using light microscopy, pathological changes were found primarily in the pia mater of the brain, ventricular ependyma, vascular walls and in adjacent areas of brain tissue—foci of necrosis of various sizes.

Since the changes in all experiments were similar, we will give the most typical example from light microscopy (Fig. 10.1).

In electron microscopic examination of the superficial layers of the cerebral cortex with intracerebral infection, myelinopathy was often observed in the myelin fibres in the form of adhesion, delamination and thinning (or pronounced swelling) of the myelin lamellae (Fig. 10.2a, b). In the axial cylinders of the myelin fibres of the central nervous system with different types of infection, a transparent ("transport") form of elementary chlamydial bodies was often observed in close proximity to the mitochondria, and at the same time, distinct signs of myelino- and axonopathy were noted, as well as changes in the structure of the mitochondria.

10.4.2 Intraperitoneal Infection (IPI)

Electron microscopy of this method of infection showed that *Chlamydiae* penetrate cells, probably by absorption of elementary bodies and their subsequent endocytosis (Fig. 10.3a). Elementary bodies of *Chlamydiae* both in cells and in fibres had either transparent or dense contents and necessarily a double membrane. The morphology of the cytoplasm of cells containing *Chlamydiae* was greatly altered. At the stage of transformation of elementary bodies into the reticular form, the disturbances of the cytostructure of infected cells and myelin fibres increased (Fig. 10.3b).

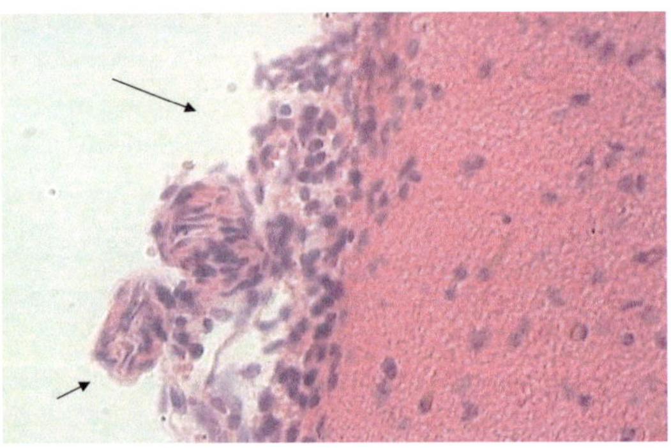

Fig. 10.1 Mouse brain with intracerebral infection with *Chlamydia*. Pia mater with a destroyed outer layer (↑) and an infiltrate of lymphoid and plasma cells penetrating into the brain tissue. Stained with haematoxylin and eosin. Magnification ×400

In the microcirculatory bed vessels of the CNS and PNS and in the experiment on mice, elementary bodies of *Chlamydia* are found both in the lumen of the capillary and endotheliocytes, and near the capillary outside of it, which indirectly indicates the exit of *Chlamydia* from the vessel and the violation of the blood-brain barrier (Fig. 10.4). The lumen of some CNS capillaries was almost entirely filled with erythrocytes. The structure of endotheliocytes is usually preserved in both the CNS and PNS, and in the endotheliocytes of the CNS capillaries, large nuclei with moderately and unevenly hyperchromic karyoplasm and very large chromatin compactions are sometimes determined, occupying a significant part of the nucleus and, possibly, replacing nucleolus-like bodies.

In all types of infection, *Chlamydia* bodies (both elementary and transitional) in brain cells were located between the organelles of the cytoplasm, and sometimes in the organelles themselves: the ER, the Golgi complex, phagosomes or in transparent vacuoles (Fig. 10.5a, b).

Microgliocytes of the central nervous system in all types of *Chlamydia* infection and especially in intranasal infection were often in a very active

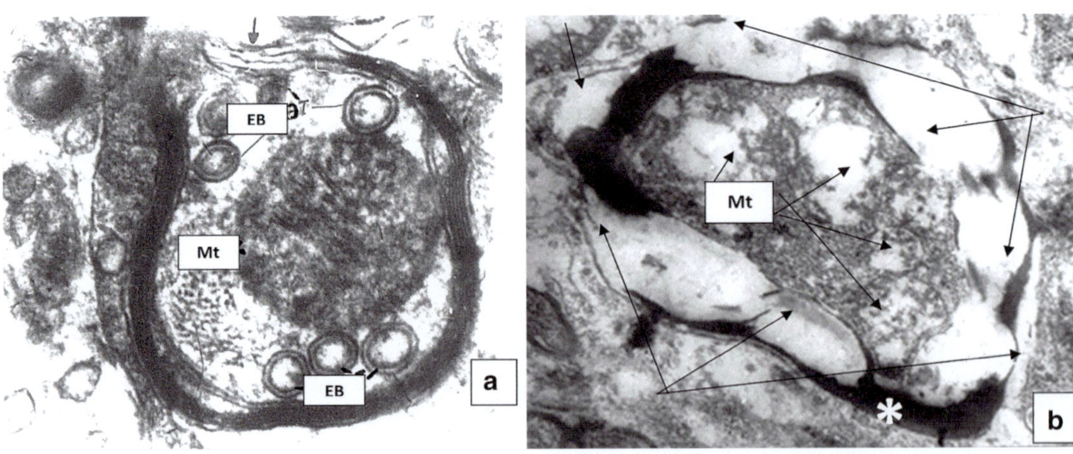

Fig. 10.2 Myelinated fibres of the brain after intracerebral infection with *Chlamydia*: (**a**) from the upper layers of the cerebral cortex; (**b**) from the brainstem. (**a**) *Mt* mitochondrion, (↓)—stratification of myelin lamellae, *EB* elementary bodies of *Chlamydia*. Magnification ×32,000. (**b**) arrows—focal swelling and disappearance of spiral lamellae (*) in the myelin sheath, *Mt* destroyed mitochondria in a compressed axial cylinder with a high density of axoplasm. Magnification ×13,000

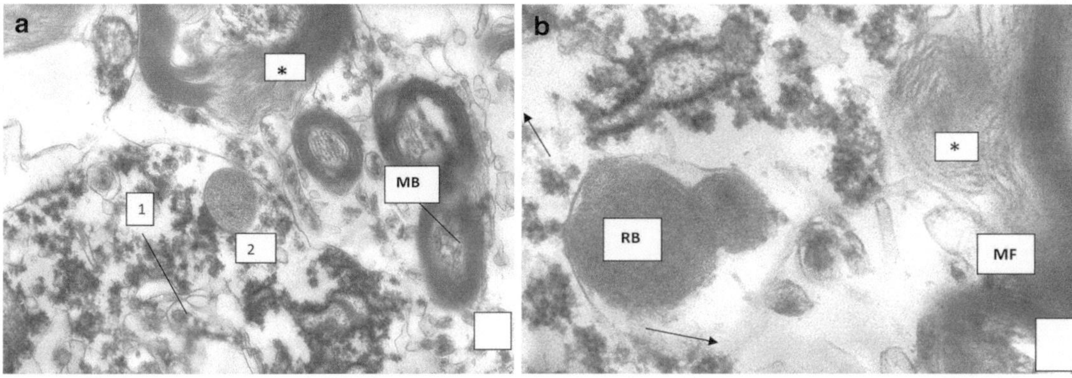

Fig. 10.3 (**a**) Neuron of the granular layer of the cerebellum of a mouse with intraperitoneal infection with *Chlamydia*. In the cytoplasm of the neuron: 1—elementary and 2—transitional body of *Chlamydia*, next to the neuron—myelin fibres (Mf) with stratification (*) and adhesion of lamellae. Magnification ×16,000. (**b**) Binary reticular body of *Chlamydia* (RT) in the cytoplasm of a neuron with a destroyed cytolemma (↑) during intraperitoneal infection with *Chlamydia*. Next to RB—myelinated fibre (MF) with stratification of myelin lamellae (*). Magnification ×32,000

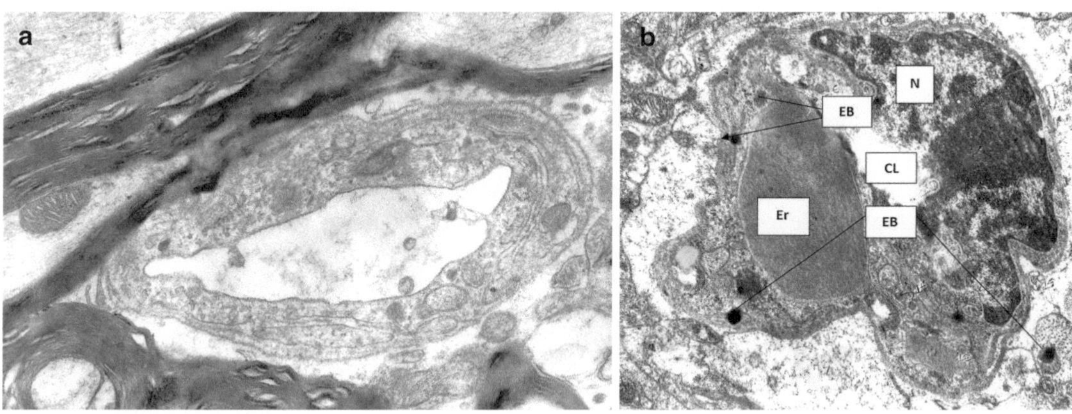

Fig. 10.4 (**a**) Capillary from the sciatic nerve of a mouse with intraperitoneal infection with *Chlamydia*. *EB* elementary bodies of *Chlamydia*, *MF* myelin fibres. Magnification ×13,000. (**b**) Capillary from the upper layer of the cerebral cortex of a mouse with intraperitoneal infection with *Chlamydia*. *EB* elementary bodies of *Chlamydia* (↑), *N* nucleus of an endotheliocyte, *Er* erythrocyte, *CL* lumen of the capillary. Magnification ×13,000

functional state, the signs of which were the presence of a large number of polysomes, heavily granulated ER tubules, lysosomes and phagosomes. In the studied parts of the central nervous system and the pia mater, elementary bodies of *Chlamydia* were often found near lysosomes and phagosomes, in which elementary bodies of *Chlamydia* were located (Fig. 10.6a) and also near large lipofuscin inclusions (Fig. 10.6b). Among the microgliocytes, lipid-overloaded cells, that is lipophages (Fig. 10.6c), were also found, which is an indirect confirmation of the active process of myelin decay with its final conversion into lipids.

In neurogliocytes of the central nervous system and lemmocytes of the central nervous system, dystrophic changes in the cytoplasm in the form of an increase in its transparency were observed in the presence of elementary bodies of *Chlamydia* during intraperitoneal infection with *Chlamydia*. They also showed changes in the nuclei by the type of apoptosis, and in lemmo-

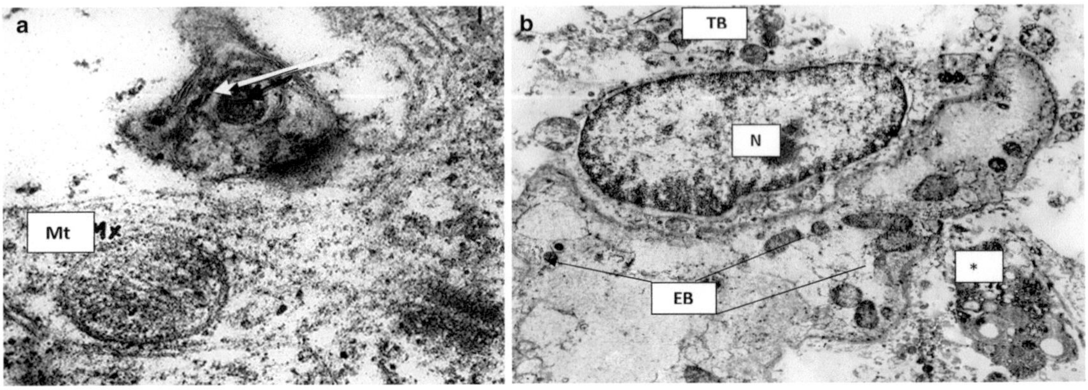

Fig. 10.5 (**a**) A section of a neuron from the cerebral cortex after intraperitoneal infection with *Chlamydia* with an elementary *Chlamydia* body (arrow) in the granular ER; *Mt* mitochondrion. Uv.—33,000. (**b**) A cell from the pia mater of a mouse with intranasal infection with *Chlamydia*. I is the nucleus. In the cytoplasm are elementary (EB) and transitional (TB) bodies of *Chlamydia* and various heteromorphic inclusions. Magnification ×10,000

cytes by the type of karyopyknosis and karyorrhexis (Fig. 10.7a, b). In the central nervous system, elementary bodies of *Chlamydia* were found not only in the cytoplasm of lemmocytes, but also near them—in the neuropil.

In addition to the above-described pictures, in the cerebral cortex with intraperitoneal infection with *Chlamydia*, clusters of "young" oligodendrocytes with a high nuclear-cytoplasmic ratio, having typically formed nuclei with nucleoli and a narrow rim of cytoplasm, were observed. Most likely, these clusters of oligodendrocytes arise as a result of their proliferation (Fig. 10.8).

In intraperitoneal infection with *Chlamydia*, the axial cylinders containing elementary *Chlamydia* bodies in myelinated and unmyelinated fibres were dystrophically changed according to the light type. In myelinated fibres, distinct myelinopathy of varying severity was observed: from swelling and adhesion of lamellae to irreversible granular disintegration of the myelin sheath (Figs. 10.9 and 10.10).

In intraperitoneal and intranasal infection with *Chlamydia*, both traces of infection in the form of organelle destruction and the elementary bodies of *Chlamydia* themselves are found in the cytoplasm of CNS oligodendrocytes. In some oligodendrocytes, a disruption of the Golgi complex structure and vacuolization (blebbing) of the cytoplasm due to the destruction of the mitochondrial structure are observed. The structure of the karyoplasm in the nucleus is noticeably altered and homogeneous, and myelino- and axonopathy occurs in nearby myelin fibres (Figs. 10.11 and 10.12).

Elementary and transitional bodies of *Chlamydia* are found in the axial cylinders of unmyelinated fibres and near them (as well as in myelinated fibres) (Fig. 10.13).

In intraperitoneal infection with *Chlamydia*, endocytosis patterns of elementary bodies of *Chlamydia* and chlamydophila were observed both in oligodendrocytes and in neurons of the cerebral cortex and hypothalamus. Not only the structure of the cytoplasm but also the nuclei were clearly disrupted by pycnosis and karyorrhexis. The nucleoli were large, but hyperosmiophilic and most likely inactive. In the cerebral cortex, in intraperitoneal infection with *Chlamydia*, the presence of elementary bodies of *Chlamydia* was noted near some dead neurons, which were in close contact with a trophic oligodendrocyte with an almost unchanged nuclear structure, and in the cytoplasm of which elementary bodies of *Chlamydia* were also found (Fig. 10.14a).

In intraperitoneal infection with *Chlamydia*, mitochondria of altered shape with a disrupted structure were found in some myelinated fibres of the spinal cord, inside of which were elementary bodies of *Chlamydia* (Fig. 10.15). In unmyelinated nerve fibres of the upper layers of

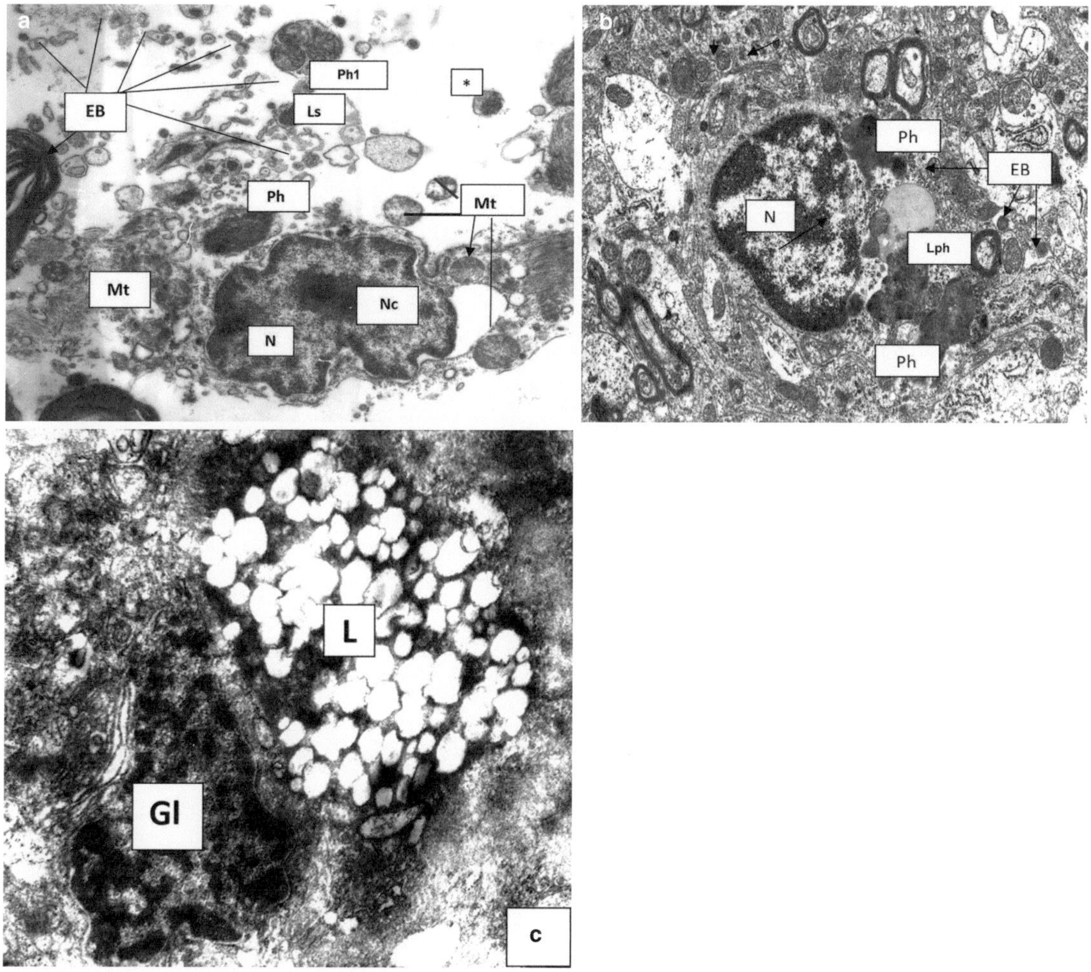

Fig. 10.6 (**a**) Microgliocyte from the semi-destroyed pia mater of a mouse after intranasal infection with *Chlamydia*. *N* nucleus, *Nc* nucleolus, *EB* elementary bodies of *Chlamydia* outside the cell, *Ph* phagosome with ET of *Chlamydia*, *Ls* lysosomes, *Mt* mitochondria; (*) transitional body of *Chlamydia*. Magnification ×10,000. (**b**) Microgliocytes from the cerebral cortex of a mouse with *Chlamydia* VBD. In (**b**) *N* nucleus, *Li* lipofuscin inclusion, Phphagosomes, *EB* elementary bodies of *Chlamydia*. In (**c**) gliocyte (Gl) in a state of apoptosis (left) and lipophage (L), completely filled with lipid droplets (right). Magnification: (**a**) ×8300; (**b**) ×6600

the cerebral cortex, very large mitochondria with disruptions in the integrity of the outer membrane and elementary bodies of *Chlamydia* inside were found (Fig. 10.16).

In intraperitoneal infection with *Chlamydia*, elementary bodies were also found in the cytoplasm of PNS lemmocytes. In this case, both the structure of their nuclei and the structure of the cytoplasm were greatly altered, and in the adjacent myelin fibres, pictures of myelino- and axonopathy were observed. Large hyperchromic phagosomes (Fig. 10.17a, b). Sometimes the structure of the lemmocyte nuclei was changed to the point of apoptoid bodies (Fig. 10.17b) or necrosis (Fig. 10.18). In the latter cases, there were severe disturbances in the lemmocyte cytoplasm, the endoneurium as a whole, and in the myelin fibres located near the lemmocyte.

The difference between the changes in the structure of some sciatic nerve lemmocytes during intranasal infection with *Chlamydia* and those already described in other types of infection was the pronounced dystrophy of the cytoplasm according to the light type and the

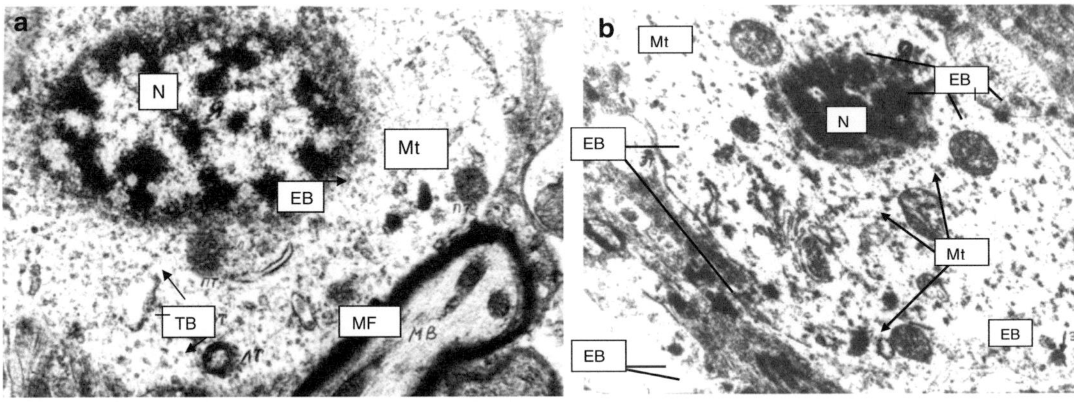

Fig. 10.7 Intraperitoneal infection with *Chlamydia*: (**a**) an astrocyte from the upper layers of the mouse cerebral cortex. *N* a nucleus with initial signs of apoptosis according to the chromatin pattern, *TB* transitional, *EB* elementary body of *Chlamydia*, *Mt* mitochondrion, *MF* myelin fibre. Magnification ×8000; (**b**) a lemmocyte from the sciatic nerve with signs of karyopyknosis and karyorrhexis. *N* nucleus. Other designations are the same as in (**a**). Magnification: ×6600

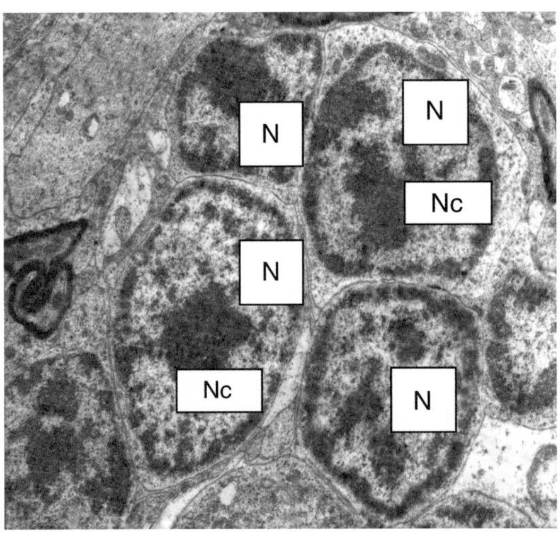

Fig. 10.8 Proliferation of oligodendrocytes in the upper layers of the mouse cerebral cortex during intraperitoneal infection with *Chlamydia*. *N* nuclei, *Nc* nucleoli with a dense fibrillar structure. Magnification: ×6600

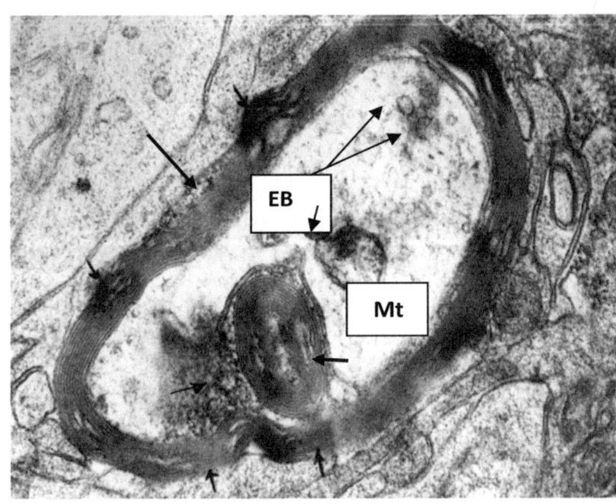

Fig. 10.9 Myelinated fibre from the upper layers of the cerebral cortex of a mouse with intraperitoneal infection with *Chlamydia*. In the almost transparent axial cylinder M t is an altered mitochondrion; EB are elementary bodies of *Chlamydia*. Arrows near the myelin sheath indicate areas of myelin change. Magnification ×10,000

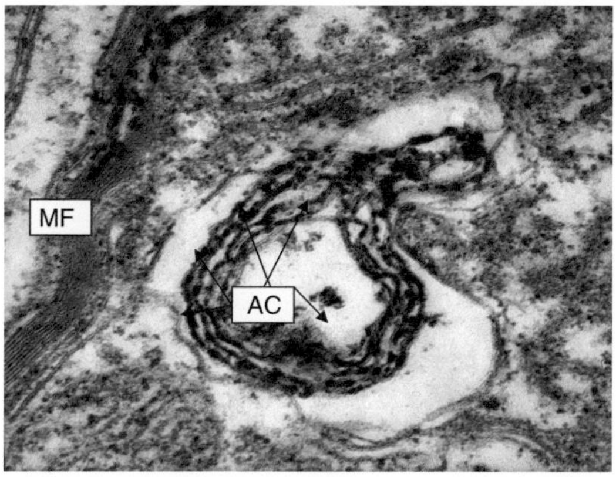

Fig. 10.10 Myelinated fibres (MF) from the pia mater of the mouse brain after intraperitoneal infection with *Chlamydia*. In the centre of the image, the axial cylinder (AC) is transparent, the myelin sheath is thinned and the myelin lamellae are sparse layers in the form of dotted lines—(arrows). Magnification ×70,000

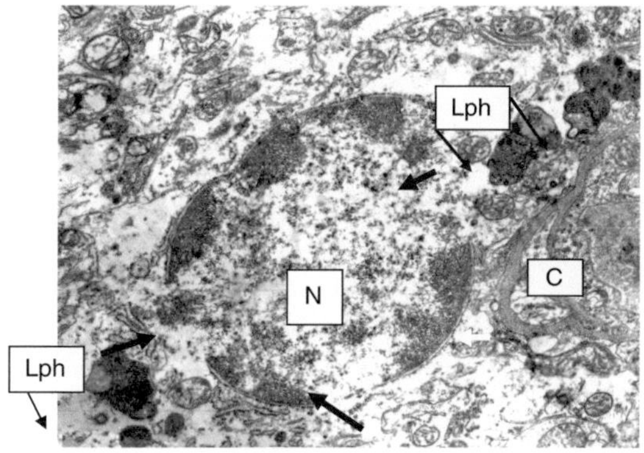

Fig. 10.12 Oligodendrocyte from the cerebral cortex of a mouse with intranasal infection with *Chlamydia* near a capillary (C). *N* nucleus with signs of apoptosis and disturbances of the karyolemma (arrows), *Lph* lipofuscin. Magnification ×10,000

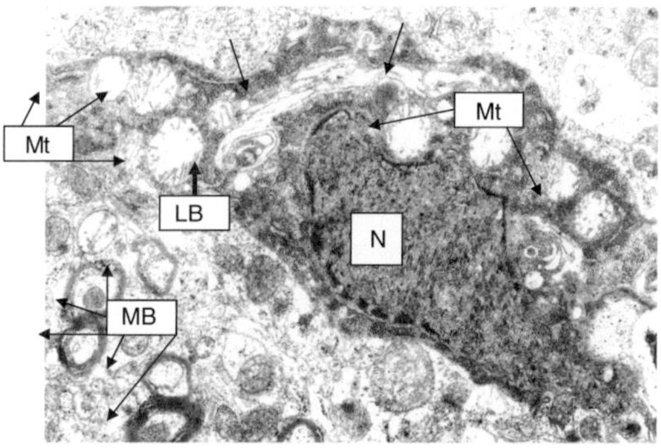

Fig. 10.11 Oligodendrocyte from the upper layers of the cerebral cortex of a mouse with intraperitoneal infection with *Chlamydia* with hyperchromic and atypically homogeneous karyoplasm in the nucleus (N) of irregular shape. In the cytoplasm—lamellar body (LB) with ET *Chlamydia* and vacuolization of organelles: mitochondria (Mx) and Golgi complex (arrows); *MF* myelin fibres with myelino- and axonopathy. Magnification ×6600

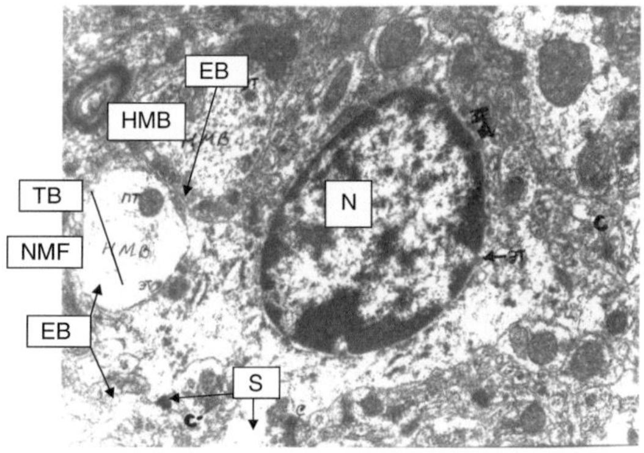

Fig. 10.13 Oligodendrocyte from the upper layers of the cerebral cortex of a mouse with intraperitoneal infection with *Chlamydia*. *N* nucleus, *EB* elementary bodies of *Chlamydia*, *TB* transitional bodies of *Chlamydia* in unmyelinated fibre, *S* synapses, *NMB* Non myelinated fibres—unmyelinated fibres. Magnification ×10,000

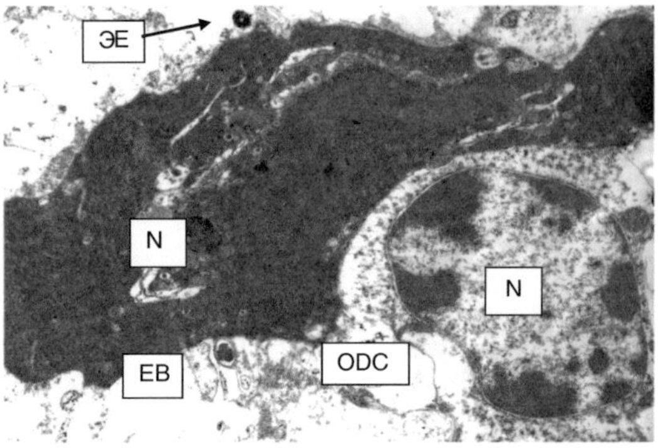

Fig. 10.14 A dead pycnomorphic neuron (N) from the cerebral cortex of a mouse infected intraperitoneally with *Chlamydia* in close contact with an almost unchanged oligodendrocyte (ODC). *N* ODC nucleus, *EB Chlamydia* elementary bodies (arrows) near the neuron and in the ODC cytoplasm. Magnification ×5000

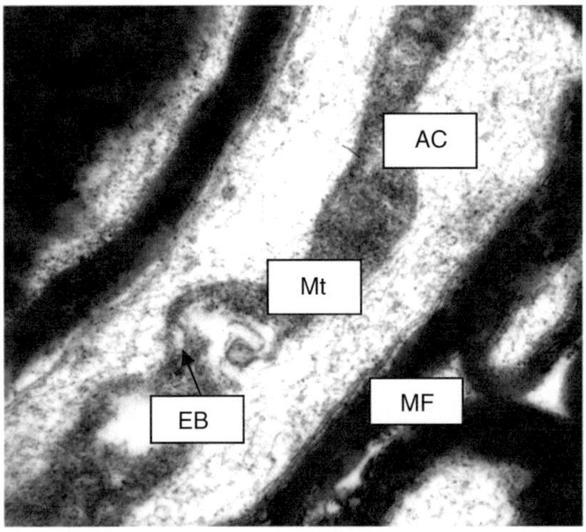

Fig. 10.15 Myelin fibres (MF) of the spinal cord in intraperitoneal infection with *Chlamydia*. *AC* axial cylinder, *Mt* large, elongated mitochondrion with areas of matrix and cristae destruction, *EB* elementary body of *Chlamydia* near the destroyed mitochondrial wall. Magnification ×16,000

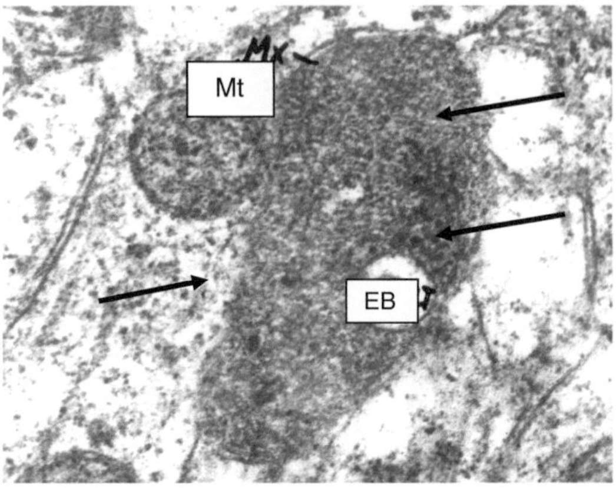

Fig. 10.16 A section of the brain from the upper layers of the cortex with intraperitoneal infection with *C. psittaci*. In the centre of the unmyelinated nerve fibre is a giant mitochondrion (Mt) with a blurred internal structure and a disruption of the outer membrane (arrows). Nearby (on the left) is a mitochondrion of normal size, but also with a blurred internal structure. In the large Mx is a transparent vacuole with an elementary body (EB) of *Chlamydia*. Magnification ×33,000

presence of elementary and transitional C bodies not only in the cytoplasm, but also in the presence of unusual outgrowths (having the appearance of a vacuole) between the outer and inner leaflets of the karyolemma (Fig. 10.19). Inside these outgrowths, as well as in narrow slit-like expansions between the outer and inner leaflets of the karyolemma, elementary bodies of *Chlamydia* with a dense structure and larger moderately osmiophilic bodies with loose contents, which sometimes came into contact with light lipid droplets, were found. It is possible that some of these bodies represented transitional forms of *Chlamydia* (from elementary bodies to reticular ones), since they also had a double membrane, like elementary bodies (Fig. 10.19).

In intranasal *Chlamydia* infection, elementary bodies of C. pneumonia were found in the neuropil of the equine tail between the myelinated fibres, sometimes in the form of large clusters (Fig. 10.20). With all types of infection, a distinct myelinopathy was observed in the form of divergence or adhesion of myelin lamellae. However, with intranasal infection, areas of complete rupture of the myelin sheath were found in individual myelinated fibres (Fig. 10.20). The axial cylinders of myelinated and unmyelinated nerve fibres were moderately or strongly destructively changed (according to the light type).

In the sciatic nerve of mice after intranasal infection with *Chlamydia*, swelling and adhesion of lamellae with their enlightenment or, on the contrary, compaction were observed in the myelin fibres.

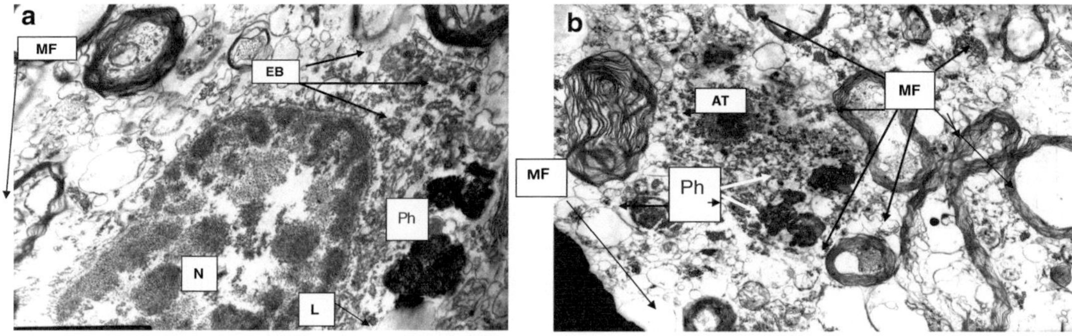

Fig. 10.17 Sciatic nerve of mouse with intraperitoneal infection with *Chlamydia*. (**a**)—lemmocyte with a strongly altered structure of the nucleus (E). In the cytoplasm: *ET* elementary bodies of *Chlamydia* (↑), *Phs* phagosomes, *L* lipid, *MV* myelin fibres. (**b**) in the centre of the image—lemmocyte with a nucleus in the form of an apoptoid body (AB); *Phs* phagosomes, *MV* myelin fibres with myelino- and axonopathy. Magnification (**a**) ×10,000; (**b**) ×5000

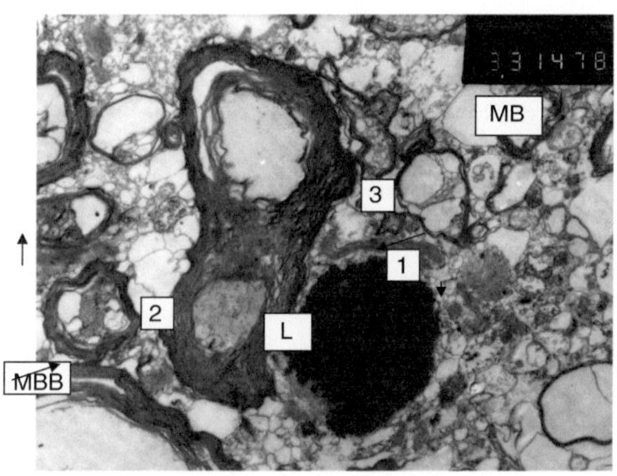

Fig. 10.18 Sciatic nerve of a mouse with intraperitoneal infection with *Chlamydia*. Necrotic lemmocyte (L) and near it—bundles of collagen fibres (1). In a large myelin fibre (MF)—axon oedema (in the upper part) In other MF—periaxonal degeneration of myelin with curvature and divergence of lamellae and formation of transparent cavities between them. 2—dense axial cylinder of MF; 3—vesicular degeneration of the axial cylinder of MF (axonopathy). Magnification ×8300

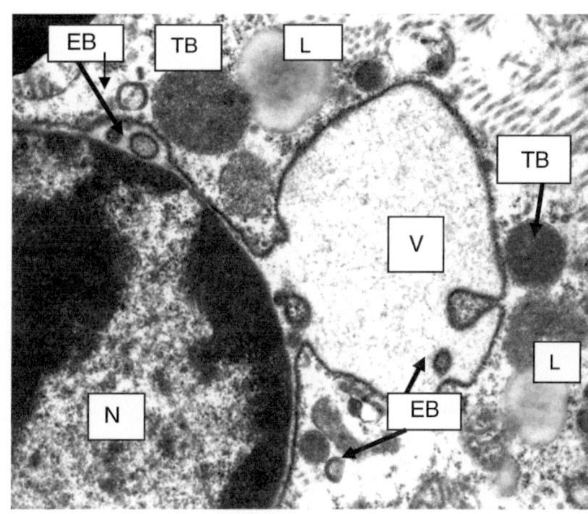

Fig. 10.19 A section of a lemmocyte from the sciatic nerve of a mouse with intranasal infection with *Chlamydia*. *EB* elementary and *TB* transitional bodies of chlamydophila *C. pneumoniae*, *I* lemmocyte nucleus, *V* vacuole from the exfoliated outer leaflet of the karyolemma, *L* lipids. Magnification ×12,500

In individual oedematous and vacuolated areas of the sciatic nerve after intraperitoneal infection. Myelin fibres in such areas of the endoneurium had various myelin disorders (myelinopathy) in the form of adhesion of lamellae, their pronounced delamination and disintegration of myelin. In myelin fibres, a distinct light-type axonopathy was also observed, that is, varying degrees of degeneration of the axial cylinders (Fig. 10.21).

It is interesting that with intraperitoneal infection with *Chlamydia*, clear signs of sclerosis were observed in the sciatic nerve. endoneurium in the form of the presence of a large number of large bundles of gliofibrils near myelin fibres with pictures of distinct myelinopathy in the form of swelling or delamination of myelin and axonopathy in the form of increased transparency of the axial cylinder (Fig. 10.22a, b).

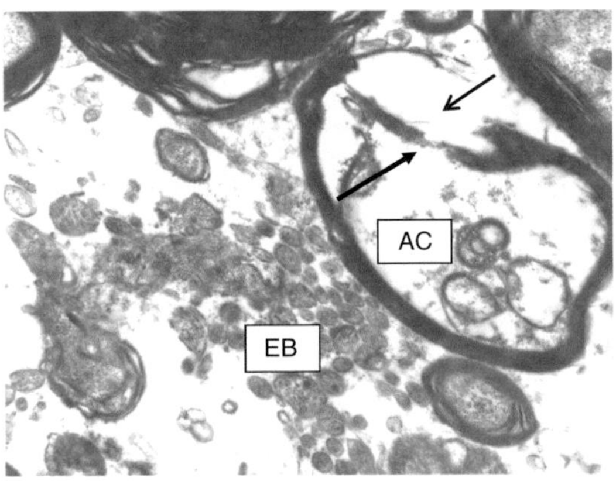

Fig. 10.20 Equine tail of a mouse with intranasal infection with *C. pneumonia*. EB is a cluster of elementary bodies near a myelinated fibre with a partially destroyed myelin sheath (↓) and a transparent axial cylinder (AC) containing vacuoles, possibly formed by mitochondria that have lost their cristae. Magnification ×16,000

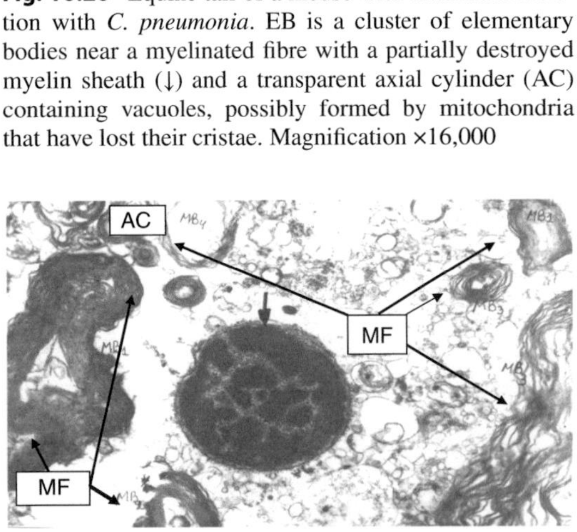

Fig. 10.21 Sciatic nerve of a mouse with intraperitoneal infection. In the centre of the image is a lymphocyte (arrow). MF are myelinated fibres with various myelinopathy. In some MFs, the transparency of the axial cylinders (AC) is increased. Magnification ×3300

In intranasal *Chlamydia* infection, elementary bodies of *C. pneumonia* were found in a number of myelinated fibres of the PNS within the area of myelin delamination surrounding the axial cylinder (Fig. 10.23). In intraperitoneal infection, elementary ("transport") bodies of *Chlamydia* were found in large myelinated fibres of the sciatic nerve with pronounced signs of light-type axonopathy in the form of increased transparency of the axial cylinders and myelinopathy in the form of both adhesion and delamination of lamellae in areas of myelin delamination near the axial cylinder (Fig. 10.24).

In intraperitoneal *Chlamydia* infection in the nodes of Ranvier of the sciatic nerve, changes in the structure of myelin notches such as an increase in their transparency were observed, and elementary *Chlamydia* bodies and altered organelles were found in the axial cylinder near the node (Figs. 10.25 and 10.26). Sometimes, with intraperitoneal *Chlamydia* infection, very severe disturbances were observed in some myelin fibres of the equine rootlets in the area of the nodes of Ranvier, up to the exposure of the axial cylinders over a large area, and a distinct dystrophy of the light type was observed in the axoplasm. Pictures of myelinopathy in the form of myelin stratification were revealed near the exposed axons of the myelin fibres in the areas of myelin notches (Fig. 10.25).

In intranasal and intraperitoneal infection with *Chlamydia*, in a number of myelinated fibres of the sciatic nerve, elementary bodies of *Chlamydia* near the node of Ranvier were sometimes found both in the axial cylinder of nerve fibres and inside the detached section of myelin lamellae (Fig. 10.25).

The capillaries of the microcirculatory bed of the PNS often had a swollen basement membrane with ruptures. The endothelial cells and pericytes lacked nuclei, but dark-type cytoplasmic dystrophy was revealed with numerous dense bodies representing the breakdown products of organ-

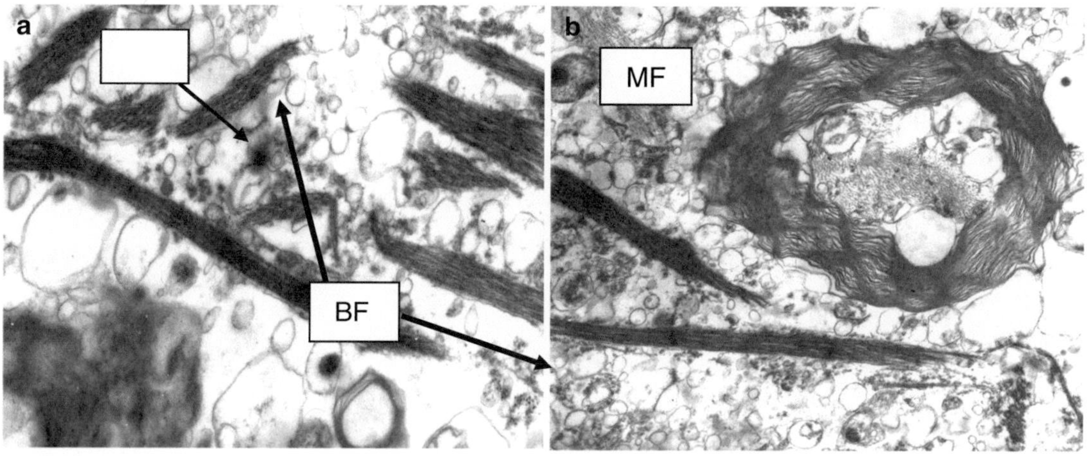

Fig. 10.22 (**a**, **b**) Sciatic nerve of a mouse with intraperitoneal infection with *Chlamydia* with signs of sclerosis endoneurium. *MV* myelinated fibres with myelino- and axonopathy, *BF* bundles of glyofibrils. Magnification: (**a**) ×8300; (**b**) ×6600

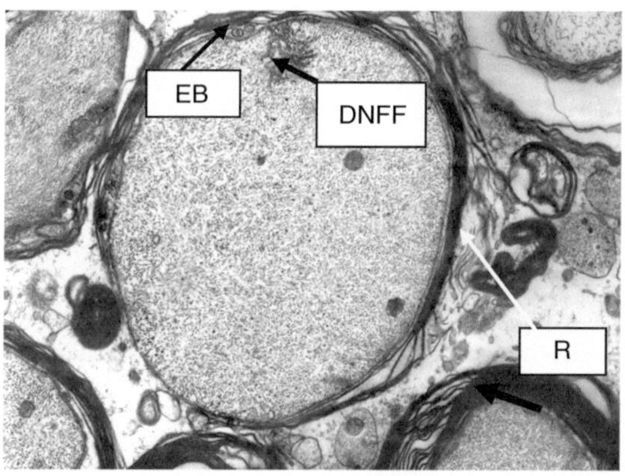

Fig. 10.23 In the centre of the image is a myelinated fibre of the sciatic nerve in intranasal infection with *Chlamydia*. *R* a strongly altered node of Ranvier, *ET* an elementary body of *Chlamydia* in the area of lamella stratification; DNFvcondensation of neurofibrils. Magnification ×13,000

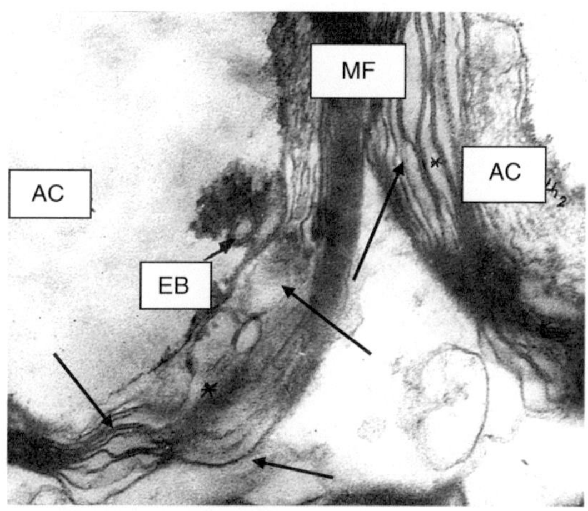

Fig. 10.24 Myelinated fibres (MFs) of the sciatic nerve in intraperitoneal infection with *Chlamydia*. *Arrows* areas of myelin lamellae delamination, *EB* elementary body inside the myelin lamella, *AC* axial cylinders with high transparency. Magnification ×20,000

elles and lysosomes. Fragments of destroyed endothelial cells were observed in the lumen of the vessel, and isolated elementary bodies of *Chlamydia* were found outside (near the basement membrane of the vessel). The latter fact indirectly indicated a violation of the blood-neural barrier. Myelinopathy was present in the myelinated fibres around the vessel—in the form of myelin thinning, delamination and adhesion of myelin lamellae, and axonopathy—in the form of increased transparency of the axial cylinders (Fig. 10.27).

In some synapses of the brain, with different types of *Chlamydia* infection, obvious dystrophic changes in the structure of synaptic terminals were found, sometimes with the typical appearance of synaptic vesicles and the synaptic cleft itself preserved. In some synapses, this was disintegration and blurring of both the synaptic cleft itself and the synaptic vesicles in the presynaptic part of the syn-

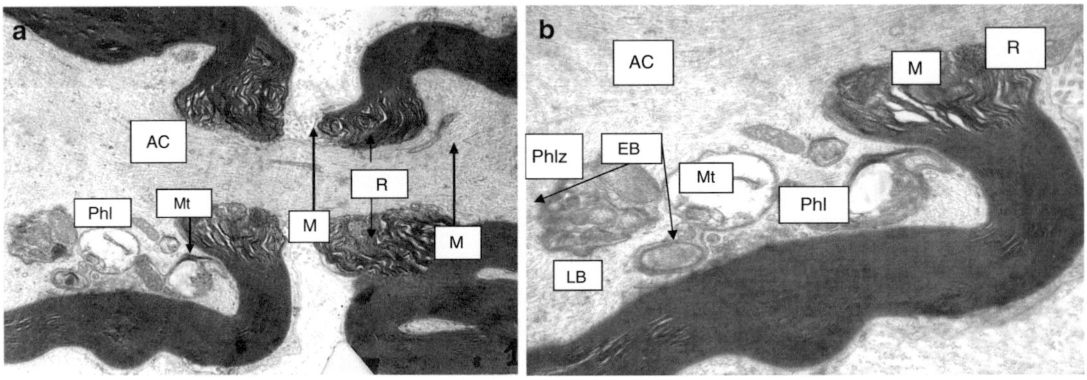

Fig. 10.25 Myelinated fibre from the sciatic nerve of a mouse after intraperitoneal infection with *Chlamydia*. (**a**) general view of the node of Ranvier; (**b**) left lower part of the node of Ranvier (R) (from **a**)—larger. *OC* axial cylinder, *Mt* vacuolated mitochondrion, *LT* lamellar body, *Flz* phagolysosomes, *H* myelin notch, *ET* elementary bodies of *Chlamydia*. Magnification: (**a**) ×10,000, (**b**) ×20,000

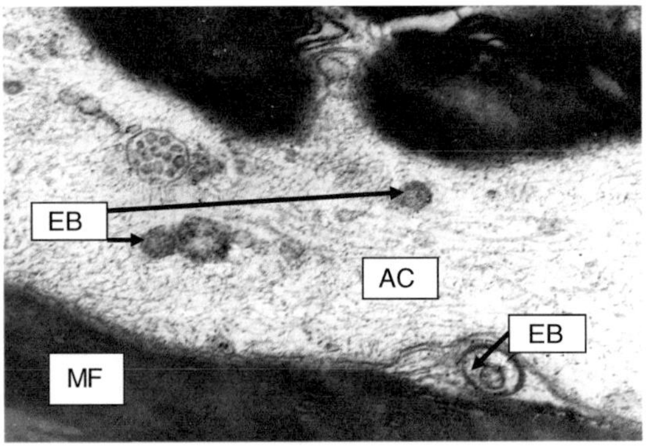

Fig. 10.26 Myelinated fibre (MF) of the sciatic nerve near the node of Ranvier after intraperitoneal infection with *Chlamydia* with chlamydial elementary bodies (EB) both in the axial cylinder (AC) and inside the area of myelin lamellae delamination. Magnification ×26,000

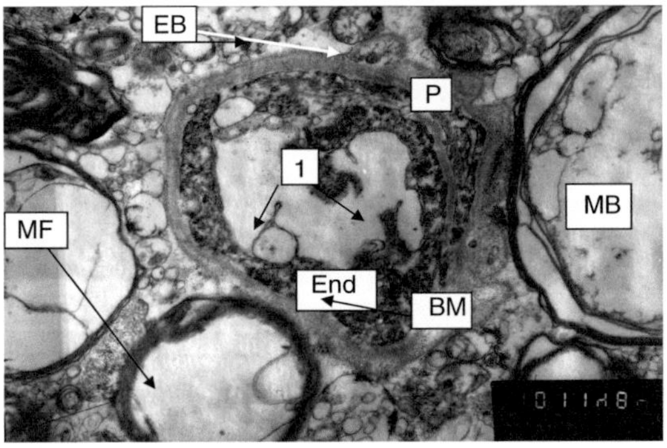

Fig. 10.27 Sciatic nerve of a mouse with intraperitoneal infection with *Chlamydia*. Capillary with swollen basement membrane (BM). In endothelial cells (End) and pericytes (P)—cytoplasmic dystrophy of the dark type. In the lumen of the vessel—areas of destroyed endothelial cells (1). Outside, near the basement membrane of the vessel: single elementary bodies of *Chlamydia* (EB) and myelin fibres (MFs) with transparent axial cylinders and myelinopathy. Magnification ×10,000

apse (Fig. 10.28a). In other synapses, on the contrary, the synaptic cleft was hyperosmiophilic (condensed) and the presynaptic terminal had increased transparency and contained a small number of vesicles with a blurred structure near the contact area of the synapse (Fig. 10.28b).

In intraperitoneal infection with *Chlamydia*, dystrophic changes of the light type were observed in the synapses of the lumbar spinal cord, and adherent or half-destroyed synaptic vesicles were observed in their presynaptic terminals (Fig. 10.29). In large nearby unmyelinated fibres with transparent axial cylinders, very dense lamellar bodies of large sizes were found in close contact with a large mitochondrion, whose matrix and cristae were heavily destroyed.

Comparison of morphological changes detected in the structures of the nervous system during electron microscopic examination of chlamydial infection with different routes of infection

Various methods of infection with different strains and species of *Chlamydia* made it possi-

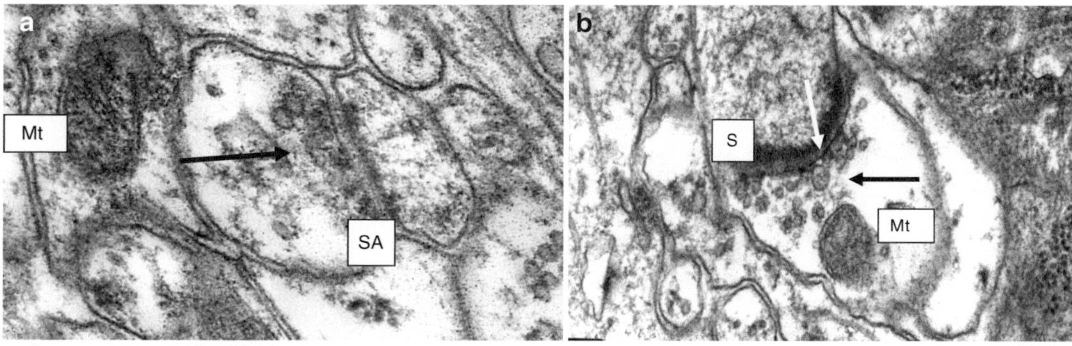

Fig. 10.28 Altered (light type) axodendritic synapses (C) in the cerebral cortex after intranasal (**a**) and intraperitoneal (**b**) infection with *Chlamydia*. Both images show an insufficient quantity and poor quality of synaptic vesicles (black arrows) in the presynaptic axonal terminal. Hyperosmophilia of the synaptic contact zone in (**b**) is indicated by a white arrow. *Mt* mitochondria with a blurred structure of the matrix and cristae. Magnification: (**a**) ×40,000; (**b**) ×33,000

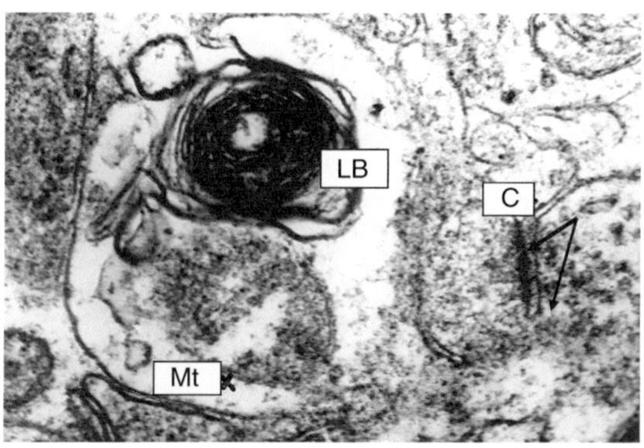

Fig. 10.29 Dystrophically altered (light type) synapse (C) in the lumbar spinal cord with intraperitoneal infection with *Chlamydia*. Adhered or semi-destroyed synaptic vesicles (↓) in the presynaptic terminal. Mt is a destroyed mitochondrion and LB is a lamellar body in a transversely cut, almost transparent large unmyelinated fibre near the synapse. Magnification ×40,000

ble, in an experiment on a model of meningoencephalopolyradiculoneuritis, to prove for the first time the fundamental possibility of *Chlamydia* penetration into all structures of the central and peripheral nervous systems through the blood-brain and blood-neural barriers.

In the presented detailed electron microscopic study of chlamydial infection, the most striking morphological changes in both the CNS and PNS were observed with intracerebral and intranasal infection. However, in general, no fundamental differences were observed with different methods of infection. The changes revealed in the CNS and PNS were identical for all methods of infection and types of *Chlamydia* at all stages of their development: elementary bodies, transitional and reticular bodies were always present. All types of *Chlamydia* affected not only the cells of the upper layers of the meninges, but also the neurons and neurogliocytes themselves. The presence of chlamydial bodies in cells and fibres was accompanied by pronounced disturbances in their structure. Thus, vacuolization of mitochondria, a large number of lysosomes of various structures and hypertrophy of the Golgi complex were observed in the CNS cells. Elementary bodies of *Chlamydia* in the cytoplasm were found in the cisterns of the Golgi complex, altered tubules of the ER and vacuoles.

In the nuclei of neuroglial cells, karyorrhexis was noted, as well as changes in chromatin by the apoptotic type. In the cerebral cortex, during intraperitoneal infection with *Chlamydia*, due to oligodendrocyte proliferation, clusters of "young" cells with a high nuclear-cytoplasmic ratio were observed, which had a narrow rim of cytoplasm around large nuclei with a normal chromatin pattern in the karyoplasm and nucleoli.

In myelin fibres of the central nervous system, in all types of *Chlamydia* infection, along with swelling and delamination of myelin, the most destructive myelinopathy in the form of granular disintegration of myelin was also noted. Axonopathy was manifested by an increase in the transparency of the axial cylinders.

In myelinated fibres of the PNS, with all types of *Chlamydia* infection, as a rule, a distinct myelinopathy was observed in the form of divergence or adhesion of myelin lamellae, and with intranasal infection, areas of complete rupture of the myelin sheath were found in individual myelinated fibres. The axial cylinders of the nerve fibres of the PNS were moderately or strongly destructively changed according to the light type in both myelinated and unmyelinated nerve fibres.

In all types of *Chlamydia* infection, changes in the Schwann cells (lemmocytes) of the PNS captured and destroyed not only the cytoplasm, but also the nucleus. The most pronounced were changes in the structure of the nuclei by the type of apoptosis up to the formation of an apoptotic body. Karyopyknosis and karyorrhexis were observed in the nuclei of individual lemmocytes. Elementary bodies of *Chlamydia* were observed in the cytoplasm of lemmocytes and in the endoneurium.

In the vessels of the microcirculatory bed of the CNS and PNS, both in the experiment on mice and in the human brain biopsy, elementary bodies of *Chlamydia* are found both in the lumen of the capillary and endothelial cells, and near the capillary outside it, which indirectly indicates the exit of *Chlamydia* from the vessel and the violation of the blood-brain and blood-neural barrier. However, no obvious violations were found in the structure of the vessels (endothelial cells, pericytes and basement membrane) of the microcirculatory bed of the CNS.

In the structure of the vessels of the microcirculatory bed of the PNS, there were changes with the appearance of ruptures in the basement membrane of the capillaries and disturbances in the structure of the cytoplasm and nuclei of the cells of the vessel wall. Thus, in the cells of the endothelium and pericytes, degenerative changes in the cytoplasm of a dark type were recorded, and the nuclei in them were often not determined. Endoluminal outgrowths of endothelial cells into the lumen of the capillaries were observed. Elementary bodies of *Chlamydia* were found near the vessels, and lymphocytes in the endoneurium of the PNS, and these facts indirectly indicate the presence of inflammation and also a violation of the haemato-neural barrier in the PNS.

In different types of *Chlamydia* infection, alterative changes in the structure of synaptic terminals were found in some synapses of both the brain and spinal cord, sometimes while maintaining the typical appearance of synaptic vesicles and compaction of the synaptic cleft itself.

References

1. Phillips S, Quigley BL, Timms P. Seventy years of chlamydia vaccine research – limitations of the past and directions for the future. Front Microbiol. 2019;10 https://doi.org/10.3389/fmicb.2019.00070.
2. Rajeevel K, Sivadasan R. Transcervical mouse infections with chlamydia trachomatis and determination of bacterial burden bio-protocol. 10(3):e3506. https://doi.org/10.21769/BioProtoc.3506.
3. Dockterman J, Coers J. Immunopathogenesis of genital Chlamydia infection: insights from mouse models. Pathog Dis. 2021;79:ftab012. https://doi.org/10.1093/femspd/ftab012.
4. Wang Y, He R, Winner H, et al. Induction of transmucosal protection by oral vaccination with an attenuated chlamydia. Infect Immun. 2023;91(5):10.1128/iai.00043-23.
5. Dockterman J, Reitano JR, Everitt JI, et al. Irgm proteins attenuate inflammatory disease in mouse models of genital Chlamydia infection. M Bio. 2024;15(4) https://doi.org/10.1128/mbio.00303-24.
6. Li S, Wang L, Zhang Y, Ma L, Zhang J, Zu J, Wu X. Role of Interleukin-4 (IL-4) in respiratory infection and allergy caused by early-life chlamydia infection. J Microbiol Biotechnol. 2021;31(8):1109–14. https://doi.org/10.4014/jmb.2104.04028.
7. Boyko EV, Poznyak AL, Nuralova IV, et al. On the development of multiorgan chlamydial lesions in primary local infection of the eye in an experiment. Arch Pathol. 2011;6:15–8.
8. Lobzin YV, Poznyak AL, Sidorchuk SN. Chlamydial infections: diagnostics, clinical picture, treatment, rehabilitation: manual for doctors. St. Petersburg: Foliant; 2010. p. 484.
9. Contini C, Seraceni S, Cultrera R, Castellazzi M, Granieri E, Fainardi E. Chlamydophila pneumoniae infection and its role in neurological disorders. Interdiscip Perspect Infect Dis. 2010.
10. Levitt D, Danen R, Levitt P. Selective infection of astrocytes by Chlamydia trachomatis in primary

mixed neuron-glial cell cultures. Infect Immun. 1986;54(3):913–6.
11. Mikhailenko AA, Nuralova IV, Pozharskaya TD, et al. Experimental morphological study of the demyelinating process of chlamydial origin. Neuroimmunol Neuroinfect Neuroimage. 1995:72–3.
12. Mikhailenko AA, Onishchenko LS, Nuralova IV, Borzenko OV. Pathology of the peripheral nervous system of chlamydial origin. Bekhterev Neurol Bull. 1996;28(1–2):5–8.
13. Vainshenker YI, Nuralova IV, Onishchenko LS. Chlamydia of the central nervous system. Laboratory diagnostics and clinical and morphological features. Arch Pathol. 2014;1:57–62.
14. Khvorik DF, Tsyrkunov VM, Konkin DE. Evaluation of the immune response in experimental chlamydia. J GrSMU. 2008;3:80–3.
15. Kochetova OV, Kumakshev AS, Tatarnikova NA. Immunomorphological diagnostics of experimental chlamydia in rats in immune organs. Vet Sci 154–7.
16. Slobodenyuk VV, Karkishchenko NN, Afanasyev SS, et al. Spontaneous chlamydia in monkeys as a model of chlamydial infection. Biomedicine. 2010;5:6–16.
17. Gladysheva IB. Morphological characteristics of the liver in experimental chlamydia.
18. Tatarnikova NA, Bekker AA. Ultrastructural changes in the liver and kidneys in chlamydial infection.
19. Sidorova KA, Tatarnikova NA, Kochetova OV. Morphological changes in the cerebellum during experimental chlamydial infection.
20. Satta A, Stivala A, Garozzo A, et al. Experimental Chlamydia trachomatis infection causes apoptosis in human sperm. Hum Reprod. 2006;21(1):134–7. https://doi.org/10.1093/humrep/dei269. Epub 2005 Aug 26
21. Patton DL, Landers DV, Schachter J. Experimental Chlamydia trachomatis salpingitis in mice: initial studies on the characterization of the leukocyte response to chlamydial infection. J Infect Dis. 1989;159(6):1105–10.
22. Darville T, Hiltke TJ. Pathogenesis of genital tract disease due to chlamydia trachomatis. J Infect Dis. 2010;201(Suppl 2):S114–25.
23. Pagliarani S, Johnston SD, Beagley KW, et al. The occurrence and pathology of chlamydiosis in the male reproductive tract of non-human mammals: a review. Rev Theriogenol. 2020;154:152–60.
24. Reinhold P. Overview of Chlamydiosis. MSD Veterinary Manual. https://www.msdvetmanual.com/generalized-conditions/chlamydiosis/overview-of-chlamydiosis.

Conclusion

Abstract
In a resulting chapter main aspects of Chlamydiosis are summarized with revealing the questions which urgently need complex study.

Due to its widespread distribution, variability of clinical manifestations and localization of lesions, high costs of diagnosis and treatment, tendency to chronicity and impact on population reproduction, chlamydial infection is currently a serious problem for international and national health services.

Since the late 1960s, urogenital forms of chlamydial infection caused by *Chlamydia trachomatis* are more prevalent now, and it is now recognized that urogenital *Chlamydia* is an important medical and social problem not only because of its high prevalence, but also due to the high frequency of complications caused by it, which negatively affect demographic indicators. Diseases caused by *C. trachomatis*, related to sexually transmitted infections, have acquired great importance, because, as a rule, they affect people during the period of greatest sexual activity, leading to serious and even irreversible consequences in the form of infertility and neonatal pathologies in the case of the birth of a child from an infected mother.

Despite more than 20 years of screening and testing for urogenital *Chlamydia* in many countries and regions, *Chlamydia* control strategies are rooted in mere assumptions rather than reliable data.

The results of a number of studies in recent decades devoted to the discovery and study of various types of *Chlamydia* have contributed to a significant transformation of the views of scientists and doctors of various specialties on this pathogen, which began to be perceived not only as a causative agent of diseases of the urogenital system.

It has now been proven that *Chlamydia* causes a significantly larger number of diseases in humans than was previously thought. Numerous studies devoted to extraurogenital and extrapulmonary forms of chlamydial infection have allowed a new assessment of the etiopathogenetic significance of *C. pneumoniae* and *C. trachomatis* in the initiation of a number of diseases of the central and peripheral nervous system, musculoskeletal system, cardiovascular system, digestive tract and eyes. Unfortunately, these studies focussed mainly on a group of people seeking medical help and did not extend to the entire population as a whole. In addition to the fact that they are few in number and fragmentary, the methodological support in many respects does not meet modern requirements and is contradictory and ambiguous.

C.pneumoniae is implicated in the development of a wide range of diseases, and their role in the development of diseases is still questionable and requires more intense study.

In our works, structural changes in human chlamydiosis are presented in the most complete

V. Zinserling et al., *Chlamydia Infections*, https://doi.org/10.1007/978-3-031-99642-9

form. Due to some reasons, the veterinarian pathologists have better opportunities to study chlamydiosis in cattle in more detail than in medical practice. Their data fully correspond with our observations in humans. The only exception is larger importance of joints lesions in animals, but we cannot exclude that in humans though they are underestimated. The detailed electron microscopic studies

Zoonotic chlamydial infections remain a serious public health problem: they cause economic and production losses in livestock production, and they pose a threat to the health of wildlife. With the discovery of new *Chlamydia* species, the risk of zoonoses in humans is definitely increasing.

The complexity, heterogeneity and insufficient knowledge of the pathogenesis of chlamydial infection dictate the need for a targeted study of its various links.

Thus, the great epidemiological danger of *Chlamydia*, the diversity of clinical forms and the diseases they cause in humans with severe consequences allow us to consider chlamydial infection as one of the most important medical and social problems, the solution of which in many countries of the world has been elevated to the rank of national programs. Despite numerous achievements in the study of chlamydial infections, many problems remain unresolved, which requires the combined efforts of both scientists and doctors of different specialties.

The above circumstances predetermined the purpose of this work, the relevance of which is beyond doubt. The authors hope that it will help to expand the circle of *Chlamydia* researchers.

MIX
Papier aus verantwortungsvollen Quellen
Paper from responsible sources
FSC® C105338

If you have any concerns about our products,
you can contact us on
ProductSafety@springernature.com

In case Publisher is established outside the EU,
the EU authorized representative is:
Springer Nature Customer Service Center GmbH
Europaplatz 3, 69115 Heidelberg, Germany

Printed by Libri Plureos GmbH
in Hamburg, Germany